# Springer Series on Social Work

## Albert R. Roberts, PhD, Series Editor

# Human Behavior and the Social Environment

## Integrating Theory and Evidence-Based Practice

John S. Wodarski, PhD
Sophia F. Dziegielewski, PhD, LCSW
Editors

 *Springer Publishing Company*

Springer Publishing Company, Inc.
536 Broadway
New York, NY 10012-3955

*Acquisitions Editor: Sheri W. Sussman*
*Production Editor: J. Hurkin-Torres*
*Cover design by Susan Hauley*

02 03 04 05 06 / 5 4 3 2 1

---

**Library of Congress Cataloging-in-Publication Data**

Human behavior and the social environment : integrating theory and evidenced-based practice / John S. Wodarski, Sophia F. Dziegielewski, editors.
    p. cm. — (Springer series on social work)
  Includes bibliographical references and index.
  ISBN 0-8261-2343-0
  1. Social service. 2. Human behavior. 3. Social ecology. I. Wodarski, John S.
II. Dziegielewski, Sophia F. III. Springer series on social work (Unnumbered)
HV40.35 .H83 2002
361.3'2—dc21

2001049016
CIP

---

Printed in the United States of America by Maple-Vail.

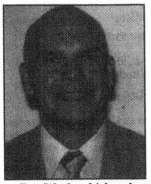
**John S. Wodarski, PhD,** received his MSSW degree from the University of Tennessee and a PhD from Washington University in Saint Louis. His main interests include child and adolescent health behavior, including research on violence, substance abuse, depression, sexuality, and employment. He is the author of over 35 texts and 355 journal publications and has presented on his research at over 249 professional meetings and conferences.

Dr. Wodarski has been the recipient of 57 Individual Awards from Federal, State, and private foundations and 21 institutional awards. He recently received the Trailblazers Award from African American Authors and currently serves as co-editor of the *Journal of Human Behavior in the Social Environment* and consulting editor of John Wiley and Sons *Series on Social Work Practice*. Dr. Wodarski served as Principal Investigator of various grants; Director or Co-Director of three research centers; Department Chair; director of two doctoral programs; and Associate Vice President for Graduate Studies and Research. He returned this year to the University of Tennessee College of Social Work as Director of Research and Development for the combined campuses at Knoxville, Nashville and Memphis.

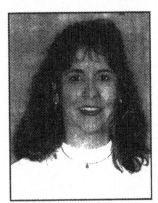
**Sophia F. Dziegielewski, PhD, LCSW,** is a professor in the School of Social Work, University of Central Florida, Orlando, FL. Her educational qualifications include a doctorate in social work from Florida State University, Tallahassee, FL and she holds a current social work license in the states of Tennessee, Georgia, and Florida. Professional honors include being named Social Worker of the Year by the National Association of Social Workers (NASW) in 1995 for the State of Tennessee.

Her professional interests focus primarily on health and mental health in the time-limited practice setting and with her nursing background is firm on the importance of social workers learning more about prescription and herbal medications and the relationship of the use of these products with psychosocial interventions. She supports her research and practice activity with over 65 journal publications, 4 books in the area of health and mental health and over 200 recent workshops and community presentations on medications, herbal preparations, and mental health assessment documentation and treatment planning in today's managed-care environment.

This book is dedicated to my wife, Lois Ann.

—*John Wodarski*

I would like to dedicate this book to two of the most influential people in shaping my life, my "second" parents, Winston and Esther Mooney.

—*Sophia F. Dziegielewski*

# Contents

## Part II: Mezzo and Macro Perspectives: Group Variables in Human Growth and Development

## Conclusions

# Contributors

**Catherine N. Dulmas, PhD, ACSW**
Assistant Professor
College of Social Work
University of Tennessee
Knoxville, TN

**Diane Dwyer, MSW**
Associate Professor/Chairperson
Department of Social Work
SUNY–Brockport
Brockport, NY

**Marvin Feit, PhD**
School of Social Work
Norfolk State University
Norfolk, VA

**Jennifer Hall, MSW**
Practicing Clinician
Lakeshore Behavioral Health
Buffalo, NY

**Carolyn Hilarski, MSW, PhD, CSW, ACSW**
Visiting Assistant Professor
Rochester Institute of
   Technology
Rochester, NY

**Janine Hunt-Jackson, MSW, CSW**
Doctoral Student
School of Social Work
SUNY–Buffalo
Buffalo, NY

**Shawn A. Lawrence, MSW**
Williamsville, NY

**Claudia M. Leo, MSW**
Jupiter, FL

**Peter Lyons, PhD**
Assistant Professor
School of Social Work
Georgia State University
Atlanta, GA

**Elaine M. Maccio, CSW**
Doctoral Student/Family
   Therapist
School of Social Work
SUNY–Buffalo
Buffalo, NY

**Gerald Moote, Jr., MSW**
School Social Worker
Williamsville Central School
   District
Williamsville, NY

**Lisa Rapp-Paglicci, MSW, PhD**
Assistant Professor
School of Social Work
University of Nevada, Las Vegas
Las Vegas, NV

**Lori A. Reyes, MSW, LCSW**
Private Practice Clinician
Delray Beach, FL

**David Skiba, MSW, CSW**
School of Social Work
SUNY–Buffalo
Buffalo, NY

**Karen D. Smith, MSW**
Program Coordinator
HOMESPACE (Housing
  Program)
Buffalo, NY

**Michael Sullivan, PhD**
Assistant Professor
College of Social Work
University of Tennessee
Memphis, TN

**Kim Zittel-Palamara, MSW, CSW,
ACSW**
Doctoral Student
UB Dental School CARES
  Program Supervisor
School of Social Work
SUNY–Buffalo
Buffalo, NY

# Acknowledgments

We remain grateful for the help and support received from the co-authors on the applications chapters included in this text. We would also like to express our sincere thanks to all the individuals who helped in the production of this book. First, we would like to thank Sheri Sussman, Managing Editor at Springer Publishing. Her high-energy level, drive, ambition and perseverance for deadlines have been invaluable.

In closing, we want to thank our family members, colleagues and friends who understood and supported us in setting priorities essential for completing this book. We have been blessed with knowing and working with so many caring and supportive family members, colleagues and friends and with that encouragement and support when you never give up—all things really are possible.

## CHAPTER 1

# Understanding Human Growth and Development: Integrating Theory and Empiricism

## Sophia F. Dziegielewski and John S. Wodarski

The world can doubtless never be well known by theory . . .
—Chesterfield, 1774 (Strachey, 1901)

Theories are methods of organizing and structuring concepts to provide a complete understanding or an insightful view of a phenomenon (Rosenhan & Seligman, 1989). Myers (1987) describes theories as, " . . . general ideas—integrated sets of principles—that explain and predict facts" (p. 9). In the field of social work there is little disagreement that some type of theoretical foundation is needed to understand human growth and development. The question remains, however, which one is the best. Theory provides this foundation, giving guidance and structure in order for facts and interventions to coincide (Brieland, 1977; Lyons, Wodarski, & Feit, 1998; Minahan, 1981; Myers & Thyer, 1997; Wodarski, 1987).

This book stresses the importance of theory along with several common prevalent human behavior theories and their relationship toward social and practice significance. Furthermore, this chapter provides a foundation for the section summaries and specific chapters within the book that cover this information in greater depth. Each chapter will attempt to integrate theory and empiricism by proposing several ques-

The editors would like to thank Mary Ann Deibel-Braun for earlier contributions to this chapter.

tions. First, what is the extent that these theories are valid in their causal explanations and predictions of behavior? Second, how much change can take place in the client? Third, what methods, techniques, and interventions does the model support in order to change a client's behavior? Last, what evaluative research is available to support the theories and their success rates?

Because there are numerous theories of human development, we should determine which theory is the most appropriate. This determination allows social workers to decide the best course of action to benefit their clients. When identifying the best approach, it is uncommon for several views to be in direct conflict with one another. However, many models remain similar and incorporate only subtle differences. Through research and through the powers of theoretical prediction, theories and the interventions utilized in the field of social work can become more accurate—presenting social workers with a more concise conceptualization of human development. Understanding the premises inherited in theories, and the evidence that validates the interventions, provides social workers with a rich selection of choices. Having this information helps social workers make more informed practice decisions, allowing for choices from practice techniques and strategies, which are proven efficient and effective.

## HUMAN BEHAVIOR THEORIES

According to Dworetzky (1987), human behavior theories are divided into two factions—the *epigenetic* and the *environmentalist*. In the epigenetic approach, interactions among individuals are directly related to the relationship of the person in the environment, in addition to the individual's inherited traits. For example, Erikson's theory is an epigenetic approach, which postulates that human behaviors are preprogrammed and evolve according to the individual's developmental phases; however, this development is constantly being interrupted by the environment (as cited in Ullrich, 1999). In an attempt to understand and improve the predictions of the complex human behaviors, this book highlights the individual traits as well as the relationship between the individual and the environment. The theoretical models that fall in this area can differ as some believe that individuals' ability to learn or think is based on their genetic predisposition (e.g., the biological model and labeling theory), while others focus on personality or social interaction (e.g., cognitive variables, life span perspective).

In comparison to the epigenetic approaches, Dworetzky (1987) warns that since individuals are social creatures it is important not to be too simplistic in approach. His point is well made because if a social worker is too narrow when defining a behavior, the results may not include an individual's social and cultural environment. When taking an environmentalist approach, social workers attempt to explain and predict behavior based on learning and past experiences. For example, it has been said that Europeans are epigenetically oriented by nature because of a strong emphasis on family. While in contrast, Americans are often viewed as more environmentally focused because of their individualistic thinking. Either way, theories and models of human behavior can differ in focus and content. Regardless of which is correct, there is no absolute theoretical framework in which the presumptions and practice implications will fall clearly into one category. Therefore, the authors' caution the reader to be careful and avoid the tendency to pigeonhole theories and their concepts, as overlapping theoretical constructs often exist.

This book highlights the theoretical and empirical findings related to many of the theories currently used in social work practice. To facilitate the presentation of these models, this book is divided into two sections. Chapters 2–5 deal with the micro aspect of social work. Here the emphasis is placed on identifying an individual's developmental issues that might affect psychosocial functioning, while enhancing the effectiveness and efficiency of the technical skills used in identifying progress and change (Barker, 1999). For example, a link is made to the biological and cognitive basis of human development, as well as the life stages approach and the effects that may occur with the use of labeling theory.

In Part II, the mezzo and macro aspects of social work, derived from system, group, or social learning theoretical models, explore human growth and development. In this section, the macro emphasis is on the intervention process used with environmental issues that relate directly to practice with families, small groups, and communities. In the final chapter of the book, a summary and synthesis is postulated, addressing the current theoretical models and how they relate to the future of social work and to the important task of mixing theory with empirically based practice.

## THEORY EVALUATION

There never comes a point where a theory can be said to be true. The most that one can claim for any theory is that it has shared the successes of all its rivals and that it has passed at least one test which they have failed. (Ayer, 1982)

All theories are conceptual generalizations that provide definition, coherence, and moral direction. Theories can give structure to the human experience; however, it is important for researchers, who are in sympathy regarding values and interests, not to develop them as their *truth* (Witkin & Gottschalk, 1988). It makes sense to question the concepts of truth. What really is it? Can theory ever be truth? Witkin and Gottschalk contend that a relevant theory needs to attend to "scientific thought and the values of the profession" (p. 211). They further suggest that a valid theory must be discriminating. It should deny myths, accept reality, and rise above a patriarchal scientific community. Additionally, a theory should recognize that individuals are able to reflect on their choices and reach goals. Behaviors are engaged because of personal regulation rather than determined by causes. "Thus conceptualizations of people as mechanically responding to stimuli (environmental or unconscious) are less desirable than theories conceiving of people as agents acting in accord with their beliefs and intentions. Humans act, not simply behave" (Witkin & Gottschalk, 1988, p. 219). Finally, theories should consider the life reality and wisdom of the individual, respect individuality, and abhor the discretionary control of one group over another (Witkin & Gottschalk, 1988). On the other hand, Slawski (1974) asserts that reliable theories must in some way include "explanatory power, informational value, predictability, and testability, or ease of application" (p. 397).

Although the use of empirical research used to support theories is growing rapidly, its application appears to be disappointing. For social workers, when and how to use empirical research to support theory and practice can at times be confusing. Decisions as how to best evaluate and scrutinize the information gathered can be perplexing. For example, what is most important in utilizing theoretical principles to guide practice? Is it acknowledging and answering the question of whether or not what we do works? And, if so, do we need more supportive information that allows the achievement of an accurate measurement? If so, how can this accurate measurement be best obtained? In addition, how are the chosen measurements to be ranked in terms of importance and contribution? For social workers, it becomes a difficult balancing act to determine which is more important: the explanation of a phenomenon or if the phenomena can be stated in concrete and measurable terms. If it is to measure the helping services provided through empirical means, measuring theory methodology would be possible. Yet, can the focus on empirically gathered data leave out significant aspects regarding the value of a theory? Last, if we assess and rank the importance of a theoretical contribution to understanding human growth and development only when it is supported by controlled experiments, will we overlook important data that can be derived from participant observation? For social workers, these issues will remain a struggle as we try to sort out the aim of social work interventions—to identify, to control, and to help individuals change troublesome human behaviors or to simply understand what an individual does and why. Perhaps, Myers (1987) can offer a suggestion to this dilemma:

> Seldom in life does one perspective give us the complete picture. Certainly our subject matter—the workings of human personality—is mysterious and complex enough to reveal different aspects when viewed from different perspectives. Thus we can do as most psychologists do today and allow each perspective to enlarge our vision. (p. 421)

## APPLYING PRACTICE TO THEORY

Selecting the most appropriate practice method based on theory requires a multitude of factors such as what approach would be best to reach efficient and effective practice. In addition to these numerous factors, selection of appropriate practice strategy supporting and recognizing the importance of counseling and the services that social workers provide concerning enhancing overall client well-being cannot be underestimated. Many times clients or their families may be resistant to counseling and remain unconvinced that this type of intervention is necessary. In addition to this, other helping professionals also may not recognize the importance of the social worker as a professional who can do more than just provide concrete referrals. It does appear, however, this view is changing because many health professionals, clients, and their families now acknowledge the importance of counseling as a service necessity that helps to ensure greater intervention success (Dziegielewski, 1998).

Although it is beyond the scope of this text to explain all theoretical and practice frameworks available to social workers, each of the chapters seeks to provide a brief presentation of several of the most common methods of practice. Before presenting this information, however, several areas need to be considered in selecting a practice method.

## Recognizing Empowerment and Diversity

In most schools of social work, students have traditionally been taught that the social work process can be defined in phases (even when not clearly established) as having a beginning, a middle, and an end. In this text several structured practice approaches are presented, yet it is not uncommon for these approaches to be met with resistance, especially when they do not appear to do what clients want or what is best for them. One of the greatest lessons that any social worker practitioner will learn is that beginnings, middles, and ends cannot always be predicted or planned. Therefore, flexibility needs to exist as sometimes even the best planned interventions can unravel. After all, there is no such thing as the one-problem client. Clients often have multiple problems, thus, clients may benefit with more options and choices for implementation of the selected methodological approaches.

When applying theoretical concepts to practice methods the term *client empowerment* cannot be underestimated. The social work dictionary defines empowerment as "the process of helping individuals, families, groups, and communities increase personal, interpersonal, socioeconomic, and political strengths and influence toward improving their circumstances" (Barker, 1999). Unfortunately, this definition is far from inclusive because implementing the concept of empowerment can vary based on social worker and situational context. In a recent study by Ackerson and Harrison (2000), these researchers found that practitioners can have various definitions for the term empowerment and, although these definitions did differ, many social workers linked empowerment to utilization of a strength's perspective. Therefore, empowerment recognizes a client's strength and reminds both the client and the practitioner of what these strengths involve. So as we approach each of these chapters and the interpretations of the basic theories of human growth and development one theme runs clear and that is "to start where the client is." This means respecting the worth and dignity of each individual as well as the diversity that makes that person special and unique. Regardless of how empowerment is defined, it is important in social work that the uniqueness of the individual must always be accentuated and highlighted in each step of the helping process. Most clients respond favorably when they are acknowledged for their strengths and challenged to maximize their own potential.

## Environmental Pressures and Practice Application

Brief and time-limited approaches to social work practice are now considered the state of the art. One major reason for this is that insurance companies will not pay for long-term treatments, and to receive reimbursement, practitioners must consider specific time-limited approaches. Furthermore, in defense of this trend many clients simply do not have the time, desire, or money for long-term treatment (especially the poor). For many social workers who believe in developing long-term and comprehensive types of clinical helping relationships, this trend is very frustrating. Today, little emphasis exists in terms of amorphous clinical judgments and vague attempts at making clients "feel better," and these efforts will no longer be allowed (Dziegielewski, 1998). In most areas of social work practice, similar to so many other areas of counseling practice, the days of insurance-covered, long-term therapy encounters have ended.

For social workers, it is now expected that services will be reflective of quality and effectiveness. A clear linkage must exist between the care provided and the resulting costs. Based on this premise, even the most seasoned social workers are now being forced to constantly battle the expectation of providing what they believe is the most beneficial and ethical practice possible, while being pressured to complete it as quickly and efficiently as reasonable. When selecting a method of practice, social workers also must defend the type of treatment offered based on promises of lower premiums and less health care expenditures. For many clients, it is not uncommon to be more interested in receiving a service that is time-limited or reimbursable, regardless of the expected benefit that they may gain from an alternate treatment strategy.

Therefore, to successfully unite theory and practice, it has become evident that practice reality based on environmental pressures will dictate brief therapy sessions, regardless of the methodology used or the orientation of the social worker (Dziegielewski, Shields, & Thyer, 1998). In social work practice, most of these therapeutic encounters generally range from 6 to 8 sessions (Wells & Phelps, 1990); however, as many as 20 have been noted (Fanger, 1984). For many social workers, one session is becoming commonplace. Because most encounters will be brief, social workers must plan and select intervention strategies based on the overall objective of bringing about positive changes in a client's current lifestyle with as little face-to-face contact as possible (Fanger, 1995). It is this emphasis on effectiveness and applicability leading to increased positive change that has helped to make time-limited, brief interventions popular. Today, time-limited approaches are the most often requested forms of practice.

## MEASURING THEORY IN PRACTICE EFFECTIVENESS

The conceptual infrastructure of social work practice is that of "interpersonal helping." Therefore, the social worker's primary responsibility and focus in the helping relationship is to effect positive change in the lives of individuals, whether it is to increase or decrease behaviors. To assist in this process the following criteria are suggested to help determine if a particular human behavior theory adds to practice knowledge.

First, does the theory lead to development of knowledge that helps to explain and predict social workers' and clients' behaviors in interactional situations in which services are to be provided to the clients? That is, are client and social worker variables identified and viewed in terms of how they might influence the interactional situation. Variables to be addressed include culture, race, gender, age, and other relevant social and cultural attributes that relate to both the client, the client system (e.g., client's family), and the social worker.

Second, does the theory lead to knowledge that explains what is involved in forming the relationship? Theory should provide a basis for understanding, thereby helping the intervener to focus on the basic features of interactional relationship. For example, how can subtle interaction effects, such as eye contact, non-verbal behavior, or gender of each participant affect the intervention process? Furthermore, once these effects are identified in a current interactional relationship, can the same incidents be expected to occur or be generalized to other relationships with the same or a different practitioner? Moreover, how does the theory assist in specifying the appropriate context for the intervention?

Third, what are the behaviors that are involved in the attempt to influence? Once identified, how and when should they be exhibited by the social worker? For example, if the social worker is involved in family therapy, are clear criteria provided as to when the different intervention techniques are to occur regarding how to proceed? At what pace should these activities continue, and when is it best to terminate services?

Fourth, there should be a direct relationship between the intervention techniques utilized and the outcomes expected to result. That is, how valid are the assumptions the theory makes about explaining and predicting behavior? How accurately measured is the amount of change that took place? Can linkage be clearly made that the intervention or treatment is directly related to any behavioral change acquired?

Fifth, if a theory provides relevant practice principles, how useful to social workers is the knowledge of the accessibility of the variables involved? Can the variables be identified and manipulated? Is the cost-benefit ratio too great? Does the knowledge violate the values of the profession?

An appropriate conceptualization and operationalization must be based on an adequate human behavior theory for intervention to achieve the development of effective programs. Social workers must be able to specify what behaviors a client will exhibit to apply a given treatment strategy. This represents a difficult requirement for many, if not most, theoretical frameworks. Therapeutic services are usually characterized on a global level and are assigned a broad label, such as transactional analysis, behavior modification, or family therapy. However, such labels are valuable only so long as they specify the operations involved in implementing the services.

For instance, the global label of behavior modification can be separated into the following distinct behavioral acts: directions, positive contact, praise, positive attention, holding, criticism, threats, punishment, negative attention, time-out, and application of a token economy (Wodarski, Feldman, & Pedi, 1974; Wodarski & Pedi, 1978). Moreover, essential attributes of the change agent that facilitate the implementation of treatment should be delineated.

Practitioners and students of social work practice should be cognizant of the values and research principles from the "womb to the tomb." As a result of intensive study regarding the attributes of behavior, the theories become inherently value-laden, which may affect the professional relationship between client and practitioner.

To facilitate the intervention process the following factors must be addressed: program rationale, duration of the intervention, an adequate specification of target behaviors and baselines, specification of information that will result in treatment efficacy, adequate treatment measures, identification of a baseline, and a method for follow-up.

First, *program rationale* should be discussed from an empirical or research perspective. In this way, a focus that links process to targeted outcomes is clear throughout the process. The resources of the program or the agency that implements the program needs to become familiar and agree to support the decision-making process. To further facilitate this process, additional questions to be answered include the following: How can the program be implemented with minimal disruption? What new communication structures need to be added? What types of measurements are used in evaluating the service? What accountability mechanisms need to be set up? What procedures can be used for monitoring execution of the program?

Second, clearly establishing the *duration* of the intervention should be done early in the planning process. As stated earlier, research supports that service provision is best when delivered in time-limited intervals. Current guidelines specify that service should be provided only until client behavior has improved sufficiently in terms of quality and quantity. This requires that outcome criteria (criteria that is reflective of the end product) be established before the service is provided with clear expectations of how the program will be evaluated. It is critical to determine how the practitioner will measure and evaluate client change behavior and determine whether the intervention meets the desired goals, which in essence determines the effectiveness and duration of treatment. After measuring intervention effectiveness, measurements of social worker effectiveness must also be undertaken. Through this type of evaluation social workers can determine whether their intervention worked. The practitioner needs to assess client change at various intervals to make this determination. The criteria should enable social workers to determine if a service is meeting the needs of the client. Moreover, assessing and evaluating these criteria consistently should assist in revealing the particular factors involved in deciding to terminate a service. The more concrete the criteria, the less this process will be based on subjective factors.

Third, each social worker must be aware of how to assess the *adequate specification of behaviors and baselines*. Observation of client behavior is one of the primary purposes of evaluation in clinical practice (Dziegielewski & Powers, 2000). Defining the purpose of evaluation will aid in answering the question of exactly how problems co-vary. An adequate treatment program must take into account the need for reliable specification of target behaviors, that is, those behaviors that are to be changed. For example, a treatment program to alleviate stress and anxiety might employ behavioral rating scales in which stressful target behaviors are concretely specified. These could include observable behaviors such as angry outbursts, leaving the room to avoid confrontation, or avoiding the places where anxiety occurs. All the above-mentioned behaviors can and should be empirically measured. In addition, a prerequisite for the adequate evaluation of any therapeutic service is securing a baseline before implementation of treatment. This enables the investigator to assess how treatment interventions compare with no treatment. Identification of a baseline behavior should be clearly identified and monitored. For a detailed description on how to measure and apply the baseline, see Dziegielewski and Powers (2000).

Fourth, the social worker should *address and identify measures of social worker and client behaviors.* This process is supported by the implementation of such measures as checklists completed by clients or significant others (e.g., group leaders, parents, referral agencies, grandparents). In this process behavioral time-sampling schedules can be utilized to assess client change. Likewise, behavioral rating scales can be used to assess the behaviors exhibited by a change agent. Although over the last 15 years there has been an emphasis for the utilization of multicriterion measurement to measure intervention success, this is rarely done. Additionally, when it has been done the few investigators who have utilized multicriterion measurement indicate that many changes secured on certain inventories do not correspond necessarily with results of other utilized measurement processes. For example, studies by Wodarski and colleagues (Wodarski & Buckholdt, 1975; Wodarski, Feldman, & Pedi, 1976; Wodarski & Pedi, 1977, 1978) found little correlation between self-inventory and behavioral rating scales. In many instances, a change can occur on one of the measurements and not on another. The strongest data are derived from behavioral observation scales simply because observers are trained for long periods of time to secure reliable and accurate data. Thus, a major question to ask of any theory is, if it does employ multicriterion measurement do these indices accurately measure and portray the behavioral problems identified.

Fifth, *criteria must be clearly identified and linked to treatment efficacy.* Any therapeutic program derived from human theory should clearly specify the criteria by which the service will be evaluated and this must be done *before* the treatment is implemented. For example, evaluation may occur by means of behavioral observations provided by trained observers or through the use of checklists completed by clients and significant others. In view of the multidimensional nature of human behavior it is necessary for professionals to evaluate more multicriterion to develop a comprehensive and rational basis for the provision of services. Moreover, highly sophisticated treatment programs will endeavor to quantify the extent of behavioral change targeted and those actually achieved along with the social relevance of changes that have occurred (i.e., do the changes really matter in terms of clients' abilities to function in their environment?).

The sixth area for integrating theory and practice research rests in *monitoring and implementing the intervention process*. Once these other conditions are met, it then becomes necessary to monitor the implementation of treatment. Such monitoring should take place periodically throughout treatment so that necessary adjustments can be made over time if the quality of treatment varies. If behavioral change is obtained and if the investigator can provide data to indicate that treatment(s) were differentially implemented, the change agents can claim with confidence that their treatment has been responsible for the observed modifications in behavior. When information cannot be provided supporting that client change has occurred, different and often rival causes (or hypotheses) can be postulated to account for the results (Wodarski & Pedi, 1977).

Last, *reliability and follow-up must be secured for all measures* used in evaluating a program. Without this basic scientific requisite, evaluative efforts may be ill spent and there can be no assurance of consistency in the data secured. See Dziegielewski and Powers (2000) for a more detailed explanation of this process. In addition, the proper assessment of any therapeutic program with clients involves follow-up. Although surprisingly few investigators now employ this procedure, it is quickly gaining in popularity due to the need of providers to prove efficacy to the funding agencies. Crucial questions answered by a follow-up include whether a therapeutic program has changed behaviors in a desired direction, how long these new behaviors were maintained, and to what other contexts they are generalized. That is, have the change agents programmed the environment to maintain the change in terms of substituting "naturally occurring" reinforcers, including training relatives or other individuals in the client's environment, gradually removing or fading the contingencies, varying the conditions of training, using different schedules of reinforcement, and using delayed gratification or reinforcement and self-control procedures (Wodarski, 1983)? Such procedures will be employed in future sophisticated and effective social service delivery systems. Pertinent questions remain concerning when and where a follow-up should occur, and who should secure the measurement. Empirical guidelines in favor of these issues do not yet exist. Failure to provide an adequate follow-up period is a major deficiency of many evaluative studies executed in the social sciences (Wodarski).

## SUMMARY

Truth is arrived at by the painstaking process of eliminating the untrue.
—Sherlock Holmes (Myers, 1987, p. 9)

This chapter has provided an introduction to many of the presumptions that undergrid the premise of this book, which is to link theoretical concepts with issues, related to empirically based practice. The following chapters address the phenomena of human growth and development from a theoretical perspective, highlighting the empirical findings related to current conceptualizations used to explain, predict, and change human behavior. Indeed, all theories can be viewed as a potential framework for creation of an atmosphere of practice that implies intervention efficiency and effectiveness.

The reader is cautioned to remember that there are few works in the literature in which theories are presented as complete logical systems. If theory is used without creative practice skill in terms of strategy selection and implementation, even the best treatment programs can fail because they have focused only on one aspect of a client's problem. Social work needs comprehensive theories of behavioral causation that include treatment paradigms specified in accordance with the theory (Daniel, Wassell, Ennis, Gilligan, & Ennis, 1997; Wodarski, 1987; Wodarski & Ammons, 1981; Wodarski & Lenhart, 1984). According to Sutton (1998), theoretical models do not always predict behavior as well as expected. Moreover, many theories seem to fall short of being able to predict the possible extent of change that can take place in a client, or, how it will be measured (Wodarski, 1987). In today's managed care environment the measurement of goals and objectives based in concrete outcomes have made empirical measurement in theory and practice essential. Concepts that are difficult to measure can complicate practice strategy. For example, functional theory is based on the concept of "freeing the will" (Dore, 1990). In terms of establishing a measurement, how can the social worker decide exactly what that is when, and if, it happens? Moreover, once identified, how might one go about measuring that? Caution needs to be given to quantify concepts that might be assumed indicative of treatment success but in today's system cannot be measured. For example, when Luiselli, Marholin, Steinman, and Steinman (1980) reviewed articles from four major journals relative to the specific dependent measures used for relaxation techniques, results showed that in 70% of the articles no indication was made regarding how the effects of relaxation were assessed (p. 663).

This places the responsibility on the social work practitioner who must decide which theory is best, and how it will contribute to the outcomes desired. Wodarski (1987) suggested that there was an urgent need to evaluate through research the effectiveness of various theoretical conceptualizations with certain clients. Yet, Downing (1996), in her judicious review of changes being made to the probation department, warned of the "dangers of misusing theory to satisfy a perceived demand for a simplistic, reductionist view . . . " (p. 65).

Clearly, as our culture becomes increasingly more diverse, consideration concerning gender and ethnic-minority variables becomes paramount (White, 1984; Wodarski, 1987).

Hoskins (1998) concurs with this view as she relates:

> Traditional psychological theories make up the core curriculum for educating helping professionals throughout a variety of academic institutions. Although these theories have contributed to contemporary approaches and have historical relevance, they also have major shortcomings when it comes to working with differences. Issues of ethnicity, economic status, and gender are for the most part absent from the dominant psychological models of helping. (p. 83)

As professionals, we are obligated to offer our clients the most empirically effective treatment at hand (Cormier & Cormier, 1991; Wodarski, 1992). Moreover, there are now treatments that have been empirically validated through research (Ammerman, Last, & Hersen, 1993; Giles, Prial, & Neims, 1993; Gorey, Thyer, & Pawluck, 1996; MacDonald, Sheldon, & Gillespie, 1992; Reid & Hanrahan, 1992; Thyer, 1995).

Contrary to the nihilistic view that "virtually any intervention can be justified on the grounds that it has as much support as alternative methods" (Witkin, 1991, p. 158), numerous outcome studies comparing various forms of psychosocial treatments regularly find that certain types of interventions work better than others for particular problems (Myers & Thyer, 1997).

Today, empirically based treatment technologies that consist of behavioral approaches are increasingly favored for their superior research designs (Thyer & Myers, 1998). More than ever, data supports the successful history of behavior modification practices with children who have been classified as hyperactive, autistic, delinquent, or retarded, as well as adults classified as antisocial, retarded, neurotic, or psychotic (Davison & Neale, 1994; Glass & Arnkoff, 1992; Goldfried, Greenberg, & Marmar, 1990; Thyer, 1995). Indeed, "behavioral therapy" may be considered the initial treatment of choice for a wide variety of disorders, including anxiety, depression, sexual dysfunction, eating disorders, schizophrenia, psychosomatic complaints, and substance abuse" (Thyer & Myers, 1998, p. 45). Technologies with accumulating empirical history include: (a) Relaxation Training, (b) Assertiveness Training, (c) Anger Management, (d) Stress Management, (e) Problem-Solving Skills, (f) Self-esteem Building, (g) Urge Control, and (h) Relapse Prevention. These types of techniques highlight the importance of the social-behavioral perspective as it builds on the foundations of well-established concepts of learning and cognitions and the power of social situations in the reality of human existence.

> Theories are created to explain observations, but what we observe is influenced by our theoretical perspective (Myers, 1987, p. 9)

It is essential for social workers to examine the client from different theoretical perspectives. It is the responsibility of each professional to assess, through the available research, the efficacy and reliability of the diverse assumptions made about the individual in these various theoretical philosophies and to embrace the appropriate intervention techniques accordingly. Utilizing theory to support a practice framework or method will never be a simple task. There will be numerous cases that will present the professional with unique challenges including making the decision regarding what practice method to use, finding a delicate balancing act between the needs of the client, understanding the demands of the environment, and recognizing the skills and knowledge available to the social worker.

Furthermore, most social workers continue to believe that social work practice is clearly more involved than simply choosing what works to satisfy empirical standards. It takes knowing the client and the strategies and methods available as well as the theoretical foundations that underlie the practice techniques selected. In today's environment there are a multitude of complicated problems that must be addressed and an urgency to address them as quickly and effectively as possible. Social workers should be trained in these methods of helping. In addition, we must realize that this training cannot be static. All social workers must continue learning and growing to anticipate the needs of our clients.

Again, we welcome the reader to look at the current theories that provide the knowledge base for human growth and development, which in turn lead to the practice approaches utilized. Social workers are needed in the practice arena to address a variety of problems, and professionals must not succumb to the pressure of only providing concrete services. The following chapters show that the number of people suffering from anxiety and depressive disorders, self-destructive acts, and life-threatening illnesses has steadily risen—and so has the need for counselors, social workers, and psychologists who engage in clinical practice. Furthermore, to receive and continue to qualify for reimbursement for such services, social workers must remain aware of and be active in the social and political climate that surrounds our practice arena. Generally, social and political changes do not happen quickly. In the meantime, social workers are encouraged to learn more about integrating theory and practice from an empirical perspective. Although unity between theories seems disquieting, it is only when practitioners address these issues that social work practice can hope to achieve the goal of helping clients to the fullest possible extent to live productive lives.

## REFERENCES

Ackerson, B. J., & Harrison, W. D. (2000). Practitioner's perceptions of empowerment. *Families in Society, 81* (3), 238–244.

Ammerman, R. T., Last, C. G., & Hersen, M. (1993). *Handbook of prescriptive treatments for children and adolescents.* Boston: Allyn and Bacon.

Ayer, A. J. (1982). *Philosophy in the twentieth century.* London: Weidenfeld and Nielson.

Barker, R. L. (1999). *The social work dictionary* (4th ed.). Washington, DC: NASW Press.

Brieland, D. (1977). Historical overview: Special issue on conceptual frameworks for social work practice. *Social Work, 22* (5), 341–346.

Cormier, W. H., & Cormier, L. S. (1991). *Interviewing strategies for helpers* (3rd ed.). Pacific Grove, CA: Brooks Cole.

Daniel, B., Wassell, S., Ennis, J., Gilligan, R., & Ennis, E. (1997). Critical understandings of child development: The development of a module for a post qualifying certificate course in child protection studies. *Child and Family Social Work, 2* (4), 209–219.

Davison, G. C., & Neale, J. M. (1994). *Abnormal psychology* (6th ed.). New York: John Wiley & Sons.

Dore, M. M. (1990). Functional theory: Its history and influence on contemporary social work practice. *Social Service Review, 64* (3), 358–374.

Downing, K. (1996). Probation training, cognition and crime: Uses and abuses of theory. *Social Work Education, 15* (4), 65–75.

Dworetzky, J. P. (1987). *Introduction to child development.* New York: West.

Dziegielewski, S. F. (1998). *The changing face of health care social work: Professional practice in the era of managed care.* New York: Springer.

Dziegielewski, S. F., & Powers, G. T. (2000). Procedures for evaluating time-limited crisis intervention. In A. Roberts (Ed.), *Crisis intervention handbook* (2nd ed.). New York: Oxford University Press.

Dziegielewski, S. F., Shields, J., & Thyer, B. A. (1998). Short-term treatment: Models and methods. In J. Williams & K. Ell, *Advances in mental health research: Implications for practice.* Washington, DC: NASW Press.

Fanger, M. T. (1995). Brief therapies. In R. L. Edwards (Ed.-in-Chief), *Encyclopedia of social work* (19th ed., Vol. 1, pp. 323–334). Washington, DC: NASW Press.

Giles, T. R., Prial, E. M., & Neims, D. M. (1993). Evaluating psychotherapies: A comparisons of effectiveness. Special series: Evaluation in treatment methods in psychiatry: 3. *International Journal of Mental Health, 22* (2), 43–65.

Glass, C. R., & Arnkoff, D. B. (1992). *Behavior therapy.* Washington, DC: American Psychological Association.

Goldfried, M. R., Greenberg, L. S., & Marmar, C. (1990). Individual psychotherapy: Process and outcome. *Annual Review of Psychology, 41,* 659–688.

Gorey, K., Thyer, B. A., & Pawluck, D. (1996). *The differential effectiveness of social work interventions: A meta-analysis.* Manuscript submitted for publication.

Hoskins, M. (1998). Constructivism and child and youth care practice: Visions for the 21st century. *Journal of Child and Youth Care, 11* (4), 83–92.

Luiselli, J. K., Marholin, D., Steinman, D. L., & Steinman, W. M. (1980). Assessing the effects of relaxation training. *Behavior Therapy, 10* (5), 663–668.

Lyons, P., Wodarski, J. S., & Feit, M. D. (1998). Human behavior theory: Emerging trends and issues. *Journal of Human Behavior in the Social Environment, 1* (1), 1–21.

MacDonald, G., Sheldon, B., & Gillespie, J. (1992). Contemporary studies of the effectiveness of social work. *British Journal of Social Work, 22* (6), 615–643.

Minahan, A. (1981). Introduction to special issue. *Social Work, 26* (1), 5–6.

Myers, D. G. (1987). *Psychology.* New York: Worth.

Myers, L. L., & Thyer, B. A. (1997). Should social work clients have the right to effective treatment? *Journal of the National Association of Social Workers, 42* (3), 288–298.

Reid, W. J., & Hanrahan, P. (1992). Recent evaluations of social work: Grounds for optimism. *Social Work, 27,* 328–340.

Rosenhan, D. L., & Seligman, M. E. P. (1989). *Abnormal psychology.* New York: W. W. Norton.

Slawski, C. (1974). Evaluating theories comparatively. *Zeitschrift fur Soziologie, 3* (4), 397–407.

Strachey, C. (Ed.). (1901). English statesman, man of letters—letter, 30 Aug. 1749 (first published 1774). *Letters of the Earl of Chesterfield to his son, 1* (190).

Sutton, S. (1998). Predicting and explaining intentions and behavior: How well are we doing? *Journal of Applied Social Psychology, 28* (15), 1317–1338.

Thyer, B. A. (1995). Promoting an empiricist agenda within the human services: An ethical and humanistic imperative. *Journal of Behavior Therapy and Experimental Psychiatry, 26* (2), 93–98.

Thyer, B. A., & Myers, L. L. (1998). Social learning theory: An empirically based approach to understanding human behavior in the social environment. *Journal of Human Behavior in the Social Environment, 1* (1), 33–52.

Ullrich, W. J. (1999). Depth psychology, critical pedagogy, and initial teacher preparation. *Teaching Education, 10* (2), 17–33.

Wells, R. A., & Phelps, P. A. (1990). The brief psychotherapies: A selective overview. In R. A. Wells & V. J. Giannetti (Eds.), *Handbook of the brief psychotherapies* (pp. 3–26). New York: Plenum.

White, B. W. (Ed.). (1984). *Color in a white society: Selected papers from the NASW conference Color in a white society, Los Angeles, 1982.* Silver Spring, MD: National Association of Social Workers.

Witkin, S. L. (1991). Empirical clinical practice: A critical analysis. *Social Work, 36* (2), 158–163.

Witkin, S. L., & Gottschalk, S. (1988). Alternative criteria for theory evaluation. *Social Service Review, 62* (2), 211–224.

Wodarski, J. S. (1983). Clinical practice and the social learning paradigm. *Social Work, 28* (2), 154–160.

Wodarski, J. S. (1987). *Social work practice with children and adolescents.* Springfield, IL: Charles C. Thomas.

Wodarski, J. S. (1992). Social work perspective on human behavior. *Journal of Health & Social Policy, 4* (2), 93–112.

Wodarski, J. S., & Ammons, P. W. (1981). Comprehensive treatment of runaway children and their parents. *Family Therapy, 8* (3), 229–240.

Wodarski, J. S., & Buckholdt, D. (1975). *Behavioral instruction in college classrooms: A review of methodological procedures.* Springfield, IL: Charles C. Thomas.

Wodarski, J. S., Feldman, R. A., & Pedi, S. J. (1974). Objective measurements of the independent variables: A neglected methodological aspect of community-based behavioral research. *Journal of Abnormal Child Psychology, 2* (3), 239–244.

Wodarski, J. S., Feldman, R. A., & Pedi, S. J. (1976). Integrating anti-social children into pro-social groups at summer camp: A three-year study. *Social Service Review, 86,* 257–272.

Wodarski, J. S., & Lenhart, S. D. (1984). Alcohol education for adolescents. *Social Work Education, 6* (2), 69–92.

Wodarski, J. S., & Pedi, S. J. (1977). The comparison of anti-social and pro-social children on multi-criterion measures at a community center: A three-year study. *Social Work, 22,* 290–296.

Wodarski, J. S., & Pedi, S. J. (1978). The empirical evaluation of the effects of different group treatment strategies against a controlled treatment strategy on behavior exhibited by anti-social children, behavior of the therapist, and two self-ratings measuring anti-social behavior. *Journal of Clinical Psychology, 34* (2), 471–481.

# Micro and Mezzo Perspectives: Individual Approaches to Human Growth and Development

# Micro and Mezzo Perspectives: Individual Approaches to Human Growth and Development

## Carolyn Hilarski, Sophia F. Dziegielewski, and John S. Wodarski

This chapter introduces human growth and development from an individual perspective (referred to as micro) and incorporates the interplay between individuals and their environments (referred to as mezzo). To facilitate this process, the authors provide a brief summary of several different theoretical models representative of these perspectives. The presentation of these theoretical models sets the stage for human growth and development by providing background information in selected readings that can be found at the end of this section. The authors: (a) provide a brief overview of the theoretical model; (b) discuss how empiricism can be applied to the model; and (c) include a discussion of the intervention strategies in measuring the concepts. Special attention is paid to the importance of linking each of the theoretical perspectives to empirically based practice strategies and their effectiveness. The selected readings that follow exemplify several of the areas covered and provide the reader with greater depth in terms of understanding and application.

### INDIVIDUAL THEORETICAL MODELS: INTRODUCTORY CONCEPTS— THE PSYCHODYNAMIC MODELS

Historically, one of the most popular foundational methods for practice was the psychodynamic (also referred to as psychosexual) approach to understanding individual growth and human development. Essentially this began with the work of a Viennese practitioner, Sigmund Freud, 1856–1939 (Rosenhan & Seligman, 1989). Freud focused his understanding of human development on a system of psychic energy (or libido) that continuously shifted between sexual and aggressive drives. He believed that psychic energy or libido was fueled by a motivated set of instincts. Freud believed that an instinct is a mental representation of a physical or bodily need. According to this psychodynamic theory no behavior is accidental, but instead each behavior is related directly to reducing an internal state of tension (Carducci, 1998). In this model, inherent forces are either conscious (known to the individual) or unconscious (beyond the awareness of the individual). Freud coined the term *psychic determinism* to explain how behavior is governed by some purpose and meaning. The influence of the unconscious is unknown to the individual; however, these unconscious forces *do* contain thoughts, ideas, desires, and impulses that ultimately determine resulting behaviors. The conscious has sensory awareness that is limited to seeing, hearing, smelling, touching, tasting, and thinking. In this approach an individual strives to achieve homeostasis by relieving the tension built between instincts (conscious needs) and the desires of the unconscious. The tension or expression of trying to achieve balance can bring acceptance or anxiety to the individual (Carducci). When nonexpression arises, ambiguity results and the anxiety created must be *psychically* defended and can often result in thoughts of an obsessive nature with behaviors or compulsions designed to relieve the anxiety (Rosenhan & Seligman). (See Figure 1 for Freud's understanding of the human mind.)

Freud's developmental theory is generally credited with designating the terms *unconscious, preconscious,* and the *conscious* mind. It is the unconscious and preconscious domains that are thought to hold most of our thoughts, feelings, impulses, and struggles (Zastrow & Kirst-Ashman, 1990). Although thoughts and resulting issues in the preconscious area of the mind have *some* chance of reaching the conscious mind, those in the unconscious mind remain hidden to the individual. Freud felt that individuals were limited in what they know about their own feelings and emotions. The repressed barrier, or unconscious forgetting of anxious feelings or memories, becomes a *holding* place for all negative issues (Schwartz & Johnson, 1988). The events repressed within this area possess energy, which is motivated to reject negative thoughts and behaviors (Zastrow & Kirst-Ashman, 1990).

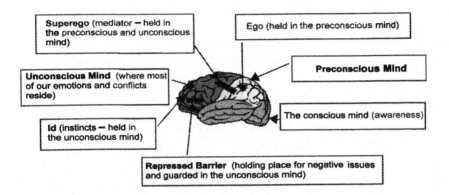

**FIGURE 1** Freud's understanding of the mind incorporated two major concepts, the conscious and unconscious.

Freud explained the structure of personality as containing three intrapsychic parts: the id, the ego, and the superego. The *id* is present at birth and is the source of instincts and impulses that is ruled by the pleasure principle (or the demand for immediate satisfaction). The ego helps to meet the needs of the id, by using cognitive processes such as perception, learning, memory, judgment, and self-awareness. The ego is ruled by the reality principle, which involves delaying gratification as well as working to meet the demands of the environment (Newman & Newman, 1995). The *superego* represents ideals, morals, and conscience (Rosenhan & Seligman, 1989). The superego's task is to ensure that the individual's thoughts, feelings, and behaviors stay within the moral standards of society (Carducci, 1998). The ego works toward satisfying and mediating conflicts between the demands of the id for gratification and the demands of the superego's desire for appropriate (good) behavior. This is all done outside of the person's awareness (Newman & Newman, 1995).

In Freud's psychodynamic theory it was hypothesized that the most significant developments in personality took place by resolving a series of conflicts associated with a sequence of psychosexual stages. Freud believed that the fundamental purpose of personality development was in preparing the individual to cope with psychic conflicts and crises in life (Carducci, 1998). He described five psychosexual stages: *Oral* (birth to 1 year), *anal* (1 to 3 years), *phallic* (3 to 6 years), *latent* (7 to 11 years), and *genital* (adolescence). According to his theory, each stage is associated with a particular body zone and is linked to the major developmental needs and challenges that are typical of various ages in childhood (Berger, 1994). Furthermore, each zone is of heightened sexual importance (Newman & Newman, 1995). The expression of libido and pleasure is associated with reducing bodily tension. For example, during the oral stage, tension is released and pleasure is received by the mouth through sucking and eating. During the anal stage tension is relieved through urinating and defecating and conflicts are thought to arise from successful or unsuccessful toilet training. Freud considered the phallic stage to be a period of heightened genital sensitivity. This stage of development is characterized by an increased sense of bodily awareness and the exploration of various body parts (Carducci, 1998). As part of the phallic stage of development children direct sexualized activity or feelings toward both sexes. In boys, psychosexual conflict arises between their desires to seek pleasure via the mother while competing against the father. Freud termed this "love triangle" the *Oedipus Complex*. In girls, the psychosexual conflict is created by their desires to seek pleasure via the father while competing against the mother; this conflict has been termed the *Electra Complex*. The *latent* stage is considered a period of reduced psychic energy (libido) in which children begin to form close relationships with same-sex groups. The genital stage occurs with the onset of puberty and secondary sex characteristics. This stage reintroduces the genital region as a source of interest. Additionally, in adolescence teenagers are becoming aware of not only meeting their own needs of pleasure, but also the needs and pleasure of others (Carducci, 1998). Individuals progress through these stages in an evolutionary manner, and it is important that at each level of development fixation does not result. For example, if an infant becomes fixated orally, then conflict could present itself later in life and the development of alcoholism could result. It is postulated that such conditions as this may occur because the resolution on issues related to weaning were never fully resolved. During the course of development conflicts must be addressed and successfully resolved. As an individual develops, the resolution of psychic conflict allows for the birth of the superego while setting the stage for later social and sexual behavior (Rosenhan & Seligman, 1989). The skills acquired for resolving these conflicts are thought to serve as the basis for resolving conflicts later in adult life.

## Empiricism and Evaluation of Psychodynamic Theory

Among many social work practitioners and researchers the psychodynamic-psychosexual theory of human development is not considered to be viable because of the lack of research to support it (Thyer & Myers, 1998). Rosenhan and Seligman (1989) suggest that the theory is not empirically supportable, as it is too complex and abstract, and it neglects the environmental aspects of the individual. Psychodynamic approaches have a long history of being attacked by those who believe in a more quantifiable approach to practice, where concepts are developed into measurable terms. For example, many behaviorists believe that it is inaccurate to make the presumption that evolution is naturally progressive. Rather, theorists who support a behavioral perspective believe that development results from respondent, operant, and observational learning. B. F. Skinner, a behaviorist (1981), clearly stated that, " . . . human development is primarily a function of selection by consequences . . . mediated of course by one's genetic endowment and biological structure and function" (Thyer & Myers, 1998, p. 41).

In contrast, other researchers and practitioners such as Kuhn (1997) have challenged the critics of psychodynamic thought, while encouraging the critics to revisit Freud's early works regarding early sexual trauma and its relationship to anxiety. Fowler (1998) also remains supportive, citing that young children often interpret information incorrectly, and it remains difficult therefore to separate an actual incident from the experience that the client reported. Supporters of the psychodynamic approaches such as Schwartz and Johnson (1988) insist that psychodynamic theory " . . . currently remains the sole example of a global psychological theory designed to account for the totality of human behavior" (p. 14). Furthermore, they consider psychodynamic theory as comprehensive, as it explains all " . . . aspects of human thought, emotion, experience, and judgment—from dreams through slips of the tongue" (Rosenhan & Seligman, 1989, p. 101). Some of the elements of the psychodynamic theory seem universal as many individuals believe in the principle of the *self* and *free will* and generally accept responsibility for creating meaning for their life.

Several theorists that are generally considered supporters of the psychodynamic approaches (see Jung & Douglas, 1997), have modified Freud's model to simplify the abstract nature of his concepts. Neo-Freudians such as the Swiss psychologist Carl Jung, 1875–1961; Erich

Fromm; Alfred Adler, 1870–1937; and Harry Stack Sullivan, 1892–1949, geared their practice and interest more toward ego and systems issues than to the principles of libido and instincts.

In summary, although it is likely history will report that the proponents of psychoanalytic or psychodynamic theory (Freudians and neo-Freudians) contributed much to our self-view, they were essentially authors and not researchers. Their contributions to human growth and development were significant for advancing understanding of and providing a framework for developmental concepts rather than hard science (Zastrow & Kirst-Ashman, 1990). Any approach that attempts to achieve prediction that explains all variables of a circumstance is almost inevitably doomed to fail, and the psychodynamic theories are no exception. However, one thing that does stand clear is that the psychodynamic theories have contributed to the demystification of abnormal behaviors by increasing practical understanding and providing hope. Application of these theories can assist to address issues that are not clearly identified or understood. In addition, this type of psychosexual model has caught the scientific community's attention to the " . . . importance of human sexuality and to the tension between our individual impulses and our social well-being" (Myers, 1987, p. 403). Empirical basis or not, relevant or not, few can argue that the psychodynamic perspective has influenced our view of human nature and changed our self-view.

## Intervention Implications

Psychodynamic intervention attempts to release the repressed elements of the unconscious mind and bring them to the forefront of the conscious mind to free negative psychic energy. In this theoretical framework, individuals strive to have control over shaping their destiny and have the capacity to do something about their individual problems. However, assessment of the client's ego strengths is crucial to understanding the depth of change that can take place and the type of treatment that will be selected (Wodarski, 1987).

Utilization of this theoretical framework can include encouraging the client to investigate dreams and thoughts for catharsis, interpretation, and ultimate self-acceptance. For example, Gestalt therapy encourages the resolution of conflicted issues with the role playing of dreams and events making this type of "looking to the self" for healing consistent with psychodynamic philosophy. Cramerus' (1998) conducted a study that hypothesized that anxiety is related to three variables inspired by the psychodynamic theory: rejection of the self, self-derogation, and fear of rejection from others. Results obtained through self-report measures from 130 adults supported that anxiety was related to negative self-perception or incongruity of the self with the perceived "ideal self." Another approach reflective of these principles is client-centered therapy that purports to give the client unconditional positive regard that allows the client to begin self-acceptance by *being accepted* in the therapeutic relationship. This relationship can also be used to examine resistance and transference. When using psychodynamic approaches to support the intervention process, the ultimate interventive goal is to reduce the amount of energy the client spends in defending and repressing unpleasant emotions and thoughts (Rosenhan & Seligman, 1989).

## Psychodynamic Theory and Functionalism

Social work is generally undertaken with very little understanding of its evolutionary metamorphosis, and seemingly having forgotten its functional school that rose in popularity along with the psychodynamic approaches (Dore, 1990). The functional perspective holds that if the client identifies the problem, then the client will ultimately decide to engage in change behavior that is designed to alter the situation. Therefore, each presenting problem is viewed as *where the client is,* "in the here and now." This model was originally based on Otto Rank's (Rank & Taft, 1924) theory of personality, developed after Rank had studied under Freud. In the 1920s, however, Rank's ideas began to take a new path when he came to believe that individual struggles pertained more to ambivalence relating to change than to internal distress relating to childhood (Dore, 1990).

Jesse Taft (1937) attempted to incorporate Rankian theory into the social work process, and his efforts resulted in the Pennsylvania School's publishing a book entitled *The Relation of Function to Process in Social Case Work* (Dore, 1990). The functional approach differs from the psychodynamic perspective in the expectation that no one understands the client's difficulty better than the client does, and the outcome of treatment is the responsibility of the client. This has an empowering effect because the client understands that any change or growth is the result of the client's decisions and actions (Smalley, 1967). This concept is different from psychoanalysis in its structure, because in psychoanalysis the therapist directs the change; in the functional school, however, it is the agency.

> The worker sets up the conditions as found in his agency function and procedure; the client representing the unknown natural forces, reacts to the limitation as well as to the possible fulfillment inherent in the function, over a period of testing it out. He tries to accept, to reject, to attempt to control, or to modify that function until he finally comes to terms with it enough to define or discover what he wants if anything, from the situation (Smalley, 1967, p. 365).

In summary, functional theory differs from psychoanalytic theory, in which the client is capable and responsible for change and the agency becomes the cultural milieu. Functional theorists focus on empowerment and active participation of the client in the change process (Grigsby, 1995). The concept of the client's *will* is respected and encouraged by the practitioner in the endeavor to help the client reach self-realization (Smalley, 1967). In this approach the therapeutic relationship forms a safe place for the negotiation of goals to pursue the resolution of the presenting problem. Clients are active participants in the process of change and help to negotiate appropriate goals to meet their needs. Goals set by the client are appropriate when they adhere to the defined purpose of the agency. The greatest criticism toward this process is that the client change depends on the degree to which the client and agency's purpose is congruent to the agency's policy and procedures, which can guide and dictate the treatment process (Smalley, 1996).

## BEHAVIORAL, COGNITIVE, AND SOCIAL LEARNING VIEWS

Philosopher John Locke (1632–1704) was the first of the classical British empiricists. He proclaimed that all knowledge is derived from experience. In his *Essay Concerning Human Understanding,* he theorized that the mind at birth is a *tabula rasa,* a blank slate (Palmer, 1994). This slate is informed only with experiences, and those experiences affect development (Schwartz & Johnson, 1988). Locke described a form of behavior therapy in writings about the practical techniques for removing a child's fear of frogs by means of graduated, nonthreatening encounters with them (Thorpe & Olson, 1997). This context postulates that we are products of our surroundings and antiquity (Bruck, 1968; Rosenhan & Seligman, 1989; Thomas, 1968). Behaviorism developed from this empiricist view, and the cognitive model grew from there (Rosenhan & Seligman, 1989).

Early in this century, psychologists were preoccupied with the study of consciousness through introspection; however, the debate continues as to whether thoughts always accurately reflect the precise content of what is experienced (Schwartz & Johnson, 1988). Behaviorism became the dominant theory in the 1920s with Watson's (1913) emerging ideas that learning is the developmental basis for all creatures (Rosenhan & Seligman, 1989). Through empirical laboratory research, behaviorists sought a global understanding of the principles of human and animal learning. These concepts incorporated several assumptions: (a) *environmentalism,* which concluded that all behaviors result from experience and are influenced by reward and punishment (Thomas, 1967); (b) *experimentalism,* wherein we look for the environmental cause of the behavior, and how we might go about changing it; and (c) *optimism,* which postulates that change can take place by changing the environment. For example, poverty is a risk factor for crime; therefore, the redistribution of wealth will help to alleviate poverty and crime (Rosenhan & Seligman, 1989). In this model, behavior is *learned* in one or more ways—Pavlovian, Respondent, or Operant conditioning (Thyer & Myers, 1998). (See Part II, chapter 6, "Learning Theories," for a more inclusive definition of how these concepts relate to practice.)

Since it is believed that thought often governs behavior, the move to include cognitions in terms of understanding human development is predictable. Piaget (1896–1980), a cognitive theorist, described cognition as the process of organizing and making meaning of experience. His emphasis was on how children think, and this process encompasses more than what knowledge had been acquired through direct behavior (Newman & Newman, 1995). Skinner (1981), a behaviorist, denies that thinking causes behavior; he asserts that thinking is connected to the cause of a certain behavior but does not always determine the action that follows. Rosenhan and Seligman (1989) offer an example that may explain this concept: "While a speedometer reflects how fast the automobile is going, it does not itself influence the speed" (p. 118).

In learning and development, the ideas of behaviorists and cognitive theorists often combine and place their emphasis on how individuals learn by experiencing associations between stimuli and reinforcement or punishment. Social learning theorist Albert Bandura (see Bandura & Walters, 1963) proposed that the description of learning gained only through classical or operant conditioning is too limited and necessitates a broader approach. See Part II, chapter 7 on social learning for a more detailed analysis and application of this model. Briefly, this model focuses on learning by imitating and is grounded in behaviorism, which philosophically encompasses thinking and the environment. For example, Bandura, Grusec, and Menlove (1967) suggested that individuals learn vicariously through observation, and this learning must involve expectations. Bandura (1977) added that all individuals possess self-efficacy and outcome expectations, or the ability to expect to achieve desired needs and goals. Thus, the social learning theory incorporates personal cognitive perceptions within a social context to explain behavior (Thomas, 1968; Thyer & Myers, 1998).

## Evaluation of Theory

Traditional postulates of the sociobehavioral theory have dramatically changed in the past 20 years with greater emphasis placed on the relationship between cognitive variables and behavior (Thyer & Myers, 1998; Wodarski, 1987). Ambiguity remains, however, in this tentative relationship. For example, Hishinuma (1998) is critical of the behaviorists and the cognitive psychologists for engaging in what he calls *separatism*. He asserts that this stance retards scientific growth and encourages the theoretical over generalization. He calls for unification between these two factions (Hishinuma, 1998, p. 1). A glimpse of this controversy is evidenced by Locke (1997), who argues with those who scoff at the concept of a causal effect for human thought. Locke asserts that conscious events are causes of action; moreover, consciousness is directly observable through an individual's introspection (p. 363). In a seeming attempt to bridge barriers between the cognitive and behavioral approaches, Dougher (1997) suggests that the cognitive behavioral debate is a paradigm clash. Moreover, that the essential disagreements are "pre-analytic" in nature and are not resolvable by data alone (p. 65).

Lyons, Wodarski, and Feit (1998) predict that behavioral theory has much to do with resolving conceptual conflicts, and the description of the controversy relating to behaviorism will likely remain ambiguous. They add that " . . . most of the demand to replace or enhance the empirical stance of behaviorism arises from poor implementation of behavioral techniques and a failure to follow recommendations made by behavioral theorists" (p. 10).

Despite this controversy, there remain many cognitive behavioral interventions cited as empirical and noteworthy (Thyer & Myers, 1998). For example, Meyers and Smith (1995) have developed a Community Reinforcement Approach (CRA) as a behavioral intervention for substance abuse. CRA was developed to use social, recreational, familial, and vocational reinforcers to assist clients in the recovery process. In place of confrontation, the program has successfully used positive reinforcement and environmental contingencies whenever possible to reward sobriety (p. 251). Fava, Rafanelli, Grandi, Conti, and Belluardo (1998) also studied the effectiveness of cognitive behavioral therapy (CBT) with chronically depressed clients. Forty clients were offered pharmacotherapy with either CBT or typical care. Results showed that CBT significantly improved residual symptoms well beyond the discontinuation of drug therapy, as opposed to the typical care group, who reported no significant changes. A two-year follow-up showed striking results—five depressive relapses in the CBT group and sixteen in the typical care group (p. 816).

When looking specifically at social learning theory, Schwartz and Johnson (1988) described a cogent structure within which to consider psychopathology and psychotherapy. "By taking into account interpretations as well as expectations, social learning theory recognizes the important role played by cognitions in determining behavior" (p. 17). After examining the effectiveness of social work intervention by reviewing 95 completed studies and client self-reports, MacDonald, Sheldon, and Gillespie (1992) relate how learning theory appears positively in the forefront of social work practice. The results were quite affirming, with "75% of those screened studies showing positive results within their different methodological conventions" (p. 615) and more than 50% were based on the social learning theory. Yet, even with this type of empirical support, Dworetzky (1987) warns against oversimplification. For example, social learning, although able to explain adequately how children learn, may still be unable to explain why at certain times children do not appear to advance cognitively as quickly as they might (p. 276).

## Interventive Implications

From a behavioral perspective, obtaining change behavior is considered limitless (Wodarski, 1987). Interventions can be varied; however, they all involve a focus on "unlearning" self-reinforcing behaviors through positive, negative, or social reinforcement (Bruck, 1968; Ellis, 1989; Thyer & Myers, 1998; Wodarski, 1987). When creating clinical conditions conducive for the development of reinforcement, four conditions are outlined to strengthen the use of positive reinforcement. They include the quality, the immediacy, and the frequency of the positive reinforcement, as well as the use of small steps for shaping the desired behavior (Thyer & Myers, 1998). Positive reinforcement is considered most effective when it is valued by the receiver and is administered consistently and close in time to the desired behavior. Shaping is used when the desired behavior needs support and this procedure involves many small steps of exposure or progress reinforced with approval and leading to the desired behavior (Thyer, 1987; Zastrow & Kirst-Ashman, 1990).

Just as reinforcement can be powerful in increasing behaviors, punishment can result in behavior decrease or extinction (Dworetzky, 1987, p. 186). Although some researchers believe that severe punishment is the most effective behavior change technique, the decision to use punishment requires careful consideration relative to the possible resulting negative consequences (Azrin & Holz, 1966). For example, punishment can often produce a negative emotional response and may initiate despondency or aggressiveness, especially if the punishment is physical and actually harms (see Dworetzky). With careful evaluation, punishment has been shown effective in decreasing the self-destructive behavior of psychotic, autistic, and developmentally disabled children (Zastrow & Kirst-Ashman, 1990). When Molm (1994) studied the use of punishment and its effectiveness, she found that, "Punishment that was both strong and consistently produced the highest frequency of reward exchange and the least negative affect toward the partner" (p. 75).

In response to the Pavlovian conditioning, systematic desensitization and flooding are two popular therapies that have been used to create behavior change. Systematic desensitization involves gradually exposing the client to the conditioned stimulus, while at the same time the client is engaged in an incompatible behavior (e.g., relaxation). Similarly, flooding is complete nonforced exposure to the conditioned stimulus for a length of time and this intervention has been used successfully with obsessive-compulsive disorders (Rosenhan & Seligman, 1989).

In this short discussion the authors have tried to highlight the virtues of cognitive-behavioral therapy. Because these methods remain sensitive to the time-limited intervention constraints often found in today's practice environment, applying the practice principles inherent in these approaches tends to be less expensive. To date, there is much evidence to support that these interventions are measurable and have been shown to be empirically effective. However, we must ask ourselves, are humans more than cognitions and behaviors? The argument can be made that in restricting analysis to discrete behaviors and cognitions, researchers/practitioners may be missing the sum and substance of the individual and thereby denying the aspect of freedom of choice? For example, if we teach an autistic child, through behavioral techniques, to hug other people, is the result more than an autistic child who has learned to hug people? Have we altered the disorder or improved the child's quality of life? Since many disorders are believed to be seriously influenced by environmental and cognitive circumstances, it stands to reason that these methods can be considered the intervention of choice in order to alleviate them by applying behavioral techniques, especially if the likelihood increases the potential for the individual to lead a more productive life.

## SUMMARY

This overview has given the reader a summary of several of the most popular theories that look directly at individuals or the interactions between individuals and their environment. The following selected readings are provided to help further explain and expand on several of these selected theories.

In chapter 2, the biological aspects that express the interplay between genetics and the environment are discussed. Biological research in the field of social work and psychology remains a focus for understanding the advances that have occurred in human behavior; this understanding has resulted in the identification of certain mental disorders. Probably the most significant aspect of the biological approach is that it allows for an interdisciplinary approach to emerge that can unite previously different fields (psychobiology, behavioral medicine, sociobiology, biological psychiatry, and neuropsychiatry) and integrates each of these respective bodies of knowledge. The chapter authors examine human growth and development by addressing the interplay between biology and behavior. Additionally, empirical research is presented on how humans respond in terms of stress and aggression. Once identified, these factors are related to different personality types. To explicate the influence of the biological role in human development certain mental disorders such as schizophrenia, the mood disorders, and substance abuse are highlighted. The role and importance of prevention are discussed as well as the implications for social workers engaging in empirically based practice.

Chapter 3 highlights the importance of identifying selected cognitive variables relative to the development of human behavior. Areas covered include cognitive theory and cognitive-behavioral therapy that designates cognitive variables as a significant factor in the empirical treatment of human behavior. Specific applications that link theory to the empirical foundation are explored and related to practice and policy implications.

The life-span development perspective is discussed in chapter 4 and represents a relatively recent addition to the body of human behavior theory. As summarized earlier in this section, while Freud and other psychoanalytic theorists propose developmental stages in early life, the life-span perspective expands this perspective by exploring the developmental changes that transpire in the individual from conception through old age. These perspectives highlight the biological, psychological, and social processes and influences that account for changes in human behavior also are outlined. These changes are considered continuous throughout the life span. This chapter elucidates the relevance of the life-span developmental approach to social work practice, and each developmental period will be discussed in terms of its critical biological, psychological, and social aspects along with the appropriate interventions and implications for social work practitioners.

In conclusion of Part I, chapter 5 highlights the fact that a social worker's assessment and diagnostic skills are what determine the explicit or implicit understanding of the client's status. This interpretation is critical because it results in the behaviors targeted for change. This chapter provides an excellent conclusion to Part I because regardless of whether the social worker's interpretation is based on a biological, analytic, cognitive-behavioral, life cycle approach, or otherwise, the assessment of the client's existing condition will always form the basis for later interventions. Thus, the authors explore the necessity for accuracy in assessment as a prerequisite for effective intervention.

## REFERENCES

Azrin, N. H., & Holz, W. C. (1966). Punishment. In W. K. Honig (Ed.), *Operant behavior*. New York: Appleton-Century-Crofts.

Bandura, A. (1977). *Social learning theory.* Englewood Cliffs, NJ: Prentice-Hall.

Bandura, A., Grusec, J. E., & Menlove, F. L. (1967). Vicarious extinction of avoidance behavior. *Journal of Personality and Social Psychology, 5,* 16–23.

Bandura, A., & Walters, R. (1963). *Social learning and personality development.* New York: Holt, Rinehart, & Winston.

Berger, K. (1994). *The developing person through the life span* (3rd ed., pp. 37–39). New York: Worth.

Bruck, M. (1968). Behavior modification theory and practice: A critical review. *Social Work, 13* (2), 43–55.

Carducci, B. (1998). *The psychology of personality, viewpoints, research, and applications.* Pacific Grove, CA: Brooks/Cole.

Cramerus, M. (1998). *A psychoanalytic model of social anxiety.* Boston: Dissertation Abstracts International 58(8-A), February 1998, 3307, US: University Microfilms International.

Dore, M. M. (1990). Functional theory: Its history and influence on contemporary social work practice. *Social Service Review, 64* (3), 358–374.

Dougher, M. J. (1997). Cognitive concepts, behavior analysis, and behavior therapy. *Journal of Behavior Therapy & Experimental Psychiatry, 28* (1), 65–70.

Dworetzky, J. P. (1987). *Introduction to child development.* New York: West.

Ellis, A. (1989). *Why some therapies don't work.* Buffalo, NY: Prometheus Books.

Fava, G. A., Rafanelli, C., Grandi, S., Conti, S., & Belluardo, P. (1998). Prevention of recurrent depression with cognitive behavioral therapy: Preliminary findings. *Archives of General Psychiatry, 55* (9), 816–820.

Fowler, R. C. (1998). Limiting the domain account of early moral judgment by challenging its critique of Piaget. *Merrill Palmer Quarterly, 44* (3), 263–292.

Grigsby, R. K. (1995). Determinism versus creativity: A response to Peile. *Social Work, 40* (5), 706–707.

Hishinuma, E. S. (1998). Pre-unified separatism and rapprochement between behaviorism and cognitive psychology: The case of the reinforcer. *Theoretical & Philosophical Psychology, 18* (1), 1–15.

Jung, C. G., & Douglas, C. (Ed.). (1997). *Visions: Notes of the seminar given in 1930–1934 by C. G. Jung* (Vol. 1). Princeton, NJ: Princeton University Press.

Kuhn, P. (1997). Sigmund Freud's discovery of the etiological significance of childhood sexual traumas. *Journal of Child Sexual Abuse, 6* (2), 107–122.

Locke, E. A. (1997). Science, Philosophy, and man's mind. *Journal of Behavior Therapy and Experimental Psychiatry, 27* (4), 363–368.

Lyons, P., Wodarski, J. S., & Feit, M. D. (1998). Human behavior theory: Emerging trends and issues. *Journal of Human Behavior in the Social Environment, 1* (1), 1–21.

MacDonald, G., Sheldon, B., & Gillespie, J. (1992). Contemporary studies of the effectiveness of social work. *British Journal of Social Work, 22* (6), 615–643.

Meyers, R. J., & Smith, J. E. (1995). *Clinical guide to alcohol treatment: The community reinforcement approach.* New York: Guilford.

Molm, L. D. (1994). Is punishment effective? Coercive strategies in social exchange. *Social Psychology Quarterly, 57* (2), 75–94.

Myers, D. G. (1987). *Psychology.* New York: Worth.

Newman, B., & Newman, P. (1995). *Development through life: A psychosocial approach.* Brooks/Cole.

Palmer, D. (1994). *Looking at philosophy: The unbearable heaviness of philosophy made lighter* (2nd ed.). Mountain View, CA: Mayfield.

Rank, O., & Taft, J. (1924). *Forward*. New York: Julian.

Rosenhan, D. L., & Seligman, M. E. P. (1989). *Abnormal psychology*. New York: W. W. Norton.

Schwartz, S., & Johnson, J. H. (1988). *Psychopathology of childhood: A clinical experimental approach* (2nd ed.). New York: Pergamon Press.

Skinner, B. F. (1981). Selection by consequences. *Science, 213*, 501–504.

Smalley, R. E. (1967). *Theory for social work practice*. New York: Columbia University Press.

Taft, J. (1937). The relations of function to process in social casework. *Journal of Social Work Process, 1*, 1–18.

Thomas, E. J. (1967). *Behavioral science for social workers*. New York: Free Press.

Thomas, E. J. (1968). Selected sociobehavior techniques and principles: An approach to interpersonal helping. *Social Work, 13* (1), 12–26.

Thorpe, G., & Olson, S. (1997) *Behavior therapy, concepts, procedures, and applications* (2nd ed.). Allyn and Bacon.

Thyer, B. A. (1987). Behavioral social work: An overview. *Behavior Therapist, 10* (6), 131–134.

Thyer, B. A., & Myers, L. L. (1998). Social learning theory: An empirically based approach to understanding human behavior in the social environment. *Journal of Human Behavior in the Social Environment, 1* (1), 33–52.

Watson, J. B. (1913). Psychology as the behaviorist views it. *Psychological Review, 20*, 158–177.

Wodarski, J. S. (1987). *Social work practice with children and adolescents*. Springfield, IL: Charles C Thomas.

Zastrow, C., & Kirst-Ashman, K. K. (1990). *Understanding human behavior and the social environment* (2nd ed.). Chicago: Nelson-Hall.

## CHAPTER 2

# The Interplay Between Biology, Genetics, and Human Behavior

## Shawn A. Lawrence and Kim Zittel-Palamara

As we move forward in our quest to understand human growth and development, researchers desire to learn more fully the mind-body connection (Freedman, 1992). The social work profession seeks to achieve this by continuing an increased interest in the interplay between biological and psychological research. Increased attention in this field facilitates a broader understanding of both human behavior and certain mental disorders through increased knowledge in the areas of genetics, biochemistry, and neuroscience (Peele, 1981). Furthermore, the knowledge provided in these areas helps to integrate previously separate fields such as psychology, behavioral medicine, sociobiology, biological psychiatry, and neuropsychiatry.

Significant gains in understanding the relationship between human development and biological factors have been achieved through the use of neuro-imaging technology, thus helping the professional in diagnosing with empirical knowledge from the biological etiology of mental health disorders. This use of neuro-imaging has enabled scientists to examine both the structure and the function of the human brain (Kane, 1993). Examining the function of the brain has allowed for research to predict the influence that medication use can have on the human brain. Therefore, these discoveries related to drug actions and reactions have greatly enhanced our understanding of human biological development. Perhaps the most rewarding outcome of this bio-behavioral research will be that it supports the elucidation of pure study groups to study different mental disorders and possible genetic linkages.

This chapter examines human growth and development by addressing the connection between biology and behavior. The empirical research reports how humans respond to stress and aggression, relative to different personality types. In addition, the biological role of those suffering from certain mental disorders such as schizophrenia, mood disorders, and substance abuse is highlighted. The role of prevention is discussed and its implications for the professional clinician.

## NATURE VERSUS NURTURE

As biobehavioral studies continue to take greater precedence in the field of mental health, controversy and criticism are evident in this trend. Critics of the biobehavioral approach warn that reducing behavior into biologically based components threatens the continued use of self-regulating therapeutic approaches. Peele (1981), who referred to this trend as reductionistic, argued against biochemistry alone. In addition, other investigators who support this contention believe that environmental factors play a substantial role in the development of psychopathology (Bellack & Mueser, 1993; Davies, Bromet, Schulz, Dunn, & Morgenstern, 1989; Gottesman, 1991; Hollandsworth, 1990; Kendler & Diehl, 1993; Lin & Kleinman, 1988; Tsuang, 2000; Whitaker, 1992). When biochemistry is used as a catchall to explain human behavior alternative practices may not receive adequate attention. This absolute notion of genetic determinism contradicts a developing view of mental illness as a heterogeneous, multifactorial illness (see Gottesman). Furthermore, to assume genetic predisposition does imply that pathology is unresponsive to intervention; the only hope to escape it would lie in people's ability to choose their own biological parents. To view biological causes alone could leave a gap in the understanding of the causes of the varying forms of mental or emotional suffering. Therefore, the controversy in the nature-nurture debate seems to be over the relative importance of genetics versus social environment and the ways in which the two interact.

In terms of human growth and development, most professionals agree that the effects of the environment cannot be overlooked. In fact, maternal environment and attitude appear to be meaningful risk factors regarding fetal outcome (Bebbington, Walsh, & Murray, 1993; Euker & Riegle, 1973; Gennaro, Brooten, Roncoli, & Kumar, 1993; Gennaro & Stringer, 1991; Mednick et al., 1998; Moyer, Herrenkohl, & Jacobowitz, 1978; Ottinger & Simmons, 1964; Williamson, LeFevre, & Hector, 1989). Laukaran and VanDenBerg (1980) proposed that a high incidence of unwanted and, therefore, stressful pregnancies are related to an elevation in the infant mortality figures in the United States. Williamson and associates (1989) reported that stressful life change independent of risk for biomedical problems was related to serious complications of pregnancy. Over the last three years, clinical studies have been completed on pregnancy and infants affected by maternal cocaine use. Some documented effects have been high rates of spontaneous abortion, intrauterine growth retardation, neonatal neurobehavioral deficits, sudden infant death syndrome, intrauterine cerebrovascular accident, and premature labor and delivery (Lex, 1991).

Twin and adoption studies have supported the role of genetic factors in individuals that develop mental disorders; however, these studies have failed to consider this relationship as part of the full range of social conditions that can be involved. For example, the epidemiological finding of an inverse relationship between schizophrenia (schizophrenia incidence increases) and social class (when social class is lowered) is cause for testing genetic models for looking directly at social class depicting class-specific rates of the disorder (Dohrenwend, Krasnoff, Askenasy, & Dohrenwent, 1978). Gottesman (1991) suggests that stressors impacting schizophrenia, such as interpersonal stress, brain trauma, disease, and drug use are not more prevalent to any socioeconomic group in the population. Present research supports further investigation toward the linkage between the environment and genetic predisposition resulting in a phenotype characterized by schizophrenia (Bebbington, Walsh, & Murray, 1993; Mednick et al., 1998; Tsuang, 2000).

Because we understand very little about the complex relationship between genetics and environment as etiological factors in mental health and disease, the best hope may be found in collaboration between genetic and environmental investigations. Albee (1982) illustrated the important role of the environment in the transition of Russian Jews and Southern Italians as they worked their way out of poverty and into the middle class. In the early 1900s these groups displayed high rates of psychopathology and were regarded as constitutionally defective in psychiatric circles. Today the children and grandchildren of these same Jews and Italians show no greater rate of pathology than other members of the middle class do. Albee (1982) asks: "What happened to all of those bad genes?" There is a strong argument for understanding the role of traumatic experiences and excessive stress in presenting mental disorders. Perhaps future research and improved knowledge will assist in prevention and interventions.

# UNDERSTANDING STRESS AND HUMAN BEHAVIOR

As our society has become progressively more complex, more uncertain, and more demanding, the incidence of stress related physical disorders has achieved critical proportions. Studies have indicated a dramatic rise in death rates from heart disease, cancer, and stroke as well as such mental health conditions as depression (Greenberg, Stiglin, Finkelstein, & Berndt, 1993). According to the Center for Disease Control, of the 10 leading causes of death in the United States, approximately 50% are related to lifestyle (Ell & Northern, 1990). Unfortunately, preventive efforts have not followed suit and remain a low priority. Changing human behavior patterns that pertain to certain lifestyle habits has yielded great possibilities for behavioral interventions.

The human body is a fascinating, precise, and self-maintaining system that supports numerous complex actions centered on bodily functions. Regardless of external demands, the body fights to maintain a constant state. Contemplation of the body's ability to sustain a rigid 98.6-degree temperature is a simple cause for amazement. When the body perceives a threat that challenges its exacting homeostasis, it sends out a call to arms, mobilizing resources to protect homeostasis. The stress response prepares the individual in time of danger for flight or fight, by secreting supplementary hormones and by stimulating autonomic nervous system actions (Seyle, 1956). In studying the body's response in stress Seyle's contributions to the field of social stress are considered landmark studies (Ell & Northern, 1990).

Modern times do not dictate the need for escaping acute physical danger; although, the stress response remains and still has adaptive functions. Information received through higher brain centers can elicit the physical stress response and generate an adaptive confrontation to psychological and emotional stresses. The autonomic nervous system economically modifies its stress level and then reverts back to normal once the perception of threat subsides. Because the stress response is mediated through the central nervous system (CNS) and neuroendocrine pathways, the brain communicates to the other organs within the body and a number of body responses occur. Adrenocorticotropic hormone (ACTH) is released from the anterior pituitary gland and regulates secretion of adrenal corticoids, the hormones that induce modification of immune and inflammatory reactions (Brown & Birley, 1968). The secretion of brain catecholamines (serotonin and norepinephrine) is then stimulated (Frankenhauser, 1975). The end result is a mobilization of fats and an increase in oxygen and blood to the cells, reinforcing the body's strength in withstanding the demands of a stressor.

The word *stress* is derived from the Latin meaning to draw together tightly. When the individual is experiencing stress the mind tightens, narrowing perceptions and decreasing options for maintaining homeostasis. Seyle (1978) defined stress as the body's nonspecific response to any demand, unpleasant or pleasant. He described the body's stress response as the General Adaption Syndrome (GAS). This syndrome consists of three stages: alarm reaction, in which the body calls on its defenses; stage of resistance, in which the body's defenses are maintained at greater than normal levels; and stage of exhaustion, in which the body can no longer maintain the high level of preparedness. When stress is prolonged and unabated the associated chemical changes become detrimental to health.

In our society we commonly see how negative psychological stress elicits the stress response. That is, although aroused to fight or flight, most modern individuals typically do not take such actions (e.g., assaulting an individual or running away). They instead maintain the negative psychological state, and the physiological (fight/flight) response is not discharged. By maintaining this state of chronic stress, the individual can pay a high price in terms of health and well-being. Stress-induced hypersecretion of corticoids or catecholamines plays a role in the etiology of a number of what Seyle (1978) termed the "disease of adaptation." In the state of chronic stress the body's response threshold also alters, becoming more sensitive to further environmental insults (Simonton, Matthews-Simonton, & Crighton, 1978).

Stress has been linked specifically with hypertension, stroke, coronary heart disease, ulcers, migraine, depression, and in general (in varying degrees) to many physical and mental disorders. Henryk-Gritt and Rees (1973) reported that psychological stress was an important precipitant of the development of migraines. Their findings suggested that migraine sufferers are predisposed to having greater sensitivity to any given stress; and hence, scored significantly higher on neurosis, hostility, and emotionality measures than did the controls.

When looking directly at the biological basis for involving daily stressful life events in relation to tension headaches, DeBenedittis and Lorenzetti (1992) found a relationship between daily life stress and the most commonly known chronic pain syndrome (headache). The authors further found that depressed mood and anxiety may account for a third intervening variable. Additionally, people suffering from asthma have also been studied in relation to stress (Janson-Bjerklie, Ferkeitch, & Brenner, 1993). Janson-Bjerklie and associates found that when life stress was experienced asthmatic symptoms became worse.

There is rising evidence on the association between job stress and physical health of workers (Bosma, Peter, Siegrist, & Marmot, 1998). Individuals who maintain high strain jobs are at a higher risk of coronary heart disease. Strain is a result of high job demands and an individual's low sense of control over outcome performance (Sorensen, Lewis, & Bishop, 1996). Low job control and a high effort reward imbalance correlate to coronary heart disease (Bosma et al., 1998). In summary, it is clear that there is a profound relationship between the stress experienced as part of an individual's development and the biological basis for the physical manifestations of disease.

## UNDERSTANDING AGGRESSION AND HUMAN BEHAVIOR

Each day popular media saturates the public with unfortunate tales of aggressive acts and grisly violence. It is well known that the underlying phenomenon of violence is anger. Rothenburg (1975) described anger as occurring most often in relation to a perception of threat, frequently under conditions of need, love, or involvement. Clearly, the preponderance of violent crimes in which the victim is a spouse, a close friend, or a relative is substantiated by this claim.

In contrast, the animal response to threat is manifested in a primitive fight-or-flight response, whereas humans feel the emotion of anger and can employ complex communications as an alternative response. Physiologically, in a state of anger a person experiences muscle tension and vascular changes readying for motor response. Rothenburg (1975) considered anger to be an "altering phenomenon" for the individual that provides a basis for communication. Thus, the angered person can employ a verbal discharge that would serve to reduce muscle tension and to promote removal of the threat or annoyance. When anger is unexpressed or hidden, the need for motor discharge remains; however, the result is often indirect attacks at the integrity of an individual, rather than at the specific threats the individual encounters. Aggression and violence can then be viewed as destructive discharges that result from a failure to communicate effectively. Finally, Rothenburg credited the most violent individuals as often being those who have difficulty in dealing with their feelings of anger.

An explanation of anger and aggression in the simple terms of failed communication overlooks significant contributions to the understanding of these phenomena. Most advances in the biology of aggression have been made through animal studies. Goldstein (1974) reviewed a number of significant studies on aggression and reported substantial evidence suggesting that hereditary factors play a role in the variations of aggression within animal species. Evidence for genetic contributions to aggression in humans is less clear. For example, Mednick, Gabrielli, and Hutchings (1984, 1987) suggested that there was a clear genetic component for criminality of property, reporting that adoptees with both adoptive and biological fathers who were criminals were more likely themselves to be criminal or participate in criminal acts. In addition, when reviewing twin studies Dilalla and Gottesman (1991) concluded that the concordance rates suggest a high heritability for adult criminality. The average concordance rate for monozygotic (MZ) twins is 50%; for di-zygotic (DZ), 22%. Though these studies may suggest a genetic component, most scientists acknowledge that there appears to be a strong environmental influence that cannot be underestimated (Dilalla & Gottesman, 1991; Goldman & Fishbein, 2000; Mednick, Moffitt, & Stack, 1987). This biological tendency was also evident in a review of genetic studies on delinquency. Although, other research findings have found sparse findings that indicate delinquent behaviors are not significantly heritable (Dilalla & Gottesman, 1991). In summary, family and twin studies have failed to conclusively separate genetic and environmental influences on behavior.

Another earlier line of studies conducted in the 1960s examined some genetic factors associated with criminality. There was excitement in the media over the discovery of a sex chromosome abnormality (XYY) in certain individuals involved in crime (Jarvik, Klodin, & Matsuyama, 1973). Human cells usually contain 46 chromosomes, 2 of which (X and Y) are responsible for gender determination. Typically, males will have a chromosome complement of (46,XY). The presence of an extra Y chromosome (47,XYY) indicates a double amount of genetic coding for male characteristics. If males are considered to be the more aggressive gender, then one might logically deduce that an additional male sex chromosome would increase an individual's predisposition to aggressive behavior. However, the "born criminal" genotype has been challenged in the past 20 years (Akers, 1994). Akers says even major supporters of biological theories of crime reject the XYY theory as scientifically valid. More recent theories suggest that no specific criminal behavior is genetic or predetermined by physiology.

Recently, researchers have studied the correlation between the productions of the male hormone testosterone with aggression (Booth & Osgood, 1993; Coccaro, Kavoussi, & McNamee, 2000; Dilalla & Gottesman, 1991; Kreuz & Rose, 1972; Persky, Smith, & Basu, 1971). When testosterone output was measured in a population of phenotypic (47,XYY) male subject's, levels were found to be significantly higher than that of the general population of males (Ismail, Harkness, Kirkham, Lorraine, Whatmore, & Brittain, 1968). Kreuz and Rose (1972) found elevated levels of testosterone in their sample of prisoners with histories of extreme violence and crime during adolescence. The authors suggested that, within a population predisposed by virtue of social and environmental risk factors to develop antisocial behaviors, testosterone levels might be an important additional component in unlocking the mystery behind aggressive crime in adolescence.

More recent research suggests that norepinephrine, dopamine, and serotonin at varying levels in individuals may cause aggressive behavior (Coccaro, Kavoussi, & McNamee, 2000; Coscina, 1997; Goldman & Fishbein, 2000; Linnoila, Virkunen, George, & Higley, 1993; Verhoeuen & Tuinier, 1993). Research indicates that a correlation between violent outbursts by an individual under the influence of alcohol is due to its inhibiting effects. For example, it has been documented that those who express chronic aggressive outburst have shown low glucose levels in their blood, with subsequent aggressive behaviors occurring more frequently during a hypoglycemic incident (Markku, Linnoila, & Virkkunen, 1992). Markku et al. further report that low serotonin levels and brain lesions also appear to be variables related to aggressive behaviors. Apparently, excessive drinking on a continual basis creates a lower serotonin level; and lesions in the orbital frontal lobe region have been linked to impulsive aggressive acts. In addition, Markku and associates found that aggressive individuals tended to have a father who abused substances prior to acting aggressively.

Aggression circuits in the brain are sensitive to a variety of influences. For example, the activation of other neuronal systems of the brain can reduce the sensitivity of aggression circuits, and this will inhibit aggression. A neurologically incompatible system such as that involved in euphoria has its own facilitating and inhibiting mechanisms that may modulate the firing of aggression circuits (Moyer, 1971). Blood hormones can also influence the sensitivity of aggression circuits.

# PERSONALITY TYPES AND HUMAN BEHAVIOR

An individual with Type A personality is characterized as being aggressive, hard, driving, competitive, having a sense of time urgency, impatient, and tense (Bulbulian & Bitters, 1996; Monforton, Helmes, & Deathe, 1993). People with Type A personality tend to be more sensitive to stress and are not likely to incorporate positive coping methods to deal with pressure, reports Monforton et al. (1993). In addition, individuals who are Type A are less likely or more delayed in seeking medical advice for physical symptoms.

Many Americans experience some form of cardiovascular disease, and there is strong evidence linking Type A personality with coronary artery disease (CAD) (Carmelli, Rosenman, Chesney, Fabsitz, Lee, & Borhani, 1988; Espnes & Opdahl, 1999; Monforton et al., 1993; Sims, Boomsma, Carroll, Hewitt, & Turner, 1991; Smith, 1992). Monforton et al. pose that in individuals who have a Type A personality experience an increased heart rate and an increase in stress related hormones when encountering stressful situations. The increase in reactivity in these individuals then in turn hastens the development of coronary artery disease (Ohira, Watanabe, Kolicyaski, & Kawai, 1999; Smith, 1992).

Studies of parents and their children have indicated that there is a familial aggregation for Type A personality (Sims, Boomsma, Carroll, Hewitt, & Turner, 1991). However, the heritability of Type A personality has been found to be quite low, with the pattern for monozygotic twins of .2–.5 and a correlation equal to zero for dizygotic twins (Duffy, Manicavasagar, O'Connell, Silove, Tennant, & Langelludecke, 1994). These studies, however, did not control for environmental factors. Researchers Mathews and Krantz (1976) performed a study of twin girls and their mothers and twin boys and their fathers. They found a significant correlation of the daughters overall Type A scores coinciding with their mothers. The conclusions were the same of twin boys and their fathers. This suggests a sociocultural pattern rather than genetic model of transmission (Carmelli et al., 1988). The differences indicated a factor of competitiveness rather than of heredity. Duffy et al. (1994) conducted a study to determine the heritability of Type A personality in Australian twins. The authors found that there was a high correlation when using a structured interview, but a poor correlation on the Bortner (BARS) questionnaire. The study suggests that these profound differences are a result of the test's measuring different variables. The authors suggest that further studies be conducted concentrating on specific components of Type A personality (Duffy et al., 1994).

## INTERVENTIVE APPROACHES

Albee (1982) emphasizes a primary prevention model as an approach to reduce stress. This model includes reducing powerlessness and enhancing social competence, self esteem, and support networks. This approach asserts that it is possible to reduce the incidence of some mental disorders. In recent years we have seen a greater emphasis placed on empowerment and advocacy through self-help groups. Currently, research is being conducted to give empirical support to this model. Proper nutrition, exercise, recreational activities, stress management techniques, positive mental attitude, and the development of creativity are all positive strategies for coping with today's unstable society.

Physical exercise has caught the attention of researchers not only as a method for reducing stress but also an interventive method for depression. Sustained rhythmic activity such as walking jogging, cycling, or stair stepping has been associated with the reduction of anxious symptoms (DeVries, 1981) and improvements in depression (Folkins, 1976; Folkins & Sime, 1981; Greist, Klein, Eischens, Faris, Gurman, & Morgan, 1979; Merzenbacher, 1979; Sorensen, Anderssen, Hjerman, Holme, & Ursin, 1999). In fact, Folkins and Sime found that in patients who are depressed, physical exercise such as running proved to be just as effective in relieving the depression as psychotherapy. Endurance running reportedly produces a marked increase in beta-endorphin secretion (Appenzeller, Slandefer, Appenzeller, & Atkinson, 1980; Carr, Bullen, Skrinar, Arnold, Rosenblatt, Beitius, Martin, & McArthur, 1981). The secretion of the endogenous opiates may have a role in what is called a "runner's high." Exercise also aids in increasing self-concept (Hilyer & Mitchell, 1979), improvements in sleep quality, and reductions in sexual tension (Baekland, 1970), as well as an increase in perception of general happiness and well-being (Carter, 1977).

The relationship between low levels of activity and obesity is well researched. Clearly, exercise plays a crucial role in both the prevention and treatment of obesity (Wodarski, Wodarski, Nixon, & Mackie, 1991). Regular exercise lowers blood pressure, reduces risk of coronary artery disease and hypertension, can lower depression and anxiety, and permit weight loss. To achieve the optimum effect an individual should exercise for at least 20 minutes three times per week, depending on intensity level of the exercise. Low intensity exercise will require more time to reap the same benefits of moderate to intense exercise.

## SPECIAL TOPICS: MOOD DISORDERS

Depression, mania, and bipolar disorder are the most commonly diagnosed mental illnesses in the country (Narrow, Reiger, Rae, & Mandersheid, 1993). Diagnosis of mood disorders in women is twofold greater than that of men (Kaplan, Saddock, & Grebb, 1994). The exact reason for the differences in diagnosis between men and women are unknown; hypotheses include (a) hormonal differences, (b) affects of childbirth, (c) gender specific stressors, or (d) learned helplessness (Kaplan, Saddock, & Grebb, 1994). Another proposed explanation for the difference in rates of diagnosis is that men are less likely to seek help from mental health professionals when they are depressed or experiencing problems (Nesse, 1998). The actual development and etiology of the mood disorders remains unknown; however, there are many speculations, including genetic factors as well as a combination of biological and environmental factors. This section addresses the etiology of mood disorders as well as examining the relationship between alcoholism and the treatment of mood disorders.

### Biology and Etiology

In the search for the relationship between human growth and the development of mood disorders, evidence exists that there is a genetic component in the etiology of mood disorders (Kaplan, Saddok, & Grebb, 1994). To conduct an empirical evaluation of this phenomena, however, remains difficult because of the impossibility of controlling the psychosocial factors that can play a significant role in the development of mood disorders in some individuals. In search of this quest, researchers have been studying the genetics of bipolar disorder since Emile Kraeplin differentiated bipolar disorders from schizophrenia (McInnis, 1997); but so far, in trying to replicate these studies contradictory results have been found (Kaplan, Saddok, & Grebb, 1994).

Similar to the empirical research in schizophrenia, family studies, adoption, and twin studies have also been conducted with mood-disordered individuals in an attempt to better understand the biological linkages. Family studies have revealed that the likelihood of having a mood disorder decreases as the degree of relationship widens (McInnis, 1997). In addition adoption studies have found an increased risk of mood disorders in the biological parents of the adoptee, further supporting the relevance of a genetic predisposition for the development of the mood disorders (Kaplan et al., 1994). When looking specifically at twin studies, Eliot Slater found that for monozygotic (same egg) twins the bipolar concordance rate was 70% and with dizygotic (separate eggs) twins the concordance rate was much lower at 20% (cited in McInnis). Furthermore, individuals who suffered from major depressive disorders also had similar concordance rates (see Kaplan et al.).

In summary, it appears that there are many biological factors that play a role in mood disorders, including salient factors such as neurochemicals and neuroendocrine influences.Currently, most of the empirically based research studies on affective disorders offer support for the idea that the alteration of chemicals in the brain can indeed change behavior (Hollandsworth, 1990). Similar to the mental disorder known as schizophrenia, the neurotransmitter serotonin has been implicated in the development of mood disorders (Kaplan et al., 1994).

In terms of neuroendocrine influences, thyroid functioning is often tested in the evaluation of mood disorders. Basically, hyperthyroidism is a result of an excess of the thyroid hormone, and symptoms include (a) weight loss, (b) increased appetite, (c) muscle weaknesses, and (d) cardiac disturbances (Hendrick, Altshuler, & Whybrow, 1998). There also are several mood disturbances associated with hyperthyroidism including insomnia, irritability, psychomotor agitation, and mood liability. Unfortunately, however, possibly due to the heterogeneity of the samples other similar studies have not found the same results (Hendrick et al., 1998; Joyce, 1991).

Hypothyroidism results from an inadequate production of the thyroid hormone. Typically thyroid hormones are low and TSH levels are elevated. Symptoms include low energy, change in appetite and sleep patterns, cramps, weight gain, cardiac inconsistencies, and thinning hair. The use of thyroid replacement medications can correct these symptoms, though the medications normally do not begin to become effective for a couple of weeks (Hendrick et al., 1998). The symptoms of hypothyroidism and depression often mimic each other, making a diagnosis of depression difficult with an individual who has hypothyroidism. In most cases any association made between bipolar disorder and hypothyroidism is a result of the effect of lithium on the thyroid's activity (Hendrick et al., 1998). Though certain subtypes (those clients that have rapid cycling) of the bipolar disorder may be particularly vulnerable to the antithyroid activity of lithium (Cowdry, Wehr, & Zis, 1983).

## Environmental Considerations

In studying the empirical research for such mood disorders as depression some scientists conceived that this condition was clearly interrelated with the environment and the emotional support that an individual received (Nesse, 1998). For example, infants must be close to their caretaker to meet sustenance and security needs. As children grow, however, they learn to separate and develop their own identity separate from the parent. Those children who experience a troubled separation may cause their primary caretakers to develop mood disorders.

From a behavioral perspective, depression is considered a form of learned behavior. Developing individuals who receive little positive reinforcement for their actions become withdrawn and receive even less attention. The theory of "learned helplessness" suggests that people who are depressed have been subjected to conditions they see as being out of their control for so long that they have given up hope (Ness, 1998). The indication of depression in this school of thought rests in the lack of or insufficient emotional and environmental reinforcement.

## Alcoholism and the Development of Mood Disorders

Many times the occurrence of one mental disorder may become complicated by the occurrence of another. For example, recent studies have shown that lifetime diagnoses of mood disorders and alcoholism are occurring more frequently together than what could be accounted for by chance (Farren & O'Malley, 1999; Maier, Hallmeyer, Minges, & Lichtermann, 1990). If the occurrence of alcoholism and depression are independent of each other, then the probability of them occurring simultaneously is the product of their probabilities (Backon, 1990). Using this formula the probability of the two happening together should be approximately 1%; yet, in actuality the rate for these two conditions occurring together is approximately 8.6%. Abou-Saleh, Merry, and Coppen (1984) cited in Backon found that 26% of abstinent alcoholics suffered from a major depressive disorder.

The actual reason for this comorbidity of alcoholism and mood disorders is still unknown; however, it is hypothesized that alcoholism and mood disorders share a common familial risk factor or that the one condition may derive from the other as a type of complication (Maier et al., 1990). In terms of a familial risk Maier et al. found an elevated risk for comorbidity between bipolar disorder and alcoholism among relatives of patients with both disorders. Maier and colleagues reported that this familial relationship also supported a linkage to a strong genetic component. More empirical studies in this area are needed to actually determine if there is a clear relationship between these two conditions and exactly what that relationship involves.

## Interventive Approaches

There are a variety of interventions used to treat mood disorders ranging from cognitive therapy neuroendocrine supplementation to the various drugs used to treat mood disorders.

The basic principle behind the use of cognitive therapy for intervention with mood-disordered individuals is based on the stress-diathesis model (Beck, 1987). In this model it is postulated that some individuals become depressed due to early learning experience and the development of dysfunctional beliefs (Scott, 1996). The individual has negative cognitions about the self and the future, and these thoughts dominate the thinking and manifest into the symptoms of depression (see Beck). Behavioral techniques may be used to improve activity level and enhance problem-solving and coping skills according to Scott, who also states that since previous research has indicated the response rate for cognitive behavioral interventions was similar to those receiving no treatment, an argument is made to use cognitive behavioral therapy in conjunction with pharmacotherapy.

Neuroendocrine supplementation has helped patients with treatment-resistant depression and also has produced remission. It also has helped stabilize mood in clients who have rapid cycling bipolar disorder and tend to be unresponsive to conventional pharmacotherapy (Bauer & Whybrow, 1993). Therefore, neuroendocrine supplementation has shown treatment efficacy for both mania and depression, particularly when used in conjunction with mood stabilizing medications

(Bauer & Whybrow, 1993). Some studies, however, have not found such benefits and explain the discrepancies as related to differences in initial thyroid functioning (Targum et al., 1984), or that small sample sizes and subtherapeutic doses of antidepressants may have been used (Hendrick et al., 1998).

Pharmacotherapy has historically been a popular method for intervention with depressed clients for over 40 years (Kaplan, Saddok, & Grebb, 1994). Basically, the tricyclic medications are thought to promote serotonin and norepinephrine activity by potentiating the neurotransmitters upon release (Eccleston, 1973; Hollandsworth, 1990) and by blocking reuptake, a mechanism that inactivates the released neurotransmitters. Monoamine oxidase inhibitors (MAOI) are a class of drugs that prevent the destruction of serotonin and norepinephrine and, relieve depression. It is thought, however, that MAO is not causal to acute symptomatology, but may be related to medications, diet, activity, hospitalization, sex, age, or the effects of stress rather than the disorder itself. The introduction of selective serotonin reuptake inhibitiors (SSRI's) has allowed for safer and better drug therapy than in previous years. These drugs are much safer than tricyclics or MAOI's and have been shown to be equally as effective if not superior.

Drug therapy, however, is not meant to be utilized alone and it should always be used in conjunction with some form of psychotherapeutic approach to be effective (Kaplan et al., 1994). One of the most prominent problems surrounding the use of drug therapies in the treatment of depression is compliance (Scott, 1996). The use of psychotherapeutic interventions will allow for the exploration of psychosocial issues contributing to the depression, as well as serving as a reinforcing agent for compliance (see Kaplan et al., 1994).

## Suicide

An irrational and final act, suicide has become one of the major causes of death in affective disorders (Hollandsworth, 1990). Suicide in teenagers between 15 and 24 has increased dramatically over the past two decades and is the third leading cause of fatalities in this age group. As well, suicide is the 10th leading cause of fatality in the United States across all age groups. It is approximated that 2–10% of teens attempt suicide and need emergency psychiatric intervention (Brent, 1995). It is the leading cause of death among sufferers of schizophrenia, with an estimated 10% of the schizophrenic population committing suicide. This rate is 10 times greater than that for males and 18% times greater than that for females in the general population (Gottesman, 1991).

In general, women make more suicide attempts but men have four times the rate of suicide completion. Women tend to use medication as the medium of choice (Canetto, 1994), whereas males use firearms and hangings (Garland & Zigler, 1993). "Men's rate of mortality by suicide was 20.1 per 100,000, compared with women's rate of 5 per 100,000" (Canetto, 1994, p. 516). Canetto also estimates that attempted suicides without completion are two to eight times more prevalent than those who do complete the act.

Stressful experiences are risk factors for attempting or completing suicide. The medium used to express suicidal behavior is related to culture, past events, more familiar methods to the individual, and how obtainable the means are. For unsuccessful attempts, the most common medium is psychotropic drugs (Canetto, 1994). The relationship that surfaces is an increase in trauma or high stress experience that increases the likelihood of suicidal behavior (Adams & Lehnert, 1997; Brent et al., 1993; Canetto, 1994; de Wilde, Kienhorst, Diekstar, & Wolters, 1992). Based upon current information, specific kinds of stressors seem to be connected to suicide attempts. These stressors also appear to be linked to age and a DSM–IV diagnosis (Brent et al., 1993). Adult stressors that often lead to suicidal behavior include death, changes in interpersonal relationships, and losses (Brent et al., 1993). Loss stressors have been found to be particularly poignant within six weeks of the event and highly correlated in alcohol-related suicides (Brent et al., 1993). Stressors that can trigger suicidal behaviors in those under the age of 30 appear to be legal such as employment difficulties, rejection, higher occurrence of drug misuse, and separation issues (Brent et al., 1993). Stressors for individuals over 30 years of age appear to be mainly focused on intense medical problems and have a higher prevalence of depressive disorders (Brent, 1995; Brent et al., 1993). Adolescent suicidal behavior triggers appear to be greater frequency of relationship discord with parents or romantic partners, legal problems, correction difficulties, moving, parental legal problems, sexual or physical abuse, DSM–IV diagnosis, and alcohol and drug abuse (Brent, 1995; Brent et al., 1993). Those who have suicidal thoughts tend to feel alone socially (Canetto, 1994).

The literature shows an increase in susceptibility to harming oneself as part of the epigenetic effects of experiencing trauma (Adams &

Lehnert, 1997). Of particular concern are the comorbidity of sexual abuse and thoughts or attempts of suicide. Research has implicated childhood sexual abuse associated to suicidal behaviors (Briere & Runtz, 1986; de Wilde et al., 1992). In his study, Briere (1986) found "43% of 153 females clients in a community health center crisis intervention service had a history of sexual abuse before age 15, and that 51% of these survivors had made at least one suicide attempt in the past" (Briere, p. 414). Adolescents who express suicidal behaviors seem to have a greater history of high stress in childhood. De Wilde et al. found that these stressors did not appear to relent when the child reached adolescence, and when such stressors occurred concurrent to the typical stressors associated with adolescence, their risk of suicidal behavior increases.

Suicide potential has been associated with schizophrenia, alcoholism, and depression. Goodman, Istre, Jordan, Herndon, and Kelabhn (1991) studied blood alcohol levels of suicide victims and found that 24.0% of the sample had BAC's of 0.10%. In a literature review of various courses of alcohol-related individuals, Schuckit (1985, 1986) found that patients who exhibited symptoms of affective disorders and alcohol use are at a high risk for suicide attempts.

Women tend to experience suicidal thoughts, whereas their male counterparts tend to complete the suicide act (Canetto, 1994). Women who experience noncompleted suicide usually fit the following criteria: "a depressed European-American under the age of 30 who is of low socioeconomic status and educational achievement, and who has a history of troubled personal relationships" (Canetto, p. 515). The rate of uncompleted suicide tends to decrease the older an individual becomes (Canetto, 1994). Canetto reports that the rate of suicide for men tends to increase with age; conversely, the rate for women tends to decrease with age, and triggers for women typically are related to relationship difficulties, dependent problems, and love concerns. Canetto suggests, however, that these issues are not the main concerns. Of heightened importance are socioeconomic problems, employment difficulties, antagonistic and violence relationships, and family or acquaintance history of suicide.

In adolescent males who completed suicide, there tended to be evidence of adjustment disorder (Brent, 1995). Whereas adolescent females who expressed suicidal behaviors tended to express symptoms of affective disorders and show more frequencies in attempts (Brent, 1995; Canetto, 1994). When males showed symptoms of affective disorders, there was typically concomitant substance-abusing behaviors more than their female counterparts (Brent, 1995).

## Interventive Approaches

Drugs have been the preferred course of treatment, because they are less invasive. However, electroconvulsive therapy (ECT) has been utilized to decrease the risk of suicide. Although the process is unclear, it is hypothesized that ECT increases postsynaptic responsiveness to norepinephrine, serotonin, and dopamine. The result is the disruption of the balance of neurotransmitters (Hollandsworth, 1990).

With the recent popularization of holistic medicines, alternatives to traditional medications are currently being researched. One suggestion to help increase serotonin levels associated with symptoms of depression is to drink walnut tea at various times throughout the day (Chopra, 1994). Also suggested is St. John's Wort, which contains hypericum. St. John's Wort has shown improvement with symptoms of anxiety, depression, and sleep disorders, according to Chopra. Vitamin B complex supplementation has been suggested for symptoms of depression and proper brain functioning (Balch & Balch, 1990). It should be noted, however, that more research is needed in the United States in alternative medicines, and the use of such methods should be approached cautiously (Dziegielewski & Leon, 2001). Also, taking some supplements in conjunction with certain Western medicines may be potentially harmful. Therefore, none of these remedies should be attempted without the supervision of a trained practitioner (Chopra, 1994).

## SUMMARY

By developing an understanding of the biological basis to behavior, the human services professional can focus on interventions based on behavioral component versus static biological components. A focus on biological risk factors does not have to imply emphasis on defect. With those diagnosed with a mental disorder, an elucidation of biological markers may help in the identification of vulnerable individuals, assisting in prevention and relapse rates (Zubin & Steinhauer, 1981).

Detection of early risk factors in children who have parent(s) diagnosed with a mental disorder may lead to the establishment of markers that can be used to screen the general population in order to prevent initial episodes. If the reduction of stress is a means to prevent episodes of illness, those with vulnerabilities for mental disorders may benefit from awareness. Interventions could be planned to enhance the vulnerable individual's competence and ability to cope with the demands of everyday life. Genetic counseling has been advocated by some as a preventative mechanism. With the improvement in the treatment of such mental disorders as the mood disorders the social worker can assist clients in the development of personal responsibility for health and lifestyle change. This can take place in promoting stress management techniques, such as relaxation and exercise. Intervention should also focus on the development of secure, sustaining interpersonal relationships. These techniques and relationships will serve as a buffer in times of crisis. Relaxation and exercise will aid the relief of built-up tensions. Individuals with Type A personalities should be encouraged to reorganize their lifestyles and learn ways to reduce actual or perceived pressure. "Hurry-sickness" requires drastic change in habits that can best be facilitated with planned systematic intervention (Freidman & Rosenman, 1974).

A major barrier to positive behavior is our culture, which rewards and reinforces negative health practices. For example, in the workplace the boss is much more likely to reward competitive drive and overtime, rather than an employee taking a 10-minute "meditation break." Society must provide positive reinforcement for healthy behaviors if positive behavior change is going to occur.

Social and political changes will be necessary to improve the quality and prevention that necessitates changing major social structures. A positive, progressive public health approach mandates the reduction of major stressors such as the powerlessness associated with low socioeconomic status, gender inequality, and member of a minority group or unemployed.

Rather than a continued emphasis on individual therapy, which may reach only a small percentage of the population, social workers may utilize their optimal potential as advocates. Advocating at a macrolevel for self-care and establishing networks using existing resources will aid in empowering those individuals who feel stigmatized and powerless in this society. Prevention on a larger scale will be accomplished only through community organization and social action.

This chapter has summarized some of the latest, empirically based biological research and how this information impacts social work practice. The chapter outlines the relationship between biology and behavior in the following areas: stress, aggression, and personality traits. Special topics covered that highlight the biological basis of human development are the mental health problems related to mood disorders as well as suicide. This chapter also discusses prevention and its impact on today's society. Current empirical research is reviewed in terms of intervention strategies and their efficacy towards improving social work practice.

# REFERENCES

Adams, D. M., & Lehnert, K. L. (1997). Prolonged trauma and subsequent suicidal behavior: Child abuse and combat trauma reviewed. *Journal of Traumatic Stress, 10* (4), 619–633.

Akers, R. L. (1994). *Criminological theories: Introduction and evaluation.* Los Angeles: Roxbury.

Albee, G. W. (1982). Preventing psychopathology and promoting human potential. *American Psychologist, 37,* 1043–1050.

Appenzeller, O., Slandefer, J., Appenzeller, J., & Atkinson, R. (1980). Neurology of endurance training: V. endorphins. *Neurology, 30,* 418–419.

Backon, J. (1990). Depression among Israeli alcoholics. *Journal of Clinical Psychology, 46* (1), 96–103.

Baekland, F. (1970). Exercise deprivation: Sleep and psychological reactions. *Archives of General Psychiatry, 22,* 365–369.

Balch, J. F., & Balch, P. A. (1990). *Prescription for nutritional healing.* Garden City Park, NY: Avery.

Bauer, M. S., & Whybrow, P. C. (1993). Validity of rapid cycling as a modifier for bipolar disorder in DSM–IV. *Depression, 1* (1), 11–19.

Bebbington, P., Walsh, C., & Murray, R. (1993). The causes of functional psychosis. In C. G. Costello (Ed.), *Basic issues in psychopathology* (pp. 238–270). New York: The Guilford Press.

Beck, A. (1987). Cognitive models of depression. *Journal of Cognitive Psychotherapy, 1* (1), 5–37.

Bellack, A. S., & Mueser, K. T. (1993). Psychosocial treatment for schizophrenia. In D. Shore (Ed.), *Schizophrenia.* Washington, DC: U.S. Government Printing Office.

Booth, A., & Osgood, D. W. (1993). The influence of testosterone on deviance in adulthood: Assessing and explaining the relationship. *Criminology, 31,* 91–117.

Bosma, H., Peter, R., Siegrist, L., & Marmot, M. (1998). Two alternative job stress models and the risk of coronary heart disease. *American Journal of Public Health, 88* (1), 68–74.

Brent, D. A. (1995). Risk factors for adolescent suicide and suicidal behavior: Mental and substance abuse disorders, family environmental factors, and life stress. *Suicide and Life-Threatening Behavior, 25,* Supplement, 52–63.

Brent, D. A., Perper, J. A., Moritz, G., Baugher, M., Roth, C., Balach, L., & Schweers, J. (1993). Stressful life events, psychopathology, and adolescent suicide: A case control study. *Suicide and Life-Threatening Behavior, 23* (3), Fall, 179–187.

Briere, J. (1986). Suicidal thoughts and behaviors in former sexual abuse victims. *Canadian. Journal of Behavioral Science/Review. Canadian. Science. Comprehensive, 18* (4), 413–423.

Briere, J., & Runtz, M. (1986). Suicidal thoughts and behaviours in former sexual abuse victims. *Canadian Journal of Behavioural Science, 18* (4), 413–423.

Brown, G. W., & Birley, J. L. T. (1968). Crisis and life changes and the onset of schizophrenia. *Journal of Health and Social Behavior, 9,* 203–214.

Bulbulian, R., & Bitters, D. (1996). Blood pressure response to acute exercise in Type A and B females and males. *Physiology & Behavior, 60* (4), 1177–1182.

Canetto, S. S. (1994). Gender issues in the treatment of suicidal individuals. *Death Studies, 18,* 513–527.

Carmelli, D., Rosenman, R., Chesney, M., Fabsitz, R., Lee, M., & Borhani, N. (1988). Genetic heritability and shared environmental influences of Type A measures in the NHLBI twin study. *American Journal of Epidemiology, 127* (6), 1041–1052.

Carr, D. B., Bullen, B. A., Skrinar, G. S., Arnold, M. A., Rosenblatt, M., Beitiur, I. Z., Martin, J. B., & McArthur, J. W. (1981). Physical conditioning facilitates the exercised induced secretion of beta-endorphin and beta lipoprotein in women. *New England Journal of Medicine, 305,* 561–563.

Carter, R. (1977). Exercise and happiness. *Journal of Sports Medicine, 17* (1), 307–313.

Chopra, D. (1994). *Alternative medicine: The definitive guide.* Fife, WA: Future Medicine.

Coccaro, E. F., Kavoussi, R. J., & McNamee, B. (2000). Central neurotransmitter function in criminal aggression. In D. H. Fishbein (Ed.), *The science, treatment, and prevention of antisocial behaviors: Application to the criminal justice system.* Kingston, NJ: Civic Research Institute.

Coscina, D. V. (1997). The biopsychology of impulsivity: Focus on brain serotonin. In C. D. Webster & M. A. Jackson (Eds.), *Impulsivity: Theory, assessment, and treatment* (pp. 95–115). New York: The Guilford Press.

Cowdry, R. W., Wehr, T. A., Zis, A. P., & Goodwin, F. K. (1983). Thyroid abnormalities associated with rapid cycling bipolar illness. *Archives of General Psychiatry, 40,* 414–420.

Davies, M. A., Bromet, E. J., Schulz, S. C., Dunn, L. O., & Morgenstern, M. (1989). Community adjustment of chronic schizophrenic patients in urban and rural settings. *Hospital and Community Psychiatry, 40* (8), 824–830.

DeBenedittis, G., & Lorenzetti, A. (1992). Minor stressful life events (daily hassles) in chronic primary headache: Relationship with MMPI personality patterns. *Headache, 32* (7), 330–334.

DeVries, H. A. (1981). Tranquilizer effect of exercise: A critical review. *The Physician and Sports Medicine, 9,* 46–49; 52–53; 55.

de Wilde, E. J., Kienhorst, I. C. W. M., Diekstar, R. F. W., & Wolters, W. H. G. (1992). The relationship between adolescent suicidal behavior and life events in childhood and adolescence. *American Journal of Psychiatry, 149* (1), January, 45–51.

Dilalla, L. F., & Gottesman, I. I. (1991). Biological and genetic contributors to violence—Widom's untold tale. *Psychological Bulletin, 109* (1), 125–129.

Dohrenwend, B. S., Krasnoff, L., Askenasy, A. R., & Dohrenwent, B. P. (1978). Exemplification of a method for scaling life events: The PERI life event scale. *Journal of Health & Social Behavior, 19* (2), 205–229.

Duffy, D. L., Manicavasagar, V., O'Connell, D., Silove, D., Tennant, C., & Langelludecke, P. (1994). Type A personality in Australian twins. *Behavior Genetics, 24* (95), 469–475.

Dziegielewski, S. F., & Leon, A. M. (2001). *Psychopharmacology and social work practice.* New York: Springer.

Eccleston, D. (1973). The biochemistry of human moods. *New Scientist, 57,* 827.

Ell, K., & Northern, H. (1990). *Families and health care: Psychosocial practice.* New York: Aldine De Gruyer.

Espnes, G. A., & Opdahl, A. (1999). Association among behavior personality, and traditional risk factors for coronary heart disease: A study at a primary health center in mid-Norway. *Psychological Reports, 85* (2), 505–517.

Euker, J. S., & Riegle, J. D. (1973). Effect of stress on pregnancy in the rat. *Journal of Reproduction and Fertility, 34,* 343–346.

Farren, C. K., & O'Malley, S. S. (1999). Occurrence and management of depression in the context of Naltrexone treatment of alcoholism. *American Journal of Psychiatry, 156* (8), 1258–1262.

Folkins, C. H. (1976). Effects of physical training on mood. *Journal of Clinical Psychology, 32,* 373–379.

Folkins, C. H., & Sime, W. E. (1981). Physical fitness training and mental health. *American Psychologist, 36* (4), 373–389.

Frankenhauser, M. (1975). Experimental approaches to the study of catecholamines and emotion. In L. Levi (Ed.), *Emotions: Their parameter and measurements.* New York: Raven.

Freedman, D. X. (1992). The search: Body, mind and human purpose. *American Journal of Psychiatry, 149* (7), 858–866.

Friedman, M., & Rosenman, R. H. (1974). *Type A behavior and your heart.* New York: Fawcett Crest.

Garland, A. F., & Zigler, E. (1993). Adolescent suicide prevention: Current research and social policy implications. *American Psychologist, 48* (2), 169–182.

Gennaro, S., Brooten, D., Roncoli, M., & Kumar, S. (1993). Stress and health outcomes among mothers of low-birthweight infants. *Western Journal of Nursing Research, 15* (1), 97–113.

Gennaro, S., & Stringer, M. (1991). Stress and health in low birthweight infants: A longitudinal study. *Nursing Research, 40* (5), 308–311.

Goldman, D., & Fishbein, D. H. (2000). Genetic basis for impulsive and antisocial behaviors—Can their course be altered? In D. H. Fishbein (Ed.), *The science, treatment, and prevention of antisocial behaviors: Application to the criminal justice system.* Kingston, NJ: Civic Research Institute.

Goldstein, M. (1974). Brain research and violent behavior. *Archives of Neurology, 30,* 8–31.

Goodman, R. A., Istre, B. R., Jordan, F. B., Herndon, J. L., & Kelabhn, J. (1991). Alcohol and fatal injuries in Oklahoma. *Journal of Studies on Alcohol, 52* (2), 156–161.

Gottesman, I. I. (1991). *Schizophrenia Genesis: The origins of madness.* New York: Freeman.

Greenberg, R. E., Stiglin, L. E., Finkelstein, S. N., & Berndt, E. R. (1993). The economic burden of depression in 1990. *Journal of Clinical Psychiatry, 54* (11), 405–418.

Greist, J., Klein, M. H., Eischens, R. R., Faris, J., Gurman, A. S., & Morgan, W. P. (1979). Running as a treatment for depression. *Comprehensive Psychiatry, 20* (1), 41–53.

Hendrick, V., Altshuler, L., & Whybrow, P. (1998). Psychoneuroendocrinology of mood disorders: The hypothalamic-pituitary-thyroid axis. *Psychneuroendocrinology, 21* (2), 277–292.

Henryk-Gritt, S., & Rees, W. L. (1973). Psychological aspects of migraine. *Journal of Psychosomatic Research, 17,* 140–153.

Hilyer, J. C., & Mitchell, W. (1979). Effect of systematic physical fitness training combined with counseling on the self-concept of college students. *Journal of Counseling Psychology, 26,* 427–436.

Hollandsworth, J. G., Jr. (1990). *The physiology of psychosocial disorders: Schizophrenia, depression, anxiety, and substance abuse.* New York: Plenum.

Ismail, A. A. A., Harkness, R. A., Kirkham, D. E., Lorraine, J. A., Whatmore, P. B., & Brittain, R. P. (1968). Effects of abnormal sex-chromosome complements on urinary testosterone levels. *Lancet, 1,* 220–222.

Janson-Bjerklie, S., Ferkeitch, S., & Benner, P. (1993). Predicting the outcomes of living with asthma. *Research in Nursing and Health, 16* (4), 241–250.

Jarvik, L. F., Klodin, V., & Matsuyama, S. S. (1973). Human aggression and the extra Y chromosome. *American Psychologist, 29,* 674–682.

Joyce, R. R. (1991). The prognostic significance of thyroid function in mania. *Journal of Psychiatric Research, 25* (1), 1–6.

Kane, J. (1993). Future directions in schizophrenia research. *Psychiatric Annals, 23* (4), 222–225.

Kaplan, H. I., Saddock, B. J., & Grebb, J. A. (1994). *Synopsis of psychiatry: Behavioral sciences clinical psychiatry* (pp. 516–563). Baltimore: Williams & Wilkins.

Kendler, K. S., & Diehl, S. R. (1993). The genetics of schizophrenia: A current, genetic epidemiological perspective. *Schizophrenia Bulletin, 19* (2), 261–286.

Kreuz, L. E., & Rose, R. M. (1972). Assessment of aggressive behavior and plasma testosterone in a young criminal population. *Psychosomatic Medicine, 34* (4), 321–331.

Laukaran, V. H., & VanDenBerg, B. J. (1980). The relationship of maternal attitude to pregnancy outcomes and obstetric complications. *American Journal of Obstetrics and Gynecology, 136,* 374–379.

Lex, B. W. (1991). Gender differences in substance abuse. In N. K. Mello (Ed.), *Advances in substance abuse: Behavioral and biological research.* London: Jessica Kingsley.

Lin, K., & Kleinman, A. M. (1988). Psychopathology and clinical course of schizophrenia: A cross-cultural perspective. *Schizophrenia Bulletin, 19* (2), 371–430.

Linnoila, M., Virkknen, M., George, T., & Higley, D. (1993). Impulse control disorders. *International Clinical Psychopharmacology, 8* (Suppl. 1), 53–56.

Maier, W., Hallmeyer, J., Minges, J., & Lichtermann, D. (1990). Morbid risks in relatives of affective, schizoaffective, and schizophrenic patients—Results of a family study. In A. Maneros & M. T. Tsuang (Eds.), *Affective and schizoaffective disorders: Similarities and differences.* New York: Springer-Verlag.

Markku, V., Linnoila, I., & Virkkunen, M. (1992). Aggression, suicidality, and serotonin. *Journal of Clinical Psychiatry, 53* (10 Suppl.), 46–51.

Mathews, K. A., & Krantz, D. S. (1976). Resemblance of twins and their parents in pattern A behavior. *Psychological Medicine, 38* (1), 140–144.

McInnis, M. G. (1997). Recent advances in the genetics of bipolar disorder. *Psychiatric Annals, 27* (2), 482–488.

Mednick, S. A., Gabrielli, W. F., Jr., & Hutchings, B. (1984). Genetic influences in criminal behavior: Evidence from an adoption cohort. *Science, 224,* 891–893.

Mednick, S. A., Gabrielli, W. F., Jr., & Hutchings, B. (1987). Genetic factors in the etiology of criminal behavior. In S. A. Mednick, T. E. Moffitt, & S. A. Stack (Eds.), *Causes of crime: New biological approaches.* Cambridge, England: Cambridge University Press.

Mednick, S. A., Moffitt, T. E., & Stack, S. A. (1987). *The causes of crime.* New York-Cambridge: Cambridge University Press.

Mednick, S. A., Watson, J. B., Huttunen, M., Cannon, T. D., Katila, H., Machon, R., Mednick, B., Hollister, M., Parnas, J., Schulsinger, F., Sajaniemi, N., Voldsgaard, P., Pyhala, R., Gutkind, D., & Wang, X. (1998). A two-hit working model of the etiology of schizophrenia. In M. F. Lenzenweger & R. H. Dworkin (Eds.), *Origins and development of schizophrenia: Advances in experimental psychopathology* (pp. 27–66). Washington, DC: American Psychological Association.

Merzenbacher, C. F. (1979). A diet and exercise regimen: Its effect upon mental activity and personality—A pilot study. *Perceptual and Motor Skills, 48,* 367–371.

Monforton, M., Helmes, E., & Deathe, A. B. (1993). Type A personality and marital intimacy in amputees. *British Journal of Medical Psychology, 66* (10), 275–280.

Moyer, J. A., Herrenkohl, L. R., & Jacobowitz, D. M. (1978). Stress during pregnancy: Effect of catecholamines in discreet brain regions of offspring as adults. *Brain Research, 144,* 173–178.

Moyer, K. E. (1971). A preliminary physiological model of aggressive behavior. In B. E. Eleftherious & J. P. Scott (Eds.), *The physiology of aggression and defeat.* New York: Plenum.

Narrow, W. E., Reiger, D. A., Rae, D. S., & Mandersheid, R. D. (1993). Use of services by persons with mental and addictive disorders: Findings from the National Institute of Mental Health epidemiologic catchment area program. *Archives of General Psychiatry, 50* (2), 95–107.

Nesse, R. (1998). Mood disorders: An overview—Part II. *The Harvard Mental Health Letter, 14* (7), 1–7.

Ohira, H., Wantanabe, Y., Kolicyaski, K., & Kawai, M. (1999). The type A behavior pattern and immune reactivity to brief stress: Change of volume of secretory immunoglobulin A in Saliva. *Perceptual & Motor Skills, 89* (2), 423–430.

Ottinger, D. R., & Simmons, J. E. (1964). Behavior of human neonates and prenatal maternal anxiety. *Psychological Reports, 14,* 391–394.

Peele, S. (1981). Reductionism in the psychology of the 80's. *American Psychologist, 36,* 807–808; 818.

Persky, H., Smith, K. D., & Basu, G. K. (1971). Relation of psychologic measures of aggression and hostility to testosterone production in men. *Psychosomatic Medicine, 33,* 3.

Rothenburg, A. (1975). On anger. In S. A. Pasternak (Ed.), *On violence and victims.* New York: Spectrum.

Schuckit, M. A. (1985). The clinical implications of primary diagnostic groups among alcoholics. *Archives of General Psychiatry, 42* (11), 1043–1049.

Schuckit, M. A. (1986). Genetic and clinical implications of alcoholism and affective disorder. *American Journal of Psychiatry, 143* (2), 140–147.

Scott, J. (1996). Cognitive therapy of affective disorders: A review. *Journal of Affective Disorders, 37* (1), 1–11.

Seyle, H. (1956). *The stress of life.* Highstown, NJ: McGraw-Hill.

Seyle, H. (1978). On the real benefits of eustress. *Psychology Today, 11,* 60; 64; 69–70.

Simonton, O. C., Matthews-Simonton, S., & Crighton, J. (1978). *Getting well again.* Los Angeles: J. P. Tarche.

Sims, J., Boomsma, D. I., Carroll, D., Hewitt, J. K., & Turner, J. R. (1991). Genetics of Type A behavior in two European countries: Evidence for sibling interaction. *Behavior Genetics, 21* (5), 513–528.

Smith, T. W. (1992). Hostility and health: Current status of psychosomatic hypothesis. *Health Psychology, 11* (3), 139–150.

Sorensen, G., Lewis, B., & Bishop, R. (1996). Gender, job factors, and coronary heart disease risk. *American Journal of Health Behavior, 21* (1), 3–13.

Sorensen, M., Anderssen, S., Hjerman, I., Holme, I., & Ursin, H. (1999). The effect of exercise and diet on mental health and quality of life in middle-aged individuals with elevated risk factors for cardiovascular disease. *Journal of Sports Sciences, 17* (5), 369–377.

Targum, S. D., Greenberg, R. D., Harmon, R. L., Kessler, K., Salerian, A. J., & Fram, D. H. (1984). Thyroid hormone and the TRH stimulation test in refractory depression. *Journal of Clinical Psychiatry. 45*(8):345–6.

Tsuang, M. (2000). Schizophrenia: Genes and environment. *Biological Psychiatry, 47* (3), 210–220.

Verhoeuen, W. M. A., & Tuinier, S. (1993). Affective and aggressive behavioral disorders—Thoughts about diagnosis and etiology. *New Trends in Experimental & Clinical Psychiatry, 9* (4), 123–136.

Whitaker, L. P. (1992). *Schizophrenic disorders: Sense and non-sense in conceptualization, assessment and treatment.* New York: Plenum Press.

Williamson, H. A., LeFevre, M., & Hector, M. (1989). Association between life stress and serious prenatal complications. *The Journal of Family Practice, 29* (5), 489–496.

Wodarski, J. S., Wodarski, L. A., Nixon, S. C., & Mackie, C. (1991). Behavioral medicine: An emerging field of social work practice. *Journal of Health & Social Policy, 3* (1), 19–43.

Zubin, J., & Steinhauer, S. (1981). How to break the logjam in schizophrenia. A look beyond genetics. *Journal of Nervous & Mental Disease, 169* (8), 477–492.

## CHAPTER 3

# Cognitive Variables as Factors in Human Growth and Development

## Catherine N. Dulmus

This chapter explores the relationship between cognitions and human development. Stated simply, a cognition is defined as the process of obtaining, organizing, and using intellectual knowledge. This implies an understanding of the connection between cause and effects, which leads to the development of cognitive strategies within human growth. These strategies shape how the world is viewed and therefore assist a person to better understanding the self and the environment (Kaplan, Sadock, & Grebb, 1994). The recognition and importance of understanding how an individual's cognitive approach will affect and change human behavior has supported the shift in clinical work from a strong behavioral perspective to a more cognitive one. Though this shift has been identified as revolutionary, it remains obvious that much remains to be accomplished in the integration of cognitivism and behaviorism before a true integrative approach can result (Granvold, 1994). In this chapter, cognitive variables in relation to human behavior are explored, with specific application to cognitive theory, cognitive-behavioral theory as therapy, and related practice and policy implications.

## COGNITIVE THEORY

To understand the relationship between cognitions and human behavior, emphasis is often placed on an individual's belief system in determining thoughts, feelings, and behavior. According to Ingram (1983), an organizing framework can be formulated that divides cognition into four interrelated, but distinct major elements: (a) cognitive structure, which relates to the way in which information is organized and internally represented; (b) cognitive propositions, which refer to the content stored in the cognitive structures; (c) cognitive operations, which serve as the mechanism for information processing; and (d) cognitive products, which are the result of information processing.

Similar to what is believed in psychoanalytic theory, cognitive theory maintains that anxiety is a deliberate attempt of individuals to block undesirable ideas and feelings from their own awareness (Kendall & Hollon, 1981; Mahoney, 1974). In this model individuals attempt to reduce their anxiety through actions that are designed to prevent the feared consequences and thus provide them with a sense of control. The appraisal of threat is important in that the stress reaction mediated psychologically is determined by individuals estimation of threat and their resources to deal with it. An individual's cognitions provide a framework that organizes and operationalizes a multitude of signals, signs, and codes that contain the substance and essence of the worldview of the individual.

Generally, anxiety or anxious feelings are elicited and maintained by stimuli (Bootzin & Max, 1980), which can be actual, imagined, or anticipated (Folkman, Schaefer, & Lazarus, 1979). From a cognitive perspective, classical behaviorism or an operant model is not comprehensive enough when it implies that stimulus (S) simply triggers a response (R). For the cognitive theorist, the scenario is more extensive, adding an additional dimension that results in (S) stimulus-(C) cognition-(R) response (Bolles, 1974). Therefore, the cognitive process involves an evaluation and choice of response. Cognitive therapists, instead of supplying concrete rewards for appropriate behaviors, teach the client to assess all the information regarding antecedents and consequences, and then to determine whether satisfying consequences outweigh negative ones (Wodarski, 1982).

This cognitive approach gained in popularity when it was directly applied to different mental health conditions. For example, Beck, Rush, Shaw, and Emery's (1979) development of outcome research on depression evolved along with the work of Ellis (1971), highlighting the cognitive aspects of the treatment process. These types of cognitive therapeutic frameworks were used for the treatment of generalized anxiety disorders, major, nonpsychotic unipolar depressions, phobic disorders, obesity, chemical dependency, and chronic pain. Further, though not as clearly linked, some professionals believe that this struc-

tured cognitive approach could also help to manage the lives of schizophrenics (Kingdon & Turkington, 1994).

According to a cognitive perspective, anxiety-provoking beliefs are
processed through the faulty interpretations of the anxious client. An
essential point in this approach to clinical practice is that anxiety is
elicited and maintained by stimuli (Bootzin & Max, 1980). Types of stress
and anxiety are the result of the evaluations people make regarding the
present and future significance of the stimuli for their well-being. The
stimuli can be actual, imagined, or anticipated (Folkman, Schaefer, &
Lazarus, 1979). This coincides with the point Bootzin and Max made
that cognitions often occur in an individual who cognitively rehearses
the feared event and produces emotion. In such cases as this, the
cognitions can actually serve as the stimuli that maintain the state of
anxiety. Thus, whether or not a person reacts to a stimulus with anxiety
can be governed not only by learned behavior and associations but also
by the cognitions used to deal with the stimulus (Beck, 1976). Once
the event is over the effects may linger because of the cognitions that
have been experienced. From the viewpoint of cognitive theorists, cognitions, although they take place in the mind, are not to be confused
with psychodynamic processes, which refer to the vicissitudes of an
individual's aggressive and libidinal (sexual energy) drives. A cognition
is in itself a dispassionate appraisal, based on the data available to the
thinker of what is taking place in reality. If the data are incorrect or
insufficient, or if the appraisal does not follow from the data logically,
the result is a cognitive deficit (Marzillier, 1980).

## COGNITIVE THERAPY

The goal of cognitive therapy is to break down existing negative cognitions and replace them with more positive, functionally adaptive ones
(Goodwin & Guze, 1989). Cognitive therapy is an active, directive, time-
limited, structured approach used to treat not only depression but also
a variety of psychiatric disorders such as anxiety, phobias, and problems
with pain (Breitholtz, Johansson, & Ost, 1999; Salkovskis, 1999). It is
based on an underlying theoretical rationale that individuals' affects
and behaviors are largely determined by the way in which they structure
the world. Individuals' cognitions (verbal or pictorial) clearly affect
their stream of consciousness and are based on attitudes or assumptions
(schemas) developed from previous experiences (Beck et al., 1979).

Cognitive therapy, and the work of Aaron Beck, focuses on the cognitive distortions postulated to be present in specific mental health diagnoses. The goal of cognitive therapy is to alleviate problematic symptoms and to prevent their recurrence by helping clients identify and test negative cognitions. Furthermore, there is an emphasis on developing alternative, flexible, and positive ways of thinking, and rehearsing new cognitive and behavioral responses to address them. In an attempt to understand and interpret human thought, it is believed that through understanding the schema that surrounds the cognition that all behaviors can be brought within the therapeutic context, examined, and relearned (Wodarski & Bagarozzi, 1979). Using a procedure that Meichenbaum (1977) termed "running the movie," critical events and their accompanying cognitions can be recalled and discussed. As human thought is broken down into patterns of discrete events, the ability to make generalizations about an individual's cognitive process is facilitated. Positive reinforcements are also translated into internal processes when cognitive factors come into focus. Wodarski and Bagarozzi reported that, like pure behaviorists, cognitive theorists must assume that the consequences of behavior are perceived as somehow rewarding or the behavior will be extinguished.

The cognitive therapist helps the client to think and act more realistically and adaptively about psychological problems and thus reduces symptoms (Beck et al., 1979). Instead of supplying concrete rewards for appropriate behaviors, the therapist teaches the client to assess all of the information. The client is asked to process information in regard to the cognitive antecedents (what comes before the behavior) and consequences (what comes after the behavior) and to determine whether satisfying consequences will outweigh negative ones. If it is assumed that a cognitive approach would succeed in reducing client behaviors, it must also be assumed that deviant acts are a less rational form of behavior. When given the choice, with full knowledge of the range of alternatives and consequences, the client will choose to act prosocially.

Most cognitive therapists view human thought within the intervention process as either the "behavior" that needs to be modified or as an area that is indirectly changed when the overt behavior is treated (Meichenbaum, 1975). Therefore, the cognitive therapist attempts to alter cognitive distortions to effect a change in behavior. The belief is that the intervention should aim at reducing the frequency of the cognitions that elicit undesirable behaviors (Hulbert & Sipprelle, 1978). From this perspective, it becomes obvious that the focus is not to find fault within the client, but the focus is on the cognitive self-statements the client makes, and faulty self-statements are viewed as a result of a faulty belief system and thinking pattern (Meichenbaum, 1975).

Cognitive therapists believe there are four types of cognitive distortions:

1. *Arbitrary interference*—the process of drawing a conclusion when evidence is lacking or is actually contrary to the conclusion.
2. *Overgeneralization*—the process of making an unjustified generalization on the basis of a single incident.
3. *Magnification*—the propensity to exaggerate the meaning or significance of a particular event.
4. *Cognitive deficiency*—the disregard of an important aspect of a life situation; clients with this defect ignore, fail to integrate, or do not utilize information derived form experience, and consequently behave as though they have a defect in their system of expectations.

As part of human growth, the cognitive therapist will help the client identify and address these distortions while teaching problem-solving skills that will be used throughout the life cycle (Beck, 1976).

From an empirical perspective, to apply cognitive therapy a number of the principles directly related to behavioral therapy will be added and adapted to modify negative self-statements (Meichenbaum, 1975). For example, cognitive theorists have emphasized the following cognitive aspects of depression. Beck (1976) assigned a primary position to a cognitive triad consisting of a very negative view of the self, of the outside world, and of the future. This triad is seen as the key to the consequences of depression, such as the lack of motivation, the affective state, and other ideational and behavioral manifestations. Beck suggested that the basic treatment strategy in working with depressed individuals includes five phases:

1. Identify and monitor the dysfunctional automatic thoughts;
2. Recognize the connection between thoughts, emotion, and behavior;
3. Evaluate the reasonableness of the automatic thoughts;
4. Substitute more reasonable thoughts for the dysfunctional automatic thoughts; and
5. Identify and alter dysfunctional silent assumptions.

During human interactions, the depressed person's cognitions can lead to misinterpretations of experiences; therefore, many of the secondary responses are logical consequences of such misinterpretations. The depressed person is locked in an insoluble situation, the result of which is further despair (Calhoun, Adams, & Mitchell, 1974). Thus, the cognitive responses that the social worker can assist in altering are: (a) a sense of hopelessness, (b) self-condemnation and self-defeating thoughts, (c) low self-esteem, (d) tension, (e) death wishes, and (f) a sense of helplessness.

Most professionals agree that the ultimate goal of most cognitive intervention methods is to increase individuals' abilities to control their own thoughts. In this manner self-control is viewed as a developmental achievement linking the intervention approach and the person's attributional style (Bugenthal, Whalen, & Hienker, 1977). Therefore, individual expectations and assumptions will play a significant role in the success a person will experience in therapy (Goldfried & Goldfried, 1975). Each individual, through performance, practice, and rehearsal can achieve consistent and superior results (Bandura, Adams, & Beyer, 1977). Although cognitive restructuring, problem solving, and self-instruction are the most widely used cognitive intervention methods, the addition of techniques that involve developing coping skills training, stress-inoculation training, systematic desensitization, and thought stopping can also assist in raising intervention effectiveness (Granvold, 1994).

## THE BIRTH OF COGNITIVE-BEHAVIORAL THERAPY

After behaviorism dominated American psychology for approximately 50 years, cognitive-behavior modification techniques began appearing in the psychology literature in the mid- to late-1970s (McCarthy & Rude, 2000). This created an incredible shift for many mental health researchers who had to reorient themselves to new constructs that had not been previously considered important in behaviorism. This involved the preservation of the best clinical behavioral interventions while recognizing and incorporating the cognitive experiences of the individual. While the traditional behaviorist had focused on changing *overt* behaviors, cognitive-behavioral theorists began to focus on changing *covert* behaviors as well as helping a client to address thoughts and feelings that surrounded the behaviors. The integration and recognition that cover both overt and covert behaviors are important targets of change in cognitive-behavioral theory (Cormier & Cormier, 1985).

The principles of cognitive-behavioral therapy (CBT) note that maladaptive behaviors, just like normal behaviors, are subject to alteration and change. Cognitive-behavioral therapy "emphasizes the complex interaction among cognitive events, processes, products, and structures, affect, overt behavior, and environmental context and experiences as contributing to various facets of dysfunctional behavior" (Braswell & Kendall, 1988, p. 167). Reinforcers that enhance the likelihood that they will continue maintain all behaviors. Part of CBT's focus thus entails reinforcing positive overt behaviors, such as social interactions, and covert behaviors, such as positive thoughts and self-statements.

Cognitive-behavioral therapy has been strongly influenced by Ellis's (1971) rational emotive therapy, Beck's cognitive theory of depression (Beck et al., 1979), and Meichenbaum's (1975) self-instructional training (SIT) with impulsive children. Recent research focus has included the concepts of attribution and self-efficacy. Further refinement and research has resulted in CBT's being used with a variety of client problems including both children and adults. Hart and Morgan (1993) state that cognitive-behaviorism has descended from influential and enduring forces in psychology, introducing new features while retaining preexisting ideas. This approach reflects a shift toward a more integrative, reciprocal, and holistic picture of behavior change. CBT reflects a consistent and rational extension of the scope of behavior therapy that constitutes a significant and exciting endeavor in its early stages of development.

CBT uses performance-based and cognitive interventions to produce changes in thinking, feeling, and behavior (Kendall, 1991). It concerns itself with both the external environment and the individual's internal processing of the world (Kendall & Panichelli-Mindel, 1995). After over two decades of research, a sound empirical basis now exists for cognitive-behavioral therapy (CBT) (Gortner, Gollan, Dobson, & Jacobson, 1998; Kendall & Panichelli-Mindel, 1995; Murphy, Carney, & Knesevich, 1995). In addition, the literature clearly supports the use of CBT for a variety of mental health difficulties such as anxiety, aggression, depression, attention deficits, pain, and learning disorders.

Kendall and Panichelli-Mindel (1995) refer to the cognitive-behavioral therapist as a consultant, diagnostician, and educator. As a consultant, the therapist provides ideas for experimentation, helps sort through experiences, and promotes problem solving. As a diagnostician, the therapist gathers varied data and integrates them to determine what is best for the client based on the current situation. As an educator, the therapist participates with clients to influence them to think for themselves, maximize personal strengths, and acquire cognitive skills and behavior control (see Kendall & Panichelli-Mindel; Hollon, 1999).

Unfortunately, problems are never simple and often they are not the result of one single factor; therefore, addressing them often necessitates the use of multidimensional assessments. Cognitions and behaviors can be classified on a continuum necessitating assessment of each, which may result in various CBT approaches. Therefore the assessment is an important process that establishes the diagnosis and dictates treatment (Dulmus & Wodarski, 1998). The design of a comprehensive assessment package must cover the relevant interacting variables considered most important to the specific client (Granvold & Wodarski, 1994). The assessment phase of the evaluation should identify the presenting problem(s) from both the client's and therapist's perspective (Dulmus & Wodarski, 1996). The inclusion of cognitive elements should add flexibility and scope to the assessment and treatment of client behaviors. It is necessary to develop rapport with the client to establish a therapeutic alliance that will aid in accomplishing successful assessment and treatment.

Appropriate diagnostic testing should be completed using standardized testing materials. Finch, Nelson, and Ott (1993) state, "from our perspective a clinician's time is well spent in assessment when there is a focus to the assessment and when the clinician knows how to utilize the data generated by the assessment" (p. 91). Without a thorough assessment a clinician would be at a disadvantage in establishing a diagnosis and knowing when to administer CBT. Also, measuring treatment efficacy would be difficult. The assessment is essential and all information gathered should be utilized in establishing the diagnosis and treatment plan (Dulmus & Wodarski, 1996).

A variety of inventories have been developed for the assessment of cognitive behavior and are useful for both assessment purposes and outcome evaluation (Dulmus & Wodarski, 1998). The following is a sampling of such inventories:

- *The Automatic Thoughts Questionnaire* (ATQ), developed by Hollon and Kendall (1980) to determine negative cognitions associated with depression;
- *The Dysfunctional Attitude Scale* (DAS), developed by Weissman & Beck (1978) to assess negative attitudes associated with depression;

- *The Attributional Style Questionnaire* (ASQ), developed by Peterson et al. (1982) and designed to measure attributional style on internal-external, stable-unstable, and global-specific dimensions;
- *The Irrational Beliefs Test* (IBT), the degree to which subjects maintain their beliefs (Jones, 1969);
- *Rational Behavior Inventory* (RBI), developed by Shorkey and Whiteman (1977) to measure irrational beliefs.

The worker bases the effectiveness of the therapeutic relationship upon accurate clinical judgment and cognitive assessment. A defining feature is the effectiveness of the clinical collaboration with the client. The collaborative approach includes the definition of the problem and the contextual variables that effect change. The stabilization of change should be examined to determine the effectiveness of treatment focusing upon the cognitive variable. The evaluation process is also designed and carried out together. This could be defined as "collaborative empiricism" (Beck et al., 1979). Within the relationship, the definition of such parameters as termination and the establishment of relapse prevention procedures must be developed and followed for further reevaluation of the effectiveness of treatment (Mahoney, 1991), thus requiring ongoing assessment.

There are several dangers in the interpretation of cognitive process. These aspects include the need to avoid isolation. Cognition is only one of several variables (cognition, affect, behavior, physical, psychological, and environmental factors) that interact reciprocally. Cognitive processes relate directly to both cause and effect (Meichenbaum & Cameron 1981). This factor complicates the individual assessment techniques so that procedures must be developed for each variable. Cognitive assessment is in its infancy, and the future may hold promise to isolate cognition via mathematical and statistical calculations. Yet the question remains whether a variable that is subject to so many uncertain outcomes can be useful in assessing in isolation the outcome of human behavior. Researchers must continue to refine CBT.

Cognitive-behavioral therapy is clearly problem focused. Through gaining new knowledge and skills, individuals can change cognitions, behaviors, moods, and motivations (Persons, 1989). Cognitive-behavioral therapy may well be the treatment of choice for many client problems, with multiple strategies being available for implementation.

# COGNITIVE-BEHAVIORAL THERAPY IN PRACTICE

As stated previously, cognitive-behavioral therapy may well be the treatment of choice for many client problems, with multiple strategies being available for implementation. For example, the use of homework should be strategically formulated, individually designed, and increased gradually. A comprehensive assessment can help determine if and when clients are intellectually capable of the cognitive and behavioral change. Repetitive trials and attentiveness to the client's understanding must be considered in each session.

The inclusion of significant individuals from the client's environment, including family members, can help to achieve successful generalization. Kaufer and Schefft (1988) note that including family members can assist bridging therapeutic gains with the natural environment for the rehabilitation of clients with a chronic illness. The evidence is particularly strong for children below the age of adolescence and clients with partnership problems. When individuals are influenced by their support system, change can result in reinforcement and adaptation, or inhibition and barriers. For the most part inclusion of the family can enhance treatment effects. Also, when viewed as a social support system, cognitive-behavioral constructs can assist in work-based conflicts such as substance abuse, depression, and interpersonal problems.

In therapeutic treatment, the inclusion of the natural environment as part of the treatment context is considered ideal and allows for generalization to the client's world sphere. Treatments given in the natural environment facilitate transferability of skills in the home, workplace, school, and other relevant contextual environments. This allows the therapist and client to develop a working relationship that can address maladaptive behaviors, environmental stresses, and interpersonal dynamics. For example, in the school setting CBT has been used to treat children's behavior problems. Frequently a consultant-practitioner instructs teachers, aids, school counselors, and other cognitive-behavior treatment principles. Targeted problems are identified and interventions are tailored to a specific change variable. These change behaviors are targeted for the development of linkage and transferable skills that can be generalized and applied at the community, school, family, and individual level.

Therapeutic success has been noted when the opportunity to observe clients in their own milieu occurs as a means of improving assessment, treatment planning, and implementation (Stokes & Baer, 1977). This facilitates the effective transfer of treatment anxiety and fears while involving the practitioner (Barlow, 1988; Barlow & Waddell, 1985; Matthews, Gelder, & Johnson, 1981; Sacco, 1981). Practitioner participation may aid treatment by involving gradual exposure procedures or "prolonged in vivo exposure" (Barlow, 1988), allowing the practitioner to remain with the client in a difficult situation. This supports the importance of practitioner involvement while accompanying clients to the site of their fear.

Relapse prevention methods are strategies that can be used to prevent the deterioration of treatment gains. In demanding situations there may be a greater danger than the client anticipates and relapse can result. For example, since relapse rates for people suffering from addictive disorders continue to rise, the development of self-efficacy can help in reducing levels of relapse (Brownell, Marlatt, Lichenstein, & Wilson, 1986). The strength of clients' efficacy beliefs will influence if they will try as well as their degree of coping. Since choices are made planned avoidance of certain threatening situations can be implemented. Therefore, the development of a sense of competency and effectiveness will prevent relapse, because the perception of self-efficacy has been correlated with both cessation and maintenance of change. Extreme self-efficacy may result in optimistic cognitive bias that is usually considered adaptive. If not addressed, this bias may lead to inappropriate complacency about the adequacy of one's skills for coping with difficult situations (Haaga & Stewart, 1992). It has been proposed that moderate levels of self-efficacy have been found to be the most effective for preventing relapse (Devins, 1992; Haaga & Stewart, 1992). Establishing an understanding of relapse will inoculate against future relapse.

In addition the practitioner should educate clients that they will not always be problem free (Greenwald, 1987). Marlett and his colleagues provide valuable information on lifestyle assessment and modification in relation to relapse prevention (Marlett & Gordon, 1980; Marlett & Parks, 1982). Social support that includes family members can assist in cueing certain behaviors that trigger relapse behaviors, while governing contingencies under which the client operates can provide ongoing reinforcement of the desired responses.

Early detection of relapse cues includes training and education about relapse, and often the client and therapist work together on compiling a list of relapse cues. Relapse intervention should be self-initiated whenever possible. This allows for the avoidance of protracted relapse responses that could possibly cause individuals to lose control over their behaviors (Granvold & Wodarski, 1994). Furthermore, follow-up contacts and booster sessions assure early detection of relapse. These sessions can be conducted in a variety of settings or on the telephone or by mail. The critical element is the issue of maintenance behaviors as well as a discussion of relapse prevention behaviors. The practitioner and individual can assess the status of their maintenance phase to reduce the possibility of relapse. The concept of booster sessions should be considered as a part of the process rather than an aberration. This follow-up also provides an excellent opportunity for clinical research that focuses upon outcomes.

Overall, in CBT the participation in activities can be growth producing and help to remove barriers to behavioral changes while supporting and encouraging relapse prevention behavior. Therefore, participation in activities can indirectly lead to enhancing the quality of life for the client. The family should meet with the practitioner prior to termination to deal with these issues and, when utilized, the use of self-help groups (e.g., Alcoholics Anonymous, Overeater's Anonymous, Effective Patenting Groups, Clubs) should be clearly documented.

In training the teaching of specific coping skills has proven to be a productive endeavor. For example, being knowledgeable of multiple coping strategies has increased the likelihood of abstinence from alcohol (Bliss, Garvey, Heinold, & Hitchcock, 1989). Meichenbaum and Burstein (1975) stressed the importance of educating clients to understand how cognition works when addressing and preparing high-risk situations. Problem-solving procedures often used to assist clients are relaxation and imagery rehearsals (Goldfried, Decenteceo, & Weinberg, 1974; Langer, Janis, & Wolper, 1975; Lazarus, 1974, 1977).

In general cognitive-behavioral approaches differ from the medical model in which the client is looking for a cure. In CBT the goal is to help prepare the client for the need to cope with different circumstances. In successful therapeutic planning clients' exert greater control over their environment. Self-monitoring is done systematically and makes the client aware of high-risk thoughts and actions. This preparation for maintenance will prepare for both the stimulus and the response. The use of a journal, and carrying a beeper to track behavior patterns could be helpful for achieving improved confidence in the client's ability to handle stress. Some approaches encourage the continued use of standardized scales such as the Beck's Inventory of Depression as a means of empowering the client to monitor their current situation. Counting procedures or utilizing video or audiotapes are just some of the methods that can be used to maintain behavior.

## Implications for Policy

The mental health care industry is changing rapidly. Managed care is an inescapable element of mental health services in the United States today with many private and public insurance now utilizing this cost containment program (Appelbaum, 1993). Managed health care sometimes limits the number of outpatient mental health sessions (Foos, Otten, & Hill, 1991). This managed mental health care system has had profound effects on the delivery of mental health services and has often made practitioners accountable for client outcomes. Mental health professionals are receiving pressure from managed care companies to produce empirically based treatment with proven outcomes. In today's practice environment practitioners must provide evidence that the services provided are well supported by sound clinical research studies (Corcoran, 2000). When this is done, authorization for such treatments is enhanced. Since third parties make decisions regarding reimbursement for treatment for clients, practitioners will be forced to demonstrate outcome-based treatment.

Practitioners working without empirically based practices are at risk for increased malpractice suits. Society has begun to demand proof that interventions work (Sanderson, 1995). Campbell (1994) states, "When psychotherapists fail to maintain familiarity with the current literature, develop ill-conceived treatment plans, solicit the dependency of clients, and confuse them by creating imaginary problems, their negligence invites malpractice litigation" (p. 31).

Fortunately, many cognitive-behavioral interventions meet the rigorous empirical basis demanded by third party payees. Because they are often the treatment of choice, agencies must provide practitioners with training opportunities to acquire the knowledge and skills necessary to implement CBT when indicated. The National Association of Cognitive-Behavioral Therapists (NACBT) provides credentialing for cognitive-behavioral therapists. Since its inception in 1995, it has been promoting the empirical effectiveness of CBT and advocating its use by well-trained practitioners. By providing credentialing for cognitive-behavioral therapists, NACBT ensures that credentialed practitioners have the training and experience to deliver CBT interventions while remaining current in knowledge and applications.

It is essential that mental health professionals provide comprehensive assessments and match empirically proven treatment, as it exists, to diagnosis. This demands an ongoing quest for new knowledge and training for the practitioner to enable them to provide the most effective treatments for their clients. Cognitive-behavioral therapy would certainly fall in this category. Nothing less is ethically acceptable, with less possibly leading to legal implications. In addition it is imperative to have an outcome-based practice so clients can access treatment as needed through third party gatekeepers.

## SUMMARY

Among practitioners, new applications have arisen that stretch the boundary of the orthodox cognitive behavioral perspective. CBT has been applied with a degree of effectiveness across the diagnostic mental health spectrum and has been used in psychoeducational materials as well. This trend of broad application includes a diverse body of practice research material, although consistency in application of the original premise of treatment continues to wax and wane. There are several aspects of cognitive treatment that need further exploration. These issues include (a) questions about the generalization of therapy into the daily difficulties that clients encounter, and (b) concern about the maintenance of behavioral change. These are two key elements in outcome-based treatment.

In summary it appears clear that aspects of cognitive treatment are quantifiable and have withstood the test of proven results in modification of cognitive-behavioral patterns. In the scope of therapeutic practice for this model, empirical evidence of effectiveness has been impressive. With the surge of interest in self-help application, the collaborative element of cognitive-behavioral practice has been very responsive to a more informed middle-class clientele. The area of debate is whether the treatment has been empirically evaluated when used with different socioeconomic economic groups and in gender relatedness. These concerns become particularly difficult when the field is self-propagating at an increasingly rapid pace. When practitioners were surveyed, the skills that contribute to generalization practices and maintenance of behavior appeared to be neglected. This research should be examined further to determine the barriers perceived by practitioners in training for post-treatment effectiveness. In addition, few studies examine the generalizability of CBT to clinical settings in which treatment is open ended and less standardized and in which diagnostically complicated patients are not eliminated.

Scaling techniques are a means of quantifying and measuring the influence of therapy upon the individual. The applied use of scaling techniques contributes to the growth of clinical practice research. Through scientific method the substance of practice has a greater probability of increasing effectiveness. Effective practice requires continuous reevaluation to assure the optimal level of effectiveness. When the therapy is conducted according to empirically tested aspects and implemented accordingly, the client who has self-efficacy will have the greatest rate of success. Furthermore, in the generalization of behavior, more research should be conducted to improve effectiveness in these skills. New computer programs have helped to improve content analysis (Gottschalk, 1994). Computer programs can now provide a rapid objective measure of the magnitude of various psychobiological measures— cognitive impairment, social alienation-personal disorganization, anxiety, and three kinds of hostility. This type of computerized analysis can break down interactions mathematically to examine their structure and frequency pattern. The use of these tools could contribute toward the empirical development of the field of cognitive research. Effective, socially relevant, and resilient change is essential for success. The reenforcement of significant others is a valuable factor in establishing and maintaining new behaviors patterns.

Transfer of training methods should be initiated early in treatment rather than only at the point of termination (Stokes & Baer, 1977). Some procedures, such as simulation and rehearsal, are appropriate across settings. In this way the clients engage in a collaborative effort to determine the areas of their lives that pose the greatest problems. The mastery of relevant skills requires redundancy and persistence. These overlearning techniques, when applied, can assure that when under stress the client will be able to utilize the appropriate skills.

It has been postulated that overlearning is the greatest assurance of maximum transfer (Baer, 1981; Gottman & Lieblum, 1974). Giving attention to differential skill acquisition rates and establishing appropriate time limits for these gains to occur have accomplished this. Since clients may have different rates of learning and skill acquisition, concern of the client applying the learning and the skill in the natural setting must always be considered. The variability of rates of application is particularly problematic with increased emphasis on brief therapy. Despite these concerns, longer-term skill acquisition may be required to adequately accomplish the performance level necessary for effective, durable change and transfer to the client's natural environment.

There has been a proliferation of research on the cognitive variable in the examination of human behavior. The cognitive revolution has taken hold in some schools of thought. Ideally, the research can empirically examine the probability of success of treatment and yet the dilemma remains that there has not been empirical evidence to support the maintenance of the change process. In application the trends indicate that although cognitive-behavioral techniques are effective in comparative outcome studies, either the approach equals or is statistically more successful than other models of therapy. Yet, there has not been enough work in the field of the generalization of the change indicators to assure maintenance. Because the cognitive variable is significant in the treatment of human behavior, it cannot be considered in isolation of other dimensions of behavior. Significant contributions have been made in the treatment of depression, phobias, anxiety, and panic attacks. Treatment elements have been applied to a diverse range of conditions; however, practice research has not documented statistical evidence of the effectiveness of the results. Further study must isolate the aspect of treatment that is producing the outcome. Greater attention must be given to the generalization and maintenance of treatment.

## REFERENCES

Appelbaum, P. S. (1993). Legal liability and managed care. *American Psychologist, 24* (1), 67–90.

Baer, D. M. (1981). *How to plan for generalization.* Lawrence, KS: H & H Enterprises.

Bandura, A., Adams, N., & Beyer, J. (1977). Cognitive processes mediating behavioral change. *Journal of Personality and Social Psychology, 35,* 125–139.

Barlow, D. H. (1988). *Anxiety and its disorders: The nature and treatment of anxiety and panic.* New York: Guilford.

Barlow, D. H., & Waddell, M. T. (1985). Agoraphobia. In D. H. Barlow (Eds.), *Clinical handbook of psychological disorders: A step-by-step treatment manual.* New York: Guilford.

Beck, A. (1976). *Cognitive therapy and emotional disorders.* New York: International Universities Press.

Beck, A. T., Rush, A. J., Shaw, B. F., & Emery, G. (1979). *Cognitive therapy of depression.* New York: Guilford.

Bliss, R. E., Garvey, A. J., Heinold, J. W., & Hitchcock, J. L. (1989). The influence and coping on relapse crisis outcomes after smoking cessation. *Journal of Consulting and Clinical Psychology, 57,* 443–449.

Bolles, R. C. (1974). Cognition and motivation: Some historical trends. In B. Weiner (Ed.), *Cognitive views of human motivation.* New York: Academic.

Bootzin, R., & Max, D. (1980). Learning and behavioral theories. In I. Kutash, L. Schlesinger, & Associates (Eds.), *Handbook on stress and anxiety.* Washington, DC: Jossey-Bass.

Braswell, L., & Kendall, P. (1988). Cognitive-behavioral methods with children. In K. S. Dobson (Ed.), *Handbook of cognitive-behavioral therapies.* New York: Guilford.

Breitholtz, E., Johansson, B., & Ost, L. (1999). Cognitions in generalized anxiety disorder and panic disorder patients: A prospective approach. *Behaviour Research and Therapy, 37* (6), 533–544.

Brownell, K. D., Marlatt, A. G., Lichenstein, E., & Wilson, T. G. (1986). Understanding and preventing relapse. *American Psychologist, 41* (7), 765–782.

Bugenthal, D. B., Whalen, C. K., & Hienker, B. (1977). Causal attributions of hyperactive children and motivation assumptions of two behavior change approaches: Evidence for an interactionist position. *Child Development, 48,* 874–884.

Calhoun, K. S., Adams, H. E., & Mitchell, K. M. (1974). *Innovative treatment methods in psychopathology.* New York: Wiley.

Campbell, T. W. (1994). Psychotherapy and malpractice exposure. *American Journal of Forensic Psychology, 12* (1), 5–40.

Corcoran, J. (2000). Family treatment of preschool behavior problems. *Research on Social Work Practice, 10* (5), 547–588.

Cormier, W. H., & Cormier, L. S. (1985). *Interviewing strategies for helpers: Fundamental skills and cognitive interventions* (2nd ed.). Monterey: Brooks/Cole.

Devins, G. M. (1992). Social cognitive analysis of recovery from a lapse of smoking cessation: Comment on Haaga & Stewert 1992. *Journal of Consulting and Clinical Psychology, 60* (1), 29–31.

Dulmus, C. N., & Wodarski, J. S. (1996). Assessment and effective treatment of childhood psychopathology: Responsibilities and implications for practice. *Journal of Child and Adolescent Group Therapy, 6* (2), 75–99.

Dulmus, C. N., & Wodarski, J. S. (1998). Major depressive disorder and dysthymic disorder. In B. Thyer & J. S. Wodarski (Eds.), *Handbook of empirical social work practice* (Vol. I), 273–285.

Ellis, A. (1971). Rational-emotive psychotherapy: A comprehensive approach to therapy. In G. D. Goldman & D. S. Milman (Eds.), *Innovations in psychotherapy* (pp. 293–319). Springfield, IL: Charles C Thomas.

Finch, A. J., Nelson, W. M., & Ott, E. S. (1993). *Cognitive-behavioral procedures with children and adolescents.* Boston: Allyn and Bacon.

Folkman, S., Schaefer, C., & Lazarus, R. (1979). Cognitive processes as mediators of stress and coping. In V. Hamilton & D. Warburton (Eds.), *Human stress and cognition.* New York: Wiley.

Foos, J. A., Otten, A. J., & Hill, L. K. (1991). Managed mental health: A primer for counselors. *Journal of Counseling and Development, 69,* 332–336.

Goldfried, M. R., Decenteceo, E. T., & Weinberg, L. (1974). Systematic rational restructuring as a self-control technique. *Behavior Therapy, 5* (2), 247–254.

Goldfried, M., & Goldfried, A. (1975). Cognitive change methods. In F. Kanfer & A. Goldstein (Eds.), *Helping people change.* New York: Pergamon.

Goodwin, D. W., & Guze, S. B. (1989). *Psychiatric diagnosis.* New York: Oxford University Press.

Gortner, E. T., Gollan, J. K., Dobson, K. S., & Jacobson, N. S. (1998). Cognitive-behavioral treatment for depression: Relapse prevention. *Journal of Consulting and Clinical Psychology, 66* (2), 377–384.

Gottman, J. M., & Lieblum, S. R. (1974). *How to do psychotherapy and how to evaluate it: A manual for beginners.* New York: Holt, Rinehart & Winston.

Gottschalk, L. (1994). The development, validation, and application of a computerized measurement of cognitive impairment from the content analysis of verbal behavior. *Journal of Clinical Psychology, 50* (3), 349–361.

Granvold, D. (1994). *Cognitive and behavioral treatment: Methods and applications.* Belmont, CA: Brooks/Cole.

Granvold, D., & Wodarski, J. S. (1994). Cognitive and behavioral treatment: Clinical issues, transfer of training, and relapse prevention. In D. K. Granvold (Ed.), *Cognitive and behavioral treatment,* 253–375.

Greenwald, M. A. (1987). Programming treatment generalization. In L. Michelson & L. M. Ascher (Eds.), *Anxiety and stress disorders.* New York: Guilford.

Haaga, D., & Stewart, B. L. (1992). Self-efficacy for recovery from a lapse after smoking cessation. *Journal of Consulting and Clinical Psychology, 60* (1), 24–28.

Hart, K., & Morgan, J. (1993). Cognitive-behavioral procedures with children: Historical context and current status. In A. J. Finch, W. M. Nelson, & E. S. Ott (Eds.), *Cognitive-behavioral procedures with children: A practice guide* (pp. 1–24). Boston: Allyn and Bacon.

Hollon, S. D. (1999). Rapid early response in cognitive behavior therapy: A commentary. *Clinical Psychology: Science and Practice, 6* (3), 305–309.

Hollon, S. D., & Kendall, P. C. (1980). Cognitive self-statements in depression: Development of an automatic thoughts questionnaire. *Cognitive Therapy and Research, 4,* 109–143.

Hulbert, R. T., & Sipprelle, C. N. (1978). Random sampling of cognitions in alleviating anxiety attacks. *Cognitive Therapy and Research, 2* (2), 165–169.

Ingram, R. E. (1983). Content and process distinctions in depressive self-schemata. In L. B. Alloy (Chair), *Depression and schemeta.* Symposium presented at the meeting of the American Psychological Association, Anaheim, CA.

Jones, R. G. (1969). A factored measure of Ellis's Irrational Belief System. (Doctoral dissertation, Texas Technological College, 1968). *Dissertation Abstracts International, 29,* 4379B–4380B.

Kaplan, H. I., Sadock, B. J., & Grebb, J. A. (1994). *Synopsis of psychiatry.* Baltimore: Williams & Wilkins.

Kaufer, F. H., & Schefft, B. K. (1988). *Guilding the process of therapeutic change.* Champaign, IL: Research.

Kendall, P. C. (1991). *Child and adolescent therapy: Cognitive-behavioral procedures.* New York: Guilford.

Kendall, P. C., & Hollon, S. D. (1981). Assessing self-referent speech: Methods in the measurement of self-statements. In P. C. Kendall & S. D. Hollon (Eds.), *Assessment strategies for cognitive-behavioral interventions.* New York: Guilford.

Kendall, P. C., & Panichelli-Mindel, S. M. (1995). Cognitive-behavioral treatments. *Journal of Abnormal Child Psychology, 23* (1), 107–123.

Kingdon, D., & Turkington, D. (1994). *Cognitive behavioral therapy of schizophrenics.* New York: Guilford.

Langer, E., Janis, L., & Wolper, J. (1975). Reduction of psychological stress in surgical patients. *Journal of Experimental Social Psychology, 11,* 155–165.

Lazarus, R. S. (1974). Cognitive and coping processes in emotion. In B. Weiner (Ed.), *Cognitive views of human emotion.* New York: Academia.

Lazarus, R. S. (1977). Psychological stress and the coping process. In Z. S. Lipowski, D. R. Lipsitt, & P. C. Whybrow (Eds.), *Psychosomatic medicine: Current trends and clinical applications.* New York: Oxford University Press.

Mahoney, M. J. (1974). *Cognition and behavior modification.* Cambridge, MA: Ballinger.

Mahoney, M. J. (1991). *Human change processes: The scientific foundations of psychotherapy.* New York: Basic Books.

Marlett, G. A., & Gordon, S. G. (1980). Determinants of relapse: Implications for the maintenance of behavioral change. In P. O. Davison & S. M. Davison (Eds.), *Behavioral medicine: Changing health lifestyles.* New York: Brunner/Mazel.

Marlett, G. A., & Parks, G. A. (1982). Self-management of addictive behaviors. In P. E. Karoly & F. H. Kanfer (Eds.), *Self-management and behavior change.* New York: Pergamon.

Matthews, A. M., Gelder, M. G., & Johnson, D. W. (1981). *Agoraphobia: Nature and treatment.* New York: Guilford.

Marzillier, J. (1980). Cognitive therapy and behavioral practice. *Behavior Research & Therapy, 18* (4), 249–258.

McCarthy, C., & Rude, S. (2000). Cognitively based counseling: Current state and future directions. *TCA Journal, 28* (1), 32–40.

Meichenbaum, D. (1975). Self-instructional methods. In F. Kanfer & A. Goldstein (Eds.), *Helping people change.* New York: Pergamon.

Meichenbaum, D. (1977). *Cognitive behavior modification: An integrative approach.* New York: Plenum.

Meichenbaum, D., & Cameron, R. (1981). Issues in cognitive assessment: An overview. In T. V. Merluzzi, C. R. Glass, & M. Genest (Eds.), *Cognitive assessment.* New York: Guilford.

Meichenbaum, D., Turk, D., & Burstein, S. (1975). The nature of coping with stress. In I. G. Sarsons & C. D. Spielburger (Eds.), *Stress and anxiety* (Vol. II). New York: Wiley.

Murphy, G. E., Carney, R. M., Knesevich, M. A., & Whitworth, P. (1995). Cognitive behavioral therapy, relaxation training, and tricyclic antidepressant medication in the treatment of depression. *Psychological Reports, 77* (2), 403–420.

Persons, J. B. (1989). *Cognitive therapy in practice: A case formulation approach.* New York: W. W. Norton.

Peterson, C., Semmel, A., von Baeyer, C., Abramson, L. Y., Metalsky, G. I., & Seligman, M. E. (1982). The attributional style questionnaire. *Cognitive Therapy and Research, 6,* 287–299.

Sacco, W. P. (1981). Cognitive therapy 'in vivo.' In G. Emery, S. D. Holon, & R. C. Bedrosian (Eds.), *New directions in cognitive therapy: A casebook.* New York: Guilford.

Salkovskis, P. (1999). Understanding and treating obsessive-compulsive disorder. *Behaviour Research and Therapy, 37* (1), S29–S52.

Sanderson, W. C. (1995, March). Which therapies are proven effective? (Shared perspectives). *APA Monitor,* p. 4.

Shorkey, C., & Whiteman, V. (1977). Development of the Rational Behavior Inventory: Initial validity and reliability. *Educational and Psychological Measurement, 37,* 527–534.

Stokes, T. F., & Baer, D. M. (1977). An implicit technology of generalization. *Journal of Applied Behavioral Analysis, 10,* 345–367.

Weissman, A. N., & Beck, A. T. (1978). *Development and validation of the Dysfunctional Attitudes Scale: A preliminary investigation.* Paper presented at the annual meeting of the American Education Association, Toronto.

Wodarski, J. S. (1982). National and state appeals for energy conservation: A behavioral analysis of effect. *Behavioral Engineering, 7* (4), 119–130.

Wodarski, J. S., & Bagarozzi, D. (1979). *Behavioral social work.* New York: Human Sciences.

## CHAPTER 4

# The Life Span Perspective

## Diane Dwyer and Janice Hunt-Jackson

To understand social work practice from a human growth and development perspective knowledge must be derived and subsequently drawn from a variety of sources. These perspectives include psychoanalytic theories and stage theories, biologic facts, human behavior theories, economic reports, legal issues, and specific cultural information, as well as other sources. This makes assessment somewhat of an *art*, and the more choices the social worker has available, the more opportunities there are for adequate assessment and intervention. A relatively recent addition to the body of human behavior theory is the life span development perspective. The introduction to Part I outlined that, although Freud and other psychoanalytic and psychodynamic theorists propose developmental stages in early life, utilizing a life span perspective expands on these ideas. According to Lefrancois (1993), this unique theoretical view studies the developmental changes that transpire in the individual from conception through old age. Key to this study is the consideration given to the biological, psychological, and social processes and influences that account for changes in human behavior.

Life span development theorists posit that human development is continuous. Basseches (1984) notes that this theory is rooted in the belief that changes occurring in adulthood are similar in magnitude to those of earlier developmental periods. Therefore, human development is a continuous process, not one that ceases when the individual achieves adulthood, as previously implied by the studies of noted developmental psychologists such as Piaget, Bowlby, and Erikson. Belsky, Lerner, and Spanier (1984) outline the central beliefs that guide contemporary developmental life span research, because development of both children and adults is continuous, as is that of families, societies, and cultures. This makes development *bi-directional*. For example, children influence their parents just as much as parents influence their children and this supports the assumption that all development is influenced by the context in which it occurs.

Therefore, contemporary life span research reflects a trend away from viewing the individual in isolation toward a more ecologically based study of the person in the environment. This chapter elucidates the relevance of the life span developmental approach to social work practice. Each developmental period will be discussed in terms of its critical biological, psychological, and social aspects and appropriate interventions and the implications for social work practitioners, as they work with developing individuals. Additionally, a discussion of this perspective as it applies to persons with life-long disabilities is also included.

## PRENATAL DEVELOPMENT AT BIRTH

On average, the human organism undergoes a gestation period of 28 weeks characterized by rapid fetal biological development. Genetic factors link the fetus to the family ancestry while determining the individual characteristics that influence subsequent development. These physiological changes occur within a psychosocial context. Determinants of fetal growth and functioning can include biological, psychological, and social factors. These include the pregnant woman's age at the time of conception, hereditary characteristics, adequate nutrition, alcohol consumption, smoking habits, and ingestion of either prescribed or illicit drugs. Physical neglect or abuse plays a role in the development of a baby, as do other environmental factors such as access to medical care, adequate financial and emotional support, and exposure to hazardous chemicals. The emotional status of the mother-to-be, as well as her partner–family members has an effect on the baby too. Chemical and hormonal levels in both the brain and the bloodstream affect the biological processes of the mother and the baby when the mother experiences high amounts of stress; this may have an adverse effect on her child.

In working with the expectant mother, the social worker may need to fulfill several roles. It will sometimes be necessary to provide the mother with education regarding prenatal development and childbirth. In addition, interventions designed to help reduce stress can help the client and family deal with the changes that occur with the birth of a baby. Expectant parents may need assistance in accessing and securing the resources needed (e.g., prenatal care, good nutrition, adequate financial support, and genetic counseling). Low-income families may be particularly in need of this support relative to information and advocacy, because they may have the least access to high-quality prenatal, postnatal, and other medical care. Furthermore, the stresses associated with poverty put an added burden on a pregnant woman and her family, making the prebirth environment for the baby more hazardous than desired.

Although most babies are born healthy, when they are not parents and family members often need additional attention and support. Unfortunately, 17 in 1,000 babies in all racial and ethnic groups will have Down's syndrome, and the odds of having a child with this disability increase dramatically as the childbearing mother ages (Hayes & Batshaw, 1993). Other conditions, such as Spina Bifida (1 in 1,000 births) and cerebral palsy (approximately 4,500 cases), are diagnosed each year (Hobdell, 1995). In addition there are other prebirth disabling conditions, such as Hemophilia, Tay Sachs' disease, and Sickle-Cell Anemia. If the mother knows or suspects she may be carrying a child with one of these conditions, she should see a genetic counselor as soon as possible to learn about the disability, and how to best care for herself and her child.

When a mother is told that there is a high probability that her baby will be born disabled she may feel extreme pressure to abort or give up the child. The role of the social worker is clear in helping the mother and family understand the pros and cons of bearing and caring for all newborns, including those that suffer from disabilities. Raising either a healthy or disabled child is never an easy task, but having the proper information and supports in place can make the family experience less stressful.

Another major problem that should be addressed in prenatal development and birth is that of both street and prescription drug use. The American Academy of Family Physicians (1998) report cocaine and marijuana use is most common among persons aged 18 to 34 years, and pregnancy is most likely to occur during these years. If a pregnant woman is abusing street or illegal substances she may be resistant to ending this pattern of abuse and remain in denial about how her addiction can impact the unborn child. Furthermore, women who must take certain prescription drugs to diminish aspects of disability can be faced with the knowledge that these drugs will also adversely affect the health of a child. The decision to stop taking drugs of any kind to protect a baby is a difficult one; sometimes it is a danger to the mother, whether the drugs are legal or not. Withdrawal from street drugs can cause convulsions, while ending prescription drugs may put the mother and child in danger from seizures, toxemia, diabetic complications, or other disorders.

Abortion and infertility are two more social issues related to pregnancy that may require social work intervention. Social workers are frequently called upon to assist women make decisions about unwanted or problematic pregnancies. There are many reasons women decide to abort, including the fact they are carrying a handicapped child. It may be the social worker's role to find information about these disabilities, provide support for the parents, make referrals to medical specialists (including psychiatric care), or even assist the mother in finding a doctor who will perform an abortion. Similar services may be necessary for the woman's family or the father, regardless of the reason for the abortion.

Infertility is also a source of stress for the individual or couple. It is estimated that 10–15% of couples are unable to conceive after trying for more than a year (Zastrow & Kirst-Ashman, 1994). Assisting the infertile couple in accepting their condition and exploring options of medical treatment, surrogate parenting, or adoptions are functions for the social worker. Regardless of the option chosen, the parent(s) need supportive counseling and advocacy since both the medical and legal systems can be confusing, bureaucratic, expensive, and cumbersome.

Teen pregnancy is considered a risk factor for the mother. The teen mother may face interruptions in education, and if she drops out of school she is more likely to live in poverty. If she chooses to bear her child, her socioemotional development may be affected, as she prematurely assumes the highly demanding role of parent. At this stage in her development, the societal norm is for her to be experimenting with where she is comfortable such as her physical "looks" (hairstyle, clothing, makeup), and fitting in with her peers; in short, fulfilling the tasks of *identity versus role-confusion* (Erikson, 1963). Instead, she is forced into the next step often known as *intimacy versus isolation* because of the birth of her child. Having a baby to care for changes her life, cutting her off from her peers and the "normal" modes of interaction for this age group. The girl's health and that of her baby may also be at risk. She has a higher probability than older women of experiencing prolonged labor, toxemia, hemorrhaging, and miscarriage; and, the infant is more likely to be premature or of low birth weight. Because the percentage of births to unmarried teenage mothers is increasing (O'Hare, 1994), social workers must be ready to assist these women to realistically assess their situations and make choices. The pregnant teen will need considerable supportive counseling, referral, and advocacy.

## INFANTS AND TODDLERS (BIRTH TO 2 YEARS OF AGE)

The birth process proceeds through three stages: early labor, the birth of the child, and delivery of the placenta. Approximately 3% of all newborns have some form of disability at birth (Masters, Johnson, & Kolodny, 1988); slightly more than 7% of all U.S. births are babies with low birth weights (less than 5.5 lbs.), placing them at greater risk of infant mortality (O'Hare, 1994; U.S. Department of Health and Human Services, 1990).

During the first 6 months, a baby will move from random, ineffectual motions to accomplishments such as rolling over and beginning to crawl. The baby will begin to reach for objects, grasping them and learning about them from touch and taste. In infancy, newborns are active, constantly interacting with their environment, seeking stimulation and opportunity to perfect these competencies. Infants expend large amounts of energy trying to understand and master their world (MacTurk, McCarthy, Vietz, & Yarrow, 1987). As they enter their second year, they derive increased pleasure from their ability to affect what happens to them and to the world around them (Redding, Morgan, & Harmon, 1988). Unfortunately, a problem arises when the baby is born with a disability that precludes meeting and accomplishing these tasks. Erikson (1963) believes that this is the time babies learn to trust their environment and caregivers. This *Trust versus Mistrust* stage of life means the child learns that the parent will respond to cries with cuddling, food, and affection. Infants soon realize that they have no control over a portion of the immediate environment and are able to develop a sense of security that allows further emotional growth. However, if the child's parent(s) do not respond quickly and lovingly, the child will become mistrustful and may form an insecure or indifferent attachment to the parent. Furthermore, if a parent is not educated as how to best handle an infant who has a medical or some other disabling condition, the baby may be deprived of much of the cuddling needed (Quinn, 1998). In addition, when a child does not have the ability to make eye contact due to vision impairment, spasticity, or lack of eye control, the child may be less appealing to a parent, which in turn may result in less of this type of communication. Quinn gives detailed, concrete suggestions for ways parents can provide the needed stimulus and physical contact with children with disabilities, and social workers will find this advice helpful.

In providing services to the infant, the social worker's primary interventive efforts will be directed toward the parents, thus enabling them to provide a stimulating environment for their child. This will foster the child's cognitive, physical, and social-emotional growth. Under average circumstances, the role of the social worker is that of educator and support-treatment provider. The parents may need both education regarding the needs of the infant and support while adjusting to the demands of parenthood. Counseling may be done individually, or with a couple; however, group counseling may be especially effective because it permits mutual support (Wodarski, 1982). This is particularly true of parents who have a child with a disability. The shock of finding out the baby is disabled, combined with the extra demands of caring for a child with a disability, often leaves parents overwhelmed. A parent's support group can be of inestimable worth for these families, in which parents can talk about their experiences, frustrations, fears, and joys. It will be important for the social worker(s) involved with the family to be very active in accessing and coordinating medical, psychological, therapeutic, and remedial services. They must become forceful advocates in all these areas. The parents may not be up to fighting for their child's rights or their own at first; the social worker can provide much needed support in this role.

With increasing numbers of dual career families and single parent families, child care arrangements are required for infants and young children of working parents. The quality and quantity of available options pose problems for many working parents. Social workers may deal with stress encountered by the parent(s) as they attempt to negotiate the child care system. This is especially true of parents of children with disabilities. There may be personal care and accessibility issues with which child care agencies are unwilling to handle. With child care costs running the gamut from $300–$400 to as high as $1,000 a month for someone working a 40-hour week, low- and moderate-income families may need assistance in arranging appropriate and affordable care. As

Vander Zanden (1993) points out, "working parents in the United States are faced with a serious problem: Day care is often of poor quality, very costly, and hard to find" (p. 227). From a macro perspective, another role for the social worker is to advocate in the political arena for policies and legislation that support affordable and safe child care programs, as well as nutrition, health care, housing, and cash support for families who don't have the means to provide the necessities for their children.

## EARLY CHILDHOOD (2–6 YEARS OLD)

Between the ages of 2 and 6, children continue to enlarge their repertoires of behaviors. With improved physical coordination, the child now uses locomotion as a means of exploring the environment. The child learns to master independence-producing tasks such as dressing and toilet training. Language grows, as does expressive social interactions with family and friends. The child becomes more efficient at accumulating and processing new information, providing a foundation for the development of intellectual attributes (Bartsch & Wellman, 1989; Beal & Belgrad, 1990; Hale, 1990; Moses & Flavell, 1990). During this period, children begin to see themselves as individuals, separate from others (Kuczynski & Kochenska, 1990). Erikson (1963) describes the two crises of this stage as *autonomy versus shame and doubt* and *initiative versus guilt*. However, there appears to be some controversy regarding the cross-cultural universality of these developmental crises. Some theorists suggest that independence is a more highly valued characteristic in western cultures (Thomas, 1990), and thus more likely to spur this turbulent period. Leonore Loeb Adler (1989), in her book *Cross-Cultural Research in Human Development*, warned that on a worldwide basis, individual as well as group differences occur when behavior is observed and studied. The child grows within a social context and during this phase begins to learn the knowledge, values, and skills necessary for effective functioning when interacting in the group setting. These socially sanctioned ways of life (culture) are transmitted to the child through the socialization process, and parents are the first agents of this operation. Hence, it is within the family that the child first experiences the requirements of group life. Family circumstances and parenting styles are key variables to the child's successful adaptation to society.

It should be noted the young child's playmates augment this socialization process. Play functions provide a vehicle for cognitive stimulation

(Piaget, 1952), prepare children for later life on their own terms (Ganda & Pellegrini, 1985), and let them learn and rehearse adult roles (Howes, Unger, & Seidner, 1989). Thus, play, as the *work of children,* is critical to their development. This can create a specific problem for children with disabilities because parents may try to overprotect their children to keep them from emotional or physical harm. In turn, overprotection by the parent can impede the social and developmental progress of the child with a disability. All children, both with and without disabilities, can benefit from peer interaction. Therefore, it is vital that parents allow their child to be as *independent* as possible, starting out with feeding and dressing and allowing a certain amount of rough-and-tumble play with other children.

Parents should be consistent in their discipline patterns, regardless of whether the child is disabled or not. In a parent's efforts to support the child and help build a positive self-image, suitable limits that result in appropriate behavior must be set (Patterson, as cited in Quinn, 1998).

The social worker's interventions with young children will frequently involve working with the parents or on their behalf with other systems that have an impact on the child. Children who present symptoms ranging from temper tantrums to aggression, withdrawal, or phobias may be receiving inadequate parenting. Parenting effectiveness education provided in an individual or group setting may be useful in developing proactive parenting skills. Such intervention will be most productive when it includes appropriate reinforcement contingencies for both the parent and the child.

It is during this stage of development that children have their first experience with structured education. With support and patience, most children successfully make the transition from the security of the family to the larger school social system. Children who do not experience early school success are at greater risk for subsequently dropping out of school and becoming involved in delinquency (Feldman, Caplinger, & Wodarski, 1983). This presents a particular challenge for disabled children because they may not experience success in a traditional way and may need accommodations either in the environment or in the way they access the material to be learned. All children who appear to be struggling with school adjustment will require early assessment and intervention; by doing this early in the process school social workers can identify such children and respond with appropriate planning. Individual education plans (IEP) are required in these instances and should emphasize the coordination of the family, school, and community resources.

Finally, experiencing poverty places children at increased risk physically (inadequate health care and nutrition), psychologically (stress and self-esteem issues), and socially (homelessness and increased exposure to violence). In 1991, one in five children in the United States lived below the poverty line (O'Hare, 1994). Studies have demonstrated that poverty is correlated with a variety of negative outcomes (delinquency, academic underachievement, poor physical and mental health). With the United States facing distinct changes in the welfare, Social Security, and Medicaid systems, social workers are encouraged to acknowledge and advocate for social activism focused on supporting efforts designed to reduce poverty.

## LATER CHILDHOOD (7–12 YEARS OLD)

School experiences exert significant social and intellectual influence on children and play an important role in their development. During this time period, children begin to assess their self-worth through a comparison and evaluation of their academic abilities, athletic skills, physical appearance, and social acceptance. Erikson's stage of *industry versus inferiority* is critical as children mentally compare themselves against peers, parents, and other role models to see how well they resemble the others in their lives. Harter (1987) noted that the most important sources of support for children's self-esteem are parents and classmates, not teachers or friends. Teachers have expectations that, when transmitted to the child, can affect school performance and consequently, self-worth. Hence, schools are major contributors to the maturing child as they provide opportunities for meaningful and prolonged interactions with other significant adults and peers.

Children's interactions with their peer group during this period serve several functions. As mentioned previously, peers influence the individual's sense of self-esteem. Additionally, peers serve to reinforce key cultural norms, thereby affecting the formation of values and attitudes in the child. They are also important sources of information regarding appropriate behavior. Gender roles and their ensuing behaviors receive strong reinforcement from the child's peer group. For the most part, children want to be like their peers; they want to wear the same clothes, use the same slang terms, play the same games; however, illness, hospitalization, different physical appearance, or speaking styles can all cause the child to appear different and less acceptable to peers

(Quinn, 1998). Most children can become accustomed to these differences if they have enough contact with adults that allow contact to take place without teaching the prejudice that continues to exist in today's society.

Another concern that commands notice today is the influence of electronic media in children's development. Increasingly, television has become an important socializing force in the lives of children. Children spend approximately one third of their waking hours watching television (Lefrancois, 1993). This can have both harmful and beneficial effects depending on the choice of programming. Researchers have examined the impact of children's television viewing on aggression (Eron, Huesmann, Dubow, Romanoff, & Yarmel, 1987), prosocial behavior (Radke-Yarrow, Zahn-Waxler, & Chapman, 1983) and gender role stereotyping (Rosenwasser, Lingenfelter, & Harrington, 1989). These researchers all came to a similar assumption: Those children who rely on television viewing for entertainment and leisure time activity often do so at the expense of imagination and physical play.

At this life stage children are in almost daily contact with individuals (e.g., peers, teachers, neighbors) outside their family. At this time signs of problems adjusting socially, psychologically, or academically are noted. Here the worker's role is to design and implement a treatment plan with the child, the family, and relevant collaterals. Caution must be exerted in working with children of this age, because frequently the behavior they present has been labeled (e.g., behavior disordered, emotionally disturbed, attention deficit disorder) by the classroom teacher or family member, and this label can have detrimental impact on self-concept and social functioning.

Peer group structures provide opportunities for growth for the school-aged child, and in growth there can be pain. School social workers frequently become involved in assisting children to negotiate small group power structures, thereby learning social skills that will foster broader societal adjustment. Nowhere is this more likely than in a mainstream classroom situation with a child with a disability. The obvious (and not so obvious) differences can create a gulf between this child and the rest of the class unless someone intervenes. Teaching communication, conflict resolution, and assertiveness skills are proactive functions that can be successfully accomplished by the social worker in the small group setting.

It also is during the early school years that child abuse is most likely to be detected. The child is no longer restricted to family contact or family sanctioned contacts, and teachers and social workers who have been trained to recognize signs of abuse and neglect are expected to report cases of abuse. According to the U.S. Bureau of the Census (1992), the average age of an abused child is 7 with higher risk ratios for children younger (under 3) or older (teens). More than 2 million cases of child maltreatment (including physical injuries, neglect, sexual and emotional abuse) are reported annually (Lauer, 1994). Yet in determining actual abuse and neglect the professional must take the cultural aspects relevant to each case in consideration. The United States is a diverse population with many different types of parenting styles; Sternberg (1993) give examples of parenting styles that seem to contradict each other, but when taken in sociologic context, make sense. She includes a study conducted by Baumrind (1991) in which authoritative parenting (including children in decision making, thus encouraging independence) is most productive in white middle-class children, and an authoritarian parenting style (emphasizing compliance as a virtue and punishment an appropriate way to enforce the compliance) fosters social competence for African American children. While laws direct certain behaviors, and children must be protected, it is best to keep cultural differences in mind when determining the course to take in suspected abuse and neglect cases.

## ADOLESCENCE (13–19 YEARS OLD)

Adolescence is the life stage marking the transition from childhood to adulthood in our culture. Like those developmental phases that preceded it, distinct biological, psychological, and social changes occur within the individual. Physically, the adolescent experiences a growth spurt associated with the onset of puberty (series of correlated physical events that lead to reproductive maturity). Today, individuals tend to reach their adult height and sexual maturity faster than in the past. Known as the secular trend, this tendency to mature earlier has been attributed to better health care, better nutrition, and an increased standard of living (Chumlea, 1988; Lefrancois, 1993).

One of the important tasks for the adolescent is the development of a sense of identity. According to Erikson (1963), this sense of identity is achieved only after a period of questioning, reevaluation, and experimentation. During these teen years individuals experiment with various roles that represent possibilities for future identity development. Experimentation in academic pursuits, athletic endeavors, part-time jobs, hobbies, and dating relationships all contribute to this identity formation in a prosocial fashion. It is in adolescence that Hughes and Noppe (1985) reported that teens look ahead to a time when they will be independent adults. Rice (as cited in Hughes & Noppe) lists a series of descriptive traits of *disliked adolescents* including physical handicaps, shyness, timid, withdrawn, quiet, lethargic, listless, passive nonjoiner, recluse, pessimistic, and complaining. For the child with a physical disability it is not uncommon for traits and statements about physical limitations to be mistaken for complaints. Similarly, during this time period role confusion can lead to poorly thought out actions and behaviors that appear irresponsible, childish, or rebellious. Some adolescents become entrenched in this *acting out* behavior and seek negative reinforcement from it that can delay their transition to adulthood.

Academically, it is important that the adolescent stay in school. Alspaugh (1998) reports approximately one fourth of ninth-grade students in the United States drop out before graduating from high school. On-time high school graduation is an indicator of future success, and the technical skills required in the workforce make a high school diploma essential. Unfortunately, the trend is not moving in a positive direction; in 1991 slightly less than 69% of young people graduated on time (down 4% over 5 years) (O'Hare, 1994). The dropout rate is higher for African American, Native American, and Hispanic youth compared with Caucasian and Asian youth. At the same time the unemployment rate for high school dropouts is rising, and without a college degree it has become extremely difficult to command competitive wages.

Socially, adolescence provides a period for moving from dependence on one's parents to adult independence. Parent-adolescent relationships are frequently strained as the individual struggles to assert this independence. Conflicts often arise, according to Kaluger and Kaluger (1984), about performing chores, studying, using time appropriately, dating practices, choosing friends, and spending money. These test family socialization and communication patterns.

Social workers both in private and public practice encounter adolescent clients for a variety of reasons. Families will often seek intervention because of conflicted relationships at home. As Schulman (1992) points out, teenagers are frequently the scapegoats for family dysfunction and as such family therapy is the treatment of choice. Baumrind (1991) believes that parents who are responsive yet demanding, combine authority with reason, and have frequent communication with their child tend to have adolescents who are assertive, responsible, and independent. These qualities should be fostered in the families receiving treatment.

Social workers in mental health settings must be prepared to render treatment to adolescents experiencing a variety of problems. Since teen suicide remains the second leading cause of adolescent death, eclipsed only by accidents, accurate and timely assessments are critical (Hoffman, Paris, & Hall, 1994). Suicide attempts are most frequent among teens that have had previous psychiatric symptoms, such as depression, impulsivity, aggression, antisocial behavior, or substance abuse (Berman & Jobes, 1991). Social workers must consequently prepare to assess suicide risk when treating almost all teens. Eating disorders, most commonly anorexia and bulimia, have emerged as a major adolescent mental (and physical) health concern. The American Academy of Family Physicians (1999) report 3% of women develop anorexia and another 8% develop bulimia. Treatment options must be comprehensive and multifaceted, aimed at resolving the psychosocial issues, the medical concerns, and the nutritional needs of the client.

Substance use and abuse is another problem that leads teens to treatment. The U.S. Public Health Service (1998) found the leading cause of death for adolescents is unintentional injuries and 40% of these injuries can be related to alcohol use. Social work roles with chemically dependent adolescents and their families include counselor, group facilitator, broker, and educator. Similarly these roles can be used proactively with adolescents to prevent subsequent substance abuse. Drug use and sales can be found at all socioeconomic levels, but further complicates the lives of those living in poverty. Use and abuse distances the teen from problems, however briefly, and sales provide a risky but rapid increase in income. Given this twofold allure, it is difficult to dissuade economically disadvantaged teens from becoming involved with the drug trade.

Despite the relatively static delinquency rates of the past 10 years, the adolescent homicide rate has more than doubled since 1988 (Kroshus, 1994). The Center for Disease Control (1994) reports that almost one half of the 1991 homicide victims were males 15 to 34 years old with adolescents accounting for the greatest change in rate. Among males aged 15 to 19, homicide surpasses suicide as the second leading cause of death. Thus, there is an escalating trend of juveniles being both the perpetrators and the victims of violence. The CDC suggests that factors influencing this trend include poverty, inadequate educational and economic opportunities, social and familial instability, and exposure to violence as a preferred technique for settling disputes. According to David Hamburg (1997) "By age 17, about one quarter of all adolescents have engaged in behaviors that are harmful to themselves and others. . . . Altogether, nearly half of American adolescents are at high or moderate risk of seriously damaging their life chances." Social workers, in addition to providing direct services to perpetrators and victims of juvenile violence, have a critical role to fill in designing, monitoring, implementing, and coordinating violence prevention projects aimed at reducing this serious phenomenon.

## EARLY ADULTHOOD (20–39 YEARS OLD)

As the individual enters into the life stage of adulthood, different developmental tasks must be undertaken. These typically include entering the workforce, completing any remaining educational objectives, choosing a life partner, and deciding whether the individual should become a parent. Again this stage is not marked by a specific age but rather characterized by certain life events. Thus, although not true for all segments of society, adulthood in the United States most often is defined as the point in time an individual leaves school, takes a job, or gets married. Physiologically, most young adults are at the peak of their agility, speed, and strength. Young adulthood also signals the beginning of the loss of some functions, however. Muscle tone and strength peak between the ages of 20 and 30, then begin to decline (Hoffman, Paris, & Hall, 1994). Perlmutter and Hall (1992) note that skin cells regenerate more slowly after exposure to the ultraviolet rays of the sun, and as the skin thins, wrinkles begin to appear. Reaction times also peak and begin to ebb during these years (Schultz & Curnow, 1988). Even though many young adults do not recognize these "hallmarks of aging," the clock has begun to tick.

Erikson (1963) considers the major psychosocial task of this period to be *intimacy versus isolation.* Predicated upon the earlier development of a sense of identity, he hypothesizes that the individual now strives to establish intimacy in human relationships by learning to share, compromise, and sacrifice. The alternative is isolation that occurs when the individual feels the need to erect barriers to protect a fragile sense of self. Gilligan (1982) posits that the developmental tasks for women and men differ as a function of differential socialization practices. Women have learned to accomplish the previous developmental tasks within the context of a relationship. Hence, the establishment of intimate relationships in adulthood does not pose as much of a threat to their identities. Though men must alter their adolescent identities to meet this new task, in general women tend to address their identity and intimacy needs simultaneously.

The young adult makes several lifestyle choices. Personality, interests, skills, and opportunity influence occupational decisions. These decisions are significant because work meets more than economic needs alone. An individual's self-concept is intricately tied to the roles assumed in the workplace, as are one's opportunities for social interaction and the establishment of social relationships. Establishing independent living arrangements and the selection of a life partner are usual choices made during this life stage. While marriage is the most common of such arrangements, approximately 10% of the population of adults is single by choice (Lefrancois, 1993).

Becoming a parent, deliberately or accidentally, is another significant life event of early (and middle) adulthood. This new role requires accommodation and influences the individual's partner and occupational roles. During child rearing the adult must be involved in the moral development, education, transmission of cultural norms, peer relations, and skill development of the child. This occurs while one or both parents juggle the demands of work and family, frequently resulting in considerable individual and familial stress.

Individuals in their early adult years may seek the assistance of a social worker for a variety of reasons. The ability to assume adult roles (partner, worker, parent) can be complicated by unresolved psychological or social-emotional issues from the past. Contemporary theorists (Goncalves & Ivey, 1993; Neimeyer, 1993) espouse a cognitive treatment approach based upon a developmental constructivist view of therapy. In this model the therapist helps the client identify and change previous social developmental constructions that are obstacles to successful functioning.

Stresses within interpersonal and marital relationships often bring young adults into counseling. Financial problems resulting from lack of income or poor money management skills are typical. Difficulty in adapting to the demands of parenthood is also frequently cited. Any family that is experiencing increased stress can benefit from short-term structured therapeutic intervention. For all new parents, especially those with a child with disabilities, it is wise for the social worker to allow some extra time for the family to process what has happened so that they can realistically focus on the tasks ahead of them.

When addressing this life stage, disabilities can present additional and unique challenges for individuals to face. For example, if a person with a disability has formed a significant relationship with another person and has married or chosen to cohabit with them, the couple may also choose to become parents. This decision sometimes causes great resistance from both personal and public circles. Our society displays a paternalistic attitude toward those with disabilities and the questions "Who will take care of the baby?" and "What if the baby is handicapped too?" and "Why do you want to do *that?*" are asked with increasing volume until many couples give up the dream of parenthood. If both members of a couple are disabled or if a single disabled woman wishes to have a child, the means to *physically* care for a child for the first year or so becomes a debated topic. Persons with disabilities often live on fixed incomes, and Medicaid will not pay for aide to help with a baby. In addition, parents who were considered able-bodied prior to an accident have lost children to child protective services, as have widows or divorcees with disabilities. It may be necessary for social workers to help find supports to help disabled parents to keep their children at home with them.

Sexual orientation is not determined in adulthood; however, for those individuals who have a homoerotic preference, "coming out" is often an activity associated with later adolescence or early adulthood. The individual or family may seek social work intervention for counseling or support. To be most effective, it is advised that social workers confront their own homophobia and become familiar with the gay and lesbian lifestyle prior to working with a client's confronting decisions that relate to becoming a sexual minority (Zastrow & Kirst-Ashman, 1994).

In summary, although discrimination based on race, gender, sexual orientation, or disability is not unique to a specific life stage; it often causes particular stress in the young adult. Employment, residential, and social opportunities are negatively affected by discriminatory practices. Social workers have an ethical responsibility to combat such discrimination through case and cause advocacy.

## MIDDLE ADULTHOOD (41–60 YEARS OLD)

Middle age poses new developmental tasks for the individual as well as the opportunity to continue work on those previously unfinished. The consequences of physiological aging become more apparent in middle adulthood. Diminished visual acuity and auditory function are typical. The sex glands' secretion of hormones decreases in both men and women, leading to changes in sexual functioning in both sexes, and menopause in women. As individuals age, the incidence of several chronic health problems increases, such as heart disease, hypertension, arthritis, and diabetes (Kleinhuizen, 1991). Additionally, the peak increase in incidence of cancer occurs between the ages of 45 and 65 (Brody, 1991). While biological aging is a linear function, adult health can be influenced by heredity, nutrition, and exercise patterns.

According to Erikson (1963), the psychosocial crisis faced by the individual at this life stage is *generativity versus stagnation.* Generativity is evidenced by a commitment to the improvement of life for future generations. Stagnation occurs when this commitment is not made. A survey commissioned by the American Board of Family Practice found many individuals view middle adulthood as a time when relationships are intensified and a person becomes more compassionate to the needs of others (Goleman, 1990). Goleman posits that individuals who have solidified their marriages, families, and careers are now secure enough to empathize with and assist others. Conversely, Levinson and his associates postulate that individuals face a crisis period as they reevaluate their lives at this time (Levinson, Darrow, Klein, Levinson, & McKee, 1978). However, critics of this "mid-life crisis theory" suggest that most longitudinal studies have not verified its existence (Hoffman, Paris, & Hall, 1994).

Many middle-aged adults continue to maintain the role of parent. The nature of this role is contingent upon the age of the child and, increasingly, middle-aged parents are raising younger children as a function of either delayed childbearing or remarriage. Be it parenting a young child, teen, or young adult, stress may be encountered as the individual struggles to balance personal, occupational, and familial demands. For families that have a child with a disability, however, the traditional "moving out" or "leaving of the nest" may not occur. Because few parents plan to have their children live with them their whole lives, events like this can cause extreme stress within the family system. In other situations, adult middle-aged children may be left to care for and cope with the needs of their own aging parents, thus caring for two generations at once.

Additional stress can be placed on the middle-aged adult by the requirement to care for an aging parent. Changes in societal expectations and reductions in health coverage and welfare benefits along with spiraling inflation have squeezed elderly individuals. Nursing home entrance requirements have become increasingly stringent as well. Adding these factors together may force the elderly to become dependent on their children for personal care. The stresses involved in this situation often lead to elder abuse, another increasing social problem. Social work efforts in mobilizing community resources and support for both the aging parent and the middle-aged child are necessary.

Adults during this life stage may present social workers with a varied array of problems. Family systems and workplace-related problems might persist, as well as poverty and discrimination issues. The therapeutic approaches mentioned as useful for young adults may be useful during middle adulthood as well. Because divorce affects approximately one half of all marriages (U.S. Bureau of the Census, 1992), subsequently, marriages are at greater risk. It has become a common practice expectation for social workers to assist divorcing spouses. Partners often experience a period of grief regarding failure of the marriage, so grief counseling could be indicated. One's standard of living (especially the woman's) is decreased and options regarding legal, employment, and educational opportunities must be discussed. Social workers can be helpful in locating legal assistance provided on a sliding fee scale, role-playing potential job interviews with clients, and connecting clients with academic or employment advisors to facilitate retraining for a new or first-time career.

Many middle-aged adults may undergo a period of redefining their lives and seek assistance in resolving interpersonal relationships, life style choices, and future goals. This has been termed a "mid-life crisis" in men and "empty nest syndrome" in women. More recent research has shown that contrary to previous belief, many parents look forward to the decrease in responsibility that comes with children moving away from home. Increasingly, however, and often for economic reasons, adult children remain in the home or return home to live after brief periods of independent living. Disappointment resulting from loss of privacy together with unresolved issues from the past can complicate this arrangement and necessitate social work intervention.

## LATER ADULTHOOD (BEYOND 61 YEARS OF AGE)

Despite the inevitability of physical decline associated with age, improvements in living conditions and nutrition (for the vast majority of Americans), combined with medical advances, allow more people to reach old age. Schneider (1999) suggests as a result of the aging of current baby boomers and the continued projected increase in life expectancy, the number of Americans aged 65 and above will increase from 35 million in 2000 to 78 million in 2050.

Gerontologists now refer to three distinct phases of later adulthood: (a) the young-old (61–70), (b) the old (71–80), and (c) the old-old (80+). Developmental psychologists hypothesized that the capacity for growth in creativity and learning stopped at adulthood; however, studies now acknowledge this to be untrue. Presupposing there are no physiological impairments such as stroke or dementia, older persons can build on existing knowledge, continuing to learn up until death. Therefore, it is not uncommon for many elders to embark on new creative efforts with the advent of retirement.

The most obvious physical changes in the aging individual involve the graying and thinning of hair, wrinkling of skin, and diminishing sensory abilities. In addition, sleep patterns may change (Reynolds et al., 1991) and psychomotor skills may decline (Papalia & Olds, 1992). Although chronic conditions are aggravated, it does appear that acute illnesses appear less frequently (Lewin, 1991; Vander Zanden, 1993). Though these changes can be significant and require accommodation, most elderly individuals do not consider themselves to be seriously disadvantaged in pursuing their daily activities (Vander Zanden, 1993). Neugarten (as cited in Cassel, 1994) states that people between 65 and 75 years of age are generally independent and active, continue work if they enjoy it, and have a few, manageable medical problems. In a longitudinal study Cui and Vaillant (1996) found that negative life events affected psychological health more than physical health, with depression being noted as a frequently found illness in aging. It is important to note, however, that depression is frequently misdiagnosed in the elderly. Furthermore, signs related to depression such as fatigue, listlessness, and a reduction in extracurricular activities are overlooked as expected consequences of aging. As people age, and reach age 75 or older, health status difficulties do appear to become more problematic. Often chronic health problems such as osteoarthritis, osteoporosis, dementia, visual and hearing disorders, hypertension, diabetes, and stroke-related disability can increase the need for assistance with activities of daily living (often referred to as ADLs) (Cassel, 1994). Elderly individuals are living longer and in much healthier states than ever before. Technology regarding medical advances is at an all-time high. One sad disappointment in this area, however, is the fact that many times state-of-the-art care is not considered essential for the elderly individual. At times the improvement and invention of new drugs, surgical techniques, and the general changes in medical care are often ignored when applied to elderly individuals. This is especially disappointing if a current intervention or treatment could lead to allowing elderly individuals to "preserve their functional capacity, maintain their independence, and lower the chances of medical complications that can result in institutionalization (Falvo & Lundervold, as cited in Quinn, 1998).

It is in this stage that Erikson (1963) discussed the final psychological crisis of *ego integrity versus despair*. Integrity involves the elderly individual's gaining an acceptance of one's life as having meaning with both positive and negative aspects. This acknowledgement is derived through reflection on one's life accomplishments, without perceiving this acceptance as threatening. Contrary to integrity, despair results from regret about one's life and a desire to do things differently. This desire is coupled with the realization there is no longer enough time to make the changes desired. Although this distinction sounds simple, distinct research indicates this is not the case. Feelings of integrity or despair cannot be divided into an either-or proposition. Older people may experience some sense of regret, yet when they look at their life in total they feel life satisfaction (Goleman, 1990). Older individuals do not show dramatic shifts in personality or self-concept (Vander Zanden, 1993). Social workers must not support stereotypic depictions of elderly people as bad drivers, conservatives, crotchety, disabled, or forgetful. Most often, at least in the young-old stage, people continue physically, occupationally, mentally, and creatively as they have for most of their adult lives.

Alterations in the roles performed by the older adult require social adjustment. The individual is transitioning especially relative to moving from work to retirement. The U.S. Bureau of the Census (1992) found only 16% of men and 8% of women were working past the age of 65. Retirement is a process in which the individual moves from fantasying about and planning the end of a career to readjustment and reorientation to the reality of retirement. This is a major change that may pose personal and economic stress. Reactions to retirement vary with the individual. Although many welcome the change and have no trouble occupying their time, others can become depressed with the loss of what may be an integral part of self-esteem. In some circumstances retirement isn't possible because of economic deprivation, and individuals attempt to continue in subsistence level jobs. With the impending changes in the Social Security law, it is likely that people won't be eligible for benefits until the age of 67 rather than 62 (early retirement) or 65. With the improvements in medical care and the extension in life expectancy, there isn't necessarily a reason to have a mandatory retirement age. Today, many people can expect to live as long as 20 or more years in retirement collecting retirement benefits, rather than one or two. This, of course, is one of the reasons the Social Security system is encountering problems.

Living arrangements for the elderly may also undergo alteration. The majority of older adults live in arrangements similar to those of their previous adult life. However, by virtue of health or economic conditions, 5% live in nursing homes, 5% in retirement homes, and 21% in multigenerational families (Kane & Kane, 1990). These variations may require social and psychological modifications on the part of the older adult as well as their families. Few elderly individuals want to live in nursing homes, mostly because of the loss of autonomy involved. In a study by Langer and Rodin (as cited in Hughes & Noppe, 1985), residents of one floor of a nursing home were given choices in a number of matters, while residents of another floor were used as a control group. After 3 weeks, the staff and residents were given questionnaires to gauge the emotional well-being of both groups. The group that had been given choices (had some control over their environment) indicated a higher level of satisfaction than the control group. This indicates it is not so much a change of residence, which may distress elders, but the loss of autonomy with which they must cope.

The notion that older people are lonely and isolated from their family and friends is a myth. While such cases exist, most elderly people have strong friendship and kinship ties. Though the death of a spouse, relative, or close friend can pose emotional stress at any life stage, the probability of being confronted with this traumatic event is increased for the elderly. It can be particularly difficult for women because they have longer life spans. According to the census (U.S. Bureau of the Census, 1992), there were 8.3 million older widows in the United States compared with 1.7 older widowers. This fact also makes it harder for women to find emotional support and sexual partners than for men.

In addressing the prospect of death many believe that developing a point of view about death begins in childhood and is not resolved until later adulthood. The issue becomes more concrete as individuals see their friends and loved ones dying. Advancing physical decline and loss of capabilities similarly bring death into focus. As a highly personal matter, the meaning of death varies from individual to individual, as does anxiety about its approach. Consequently, as a developmental task, death must be resolved individually, albeit in a social context.

In working with the older adult, the social worker should know of various community resources designed to provide the individual with meaningful activities and necessary medical and social support. Counseling interventions may be needed to assist the individual in adjusting to loss of a spouse, change in living situation, or medical concerns.

Elder abuse is a form of family violence receiving increased attention. The National Center of Elder Abuse (NCEA) estimated that there were 241,000 reports of elder maltreatment in 1994 (Tatara, 1996). Like other forms of family violence, elder abuse is a hidden problem. Social workers can become knowledgeable about forms of abuse, recognize incidents of elder abuse, and refer clients to adult protective service agencies. Considering the desire for those in our society to "take care of" children, the disabled, and the elderly, it is often difficult to accept the decision of an elderly person to remain in an abusive situation; however, it is important to remember this is still an adult with the right and need to make decisions. Unless elderly persons are actively a danger to themselves or others, they must be allowed to make these decisions. The social worker can offer options for alternative living situations or for prosecution of the abuser, but should abide by the decision of the client.

Demographically, the elderly population is the most rapidly growing age group, so social workers should assist in designing and monitoring the outcomes of programs to meet elderly persons' needs, and those of their families. Given the political and economic realities of the next century, such programs must be fiscally sound and effective; otherwise cuts in funding for the elderly will be called for by society and politicians. There already exists a false notion that elders use more than their share of resources, leaving others, especially children, at risk. It is important for social workers to combat this type of thinking to protect this rapidly growing segment of our population.

## SUMMARY

This chapter has provided a summary of the life span perspective and its implication for social workers. It should be stressed that at every developmental stage the individual has strengths and competencies. Practitioners, regardless of their theoretical orientation (i.e., behavioral, cognitive, constructivist, psychodynamic) should design and implement interventions that build on the strengths present in the individual.

While this life span perspective is generalist in its application to all human development, it should be noted that individuals belonging to vulnerable groups in society might have different developmental experiences. Women, people of color, and persons with disabilities progress through the same life stages; however, they may process their experiences differently. Developmental researchers and practitioners (Berzoff, 1994; Gomes & Mabry, 1991; Miller, 1994) are beginning to consider these differences, but more work in this direction is necessary.

It is also important to note that many obstacles and crises, which bring clients to social workers, are as much a function of societal factors as they are of the individual's development. Therefore, it is imperative that responsible social workers combine their micro and macro practice skills to enhance individual functioning for their clients and societal functioning for future clients. Adjustments and accommodations must be made within the individual and within society to maximize each person's potential and the overall potential of American society.

## REFERENCES

Adler, L. L. (1989). *Cross-cultural research in human development: Lifespan perspectives.* NY: Praeger.

Alspaugh, J. (1998). The relationship of school and community characteristics to high school dropout rates. *The Clearing House, 71,* 184–189.

American Academy of Family Physicians. (1998). Prevalence and effect of illicit drug use during pregnancy. *American Family Physician, 57,* 1994.

American Academy of Family Physicians. (1999). Can the development of eating disorders be predicted? *American Family Physician, 60,* 623.

Bartsch, K., & Wellman, H. (1989). Young children's attribution of action to beliefs and desires. *Child Development, 60,* 946–964.

Basseches, M. (1984). *Dialectical thinking and adult development.* Norwood, NJ: Ablex.

Baumrind, D. (1991). The influence of parenting style on adolescent competence and substance use. *Journal of Early Adolescence, 11,* 56–95.

Beal, C., & Belgrad, S. (1990). The development of message evaluation skills in young children. *Child Development, 61,* 705–712.

Belsky, J., Lerner, R., & Spanier, G. (1984). *The child in the family.* Redding, MA: Addison-Welsey.

Berman, A., & Jobes, D. (1991). *Adolescent suicide: Assessment and intervention.* Washington, DC: American Psychological Association.

Berzoff, J. (1994). From separation to connection: Shifts in understanding women's development. In J. Schriver (Ed.), *Human behavior and the social environment.* Boston, MA: Allyn and Bacon.

Brody, J. E. (1991, January 31). Personal health: In pursuit of the best possible odds of preventing or minimizing the perils of major diseases. *New York Times,* p. B9.

Cassel, C. K. (1994). Researching the health needs of elderly people. *The British Medical Journal, 308* (6945), 1655–1656.

Center for Disease Control. (1994). Current trends. *Morbidity and Mortality Weekly Report, 3,* 725–727.

Chumlea, W. (1988). Physical growth in adolescence. In B. Wolman (Ed.), *Handbook of developmental psychology.* Englewood Cliffs, NJ: Prentice-Hall.

Cui, X., & Vaillant, G. E. (1996). Antecedents and consequences of negative life events in adulthood: A longitudinal study. *American Journal of Psychiatry, 153* (1), 21–26.

Erikson, E. (1963). *Childhood and society.* New York: Norton.

Eron, L., Huesmann, L., Dubow, E., Romanoff, R., & Yarmel, P. (1987). Aggression and its correlates over 22 years. In D. Crowell, I. Evans, & C. O'Donnell (Eds.), *Childhood aggression and violence.* New York: Plenum.

Feldman, R., Caplinger, T., & Wodarski, J. (1983). *The St. Louis conundrum: The effective treatment of antisocial youths.* Englewood Cliffs, NJ: Prentice-Hall.

Ganda, L., & Pellegrini, A. (Eds.). (1985). *Play language and stories: The development of children's literate behavior.* Norwood, NJ: Ablex.

Gilligan, C. (1982). *In a different voice.* Cambridge, MA: Harvard University Press.

Goleman, D. (1990, February 6). In midlife, not just crisis but care and comfort too. *New York Times,* pp. B5, B9.

Gomes, P., & Mabry, C. (1991). Negotiating the worked: The developmental journey of African American children. In J. Everett, S. Chipunqu, & B. Leashore (Eds.), *Child welfare.* New Brunswick, NJ: Rutgers University Press.

Goncalves, O., & Ivey, A. (1993). Developmental therapy: Clinical applications. In K. Kuelwein & H. Rosen (Eds.), *Cognitive therapies in action.* San Francisco: Jossey-Bass.

Hale, S. (1990). A global developmental trend in cognitive processing speed. *Child Development, E1,* 653–663.

Hamburg, D. A. (1997). Toward a strategy for healthy adolescent development. *American Journal of Psychiatry, 154* (6), 7–12.

Harter, S. (1987). The determinants and mediational role of global self-worth in children. In N. Eisenberg (Ed.), *Contemporary topics in developmental psychology.* New York: Wiley.

Hayes, A., & Batshaw, M. L. (1993). Down Syndrome. *Pediatric Clinics of North America, 40* (3), 523–539.

Hobdell, E. F. (1995). Perceptual accuracy and gender-related differences in parents of children with myelomeningocele. *Journal of Neuroscience Nursing, 27* (4), 240–244.

Hoffman, L., Paris, S., & Hall, E. (1994). *Developmental psychology today.* New York: McGraw-Hill.

Howes, C., Unger, O., & Seidner, L. (1989). Social pretend play and toddlers: Parallels with social play with solitary pretend. *Child Development, EO*, 77–84.

Hughes, F. P., & Noppe, L. D. (1985). *Human development across the life span.* St. Paul, MN: West Publishing.

Kaluger, G., & Kaluger, M. (1984). *Human development: The span of life.* St. Louis, MO: Mosby.

Kane, R. L., & Kane, R. A. (1990). Health care for older people: Organizational and policy issues. In R. H. Binarock & L. K. George (Eds.), *Handbook of aging and the social sciences.* San Diego, CA: Academic Press.

Kleinhuizen, J. (1991, March 14). Poor, elderly have more disabilities. *USA Today,* p. D1.

Kroshus, J. (1994). Preventing juvenile violence. *Juvenile Justice Digest, 2* (2), 5–6.

Kuczynski, L., & Kochenska, G. (1990). Development of children's noncompliance strategies from toddlerhood to age five. *Developmental Psychology, 26*, 398–408.

Lauer, R. (1994). *Social problems: The quality of life.* Madison, WI: Brown and Benchmark.

Lefrancois, G. (1993). *The lifespan.* Belmont, CA: Wadsworth.

Levinson, D. J., Darrow, C. M., Klein, E. B., Levinson, M. H., & McKee, B. (1978). *The seasons of a man's life.* New York: Knoph.

Lewin, T. (1991, May 31). As elderly population grows, so does need for doctors. *New York Times,* pp. Al, A9.

MacTurk, R. H., McCarthy, M. E., Vietz, P. M., & Yarrow, L. J. (1987). *Developmental Psychology, 23,* 199–203.

Masters, W., Johnson, V., & Kolodny, R. (1988). *Crisis: Heterosexual behavior in the age of AIDS.* New York: Grove Press.

Miller, J. (1994). The development of women's sense of self. In J Schriver (Ed.), *Human behavior and the social environment.* Boston, MA: Allyn and Bacon.

Moses, L., & Flavell, J. (1990). Inferring false beliefs form actions and reactions. *Child Development, 61,* 929–945.

Neimeyer, R. (1993). Constructivist psychotherapy. In K. Kuelwein & H. Rosen (Eds.), *Cognitive therapies in action.* San Francisco: Jossey-Bass.

O'Hare, W. (1994). *Kids count data book: A profile of child well-being.* Baltimore: Annie E. Casey Foundation.

Papalia, D. E., & Olds, S. W. (1992). *Human development* (5th ed.). New York: McGraw-Hill.

Perlmutter, M., & Hall, E. (1992). *Adult development and aging* (2nd ed.). New York: Wiley.

Piaget, J. (1952). *The origins of intelligence in children.* New York: International Universities Press.

Quinn, P. (1998). *Understanding disability: A lifespan approach.* Thousand Oaks, CA: Sage.

Radke-Yarrow, M., Zahn-Waxler, C., & Chapman, M. (1983). Children's prosocial dispositions and behavior. In P. Mussen (Ed.), *Handbook of child psychology.* New York: Wiley.

Redding, R. E., Morgan, G. A., & Harmon, R. J. (1988). Mastery motivation in infants and toddlers: Is it greatest when tasks are moderately changing? *Infant Behavior and Development, 11,* 419–430.

Reynolds, C. F., Monk, T. H., Hoch, C. C., Jennings, J. R., Buysse, D. J., Houck, P. R., Jarrett, D. B., & Kupfer, D. J. (1991). Electroencephalographic sleep in the healthy "old old": A comparison with the "young old" in visually scored and automated measures. *Journal of Gerontology, 6,* 39–46.

Rosenwasser, S., Lingenfelter, M., & Harrington, A. (1989). Nontraditional gender role portrayals on television and children's gender role perceptions. *Journal of Applied Developmental Psychology, 10,* 97–105.

Schneider, E. (1999). Aging in the third millennium. *Science, 283,* 796.

Shulman, L. (1992). *The skills of helping: Individuals, families, and groups.* Itasca, IL: P. E. Peacock.

Schultz, R., & Curnow, C. (1988). Peak performance and age among superathletes. *Journal of Gerontology, 13,* 113–120.

Sternberg, K. J. (1993). Child maltreatment: Implications for policy from cross-cultural research. In I. E. Sigel (Series Ed.), D. Cicchetti, & S. L. Toth (Vol. Eds.), *Advances in applied developmental psychology: Vol. 8. Child abuse, child development, and social policy* (pp. 191–211). Norwood, NJ: Ablex Publishing.

Tatara, T. (1996). *Elder abuse questions and answers—An informational guide for professionals and concerned citizens.* Washington, DC: National Center on Elder Abuse.

Thomas, R. (Ed.). (1990). *Encyclopedia of human development and education: Theory, research and studies.* New York: Pergamon.

U.S. Bureau of the Census. (1992). Statistical abstract of the United States (112 ed.). Washington, DC: U.S. Government Printing Office.

U.S. Department of Health and Human Services. (1990). *Health, United States 1989.* Washington, DC: U.S. Government Printing Office.

U.S. Public Health Service. (1998). Alcohol and other drug abuse in adolescents. *American Family Physician, 56,* 1737–1741.

Vander Zanden, J. W. (1993). *Human development* (5th ed.). New York: McGraw-Hill.

Wodarski, J. (1982). Single parents and children: A review for social workers. *Family Therapy, 2,* 311–320.

Zastrow, C., & Kirst-Ashman, K. (1994). *Understanding human behavior and the social environment* (3rd ed.). Chicago: Nelson-Hall.

## CHAPTER 5

# Labeling Theory and Human Development

## Michael Sullivan

A major aspect in understanding the practice of social work rests in how the social worker identifies and helps the client to choose the human behaviors that need to be altered. Most professionals agree that effective assessment and diagnosis are fundamental to the social work–helping process. The social worker's interventions are always based upon some explicit or implicit understanding of the client's status and the required change. Although client assessment is based on different criteria depending on the social worker's approach (psychoanalytic, behavioral, genetic, or otherwise), assessment of the client's existing condition is the basis for intervention. Hence, accuracy in assessment is a prerequisite for effective intervention. Moreover, a critical assumption is that, with social work training, consistency in the perception process is assured. Although there have been many studies in this area, their results are contradictory. It can be argued that professional social work training, through increasing the worker's knowledge and experience in clinical observation and judgment, improves the accuracy of worker assessments. It is also possible, however, that professional training contributes to the development of stereotypes that bias subsequent assessment of client behavior (Bieri, Atkins, Briar, Leaman, Miller, & Tripodi, 1966; Crow, 1957; Quicke & Winter, 1994).

This chapter discusses how clinical assessment is considered as one form of the general process of perceiving other people. This model

The editors would like to thank Pauline Wiegand for earlier contributions to this chapter.

of person perception is derived from the hypothesis-testing theory of perception advanced by Bruner (1951, 1957) and Postman (1951). It begins with a hypothesis or expectation that influences what the individual sees, and how the individual behaves toward the other person. The individual seldom, if ever, attends to stimuli on a pure random or objective basis. Therefore, the individual absorbs and codes information from the environment that is relevant to the perceptual hypothesis. Relevant information is that which can be used to confirm or deny a perceptual hypothesis. Afterward, the individual tries to determine whether the new information confirms the hypothesis. If it does, the perception is validated and completed, and the process is thereby concluded. If it does not, the hypothesis is revised according to the internal feedback and the learning that took place during the third, "trial-and-check" phase, and the entire process is repeated until a stable perception is formed.

In human growth and development perceptual hypotheses constitute expectancies or predispositions developed from past experiences, which serve to select, organize, and transform environmental information (Postman, 1951). Therefore, the potential influence that past experiences may exert upon the perceptual process is a function of five determinants: (a) the frequency of past confirmation; (b) monopoly, fewer competing hypotheses allow for a stronger given hypothesis; (c) cognitive consequences, a given hypothesis becomes stronger as its level of integration within a supporting system of hypotheses increases; (d) motivational consequences, the relationship of a given hypothesis to the goals of the perceiver; and (e) social consequences, the extent to which the hypothesis is in agreement with the hypotheses of other observers. According to Bruner (1951), the stronger the hypothesis the greater the likelihood that it will become aroused in the perceptual process. Moreover, relatively less congruent information will be necessary to confirm the hypothesis, and more contradictory information will be required to refute it.

The hypothesis-testing theory of perception attempts to describe primarily what occurs inside the mind of the perceiver. As a process, however, clinical assessment involves a client and a social worker, and the assessment occurs within a situational context or social ecology. Numerous writers have focused attention on the multivariate nature of clinical judgment (Moos & Clemes, 1967; Sarbin, Taft, & Bailey, 1960; Tripodi & Miller, 1966). It is also helpful when considering possible influences upon the accuracy of clinical assessment, to remain aware of how factors relating to the client, the social context, and the perceiver can influence assessment. A brief review of these factors demonstrates the scope and complexity of problems pertaining to accuracy in clinical assessment. This review also serves as a backdrop for the theoretical and empirical analysis of the effects of professional training on the accuracy of assessing human development and behavior.

## LABELING THEORY

This chapter discusses the basic assumptions of labeling theory, which include: (a) an act or behavior that is exhibited by an individual, (b) the act that is evaluated and labeled deviant by a person designated as the labeler, and (c) the individual who exhibits the act (behavior) and who is referred to as the labelee.

A diagnostic label is especially important because when clients are labeled correctly they are often eligible to receive necessary remedial services. As one more closely examines the labeling process, however, it becomes evident that many clients are labeled inaccurately, which ultimately could result in their inability to participate in mainstream American life. Thus, the purpose of this chapter is twofold: (a) to examine the conceptual problems involved in labeling theory, and (b) to delineate those crucial variables necessary to ensure validity and reliability in labeling human behavior.

The discussion in this section will be highly critical at times; therefore, the authors wish to note that their motivation for the report stems from an evaluation of a 5-year research program, which focused on group integration and behavior change. The general purpose of the program was to evaluate a community-based treatment program for antisocial children. In conjunction with this evaluation, an assessment was made of the variables among group treatment strategies, group composition, and training of group social workers that led to the greatest reduction of antisocial behavior. Three treatment strategies were evaluated: (a) social learning, (b) traditional, and (c) group-centered. Types of groups included: antisocial groups, composed solely of antisocial children referred to the project by members of the professional therapeutic community (e.g., teachers, counselors, psychologists, and social workers); mixed groups, composed of one or more antisocial children and pro-social children who were members of the community; and pro-social groups, composed solely of pro-social children. Antisocial children

($n = 291$) and pro-social children ($n = 670$) participated throughout the duration of the study. The foregoing study and other studies reported in the literature suggest that professional therapeutic agents have inaccurately labeled clients, even when criteria for referral are concretely specified (Gingerich, Feldman, & Wodarski, 1976a, 1976b).

Most studies of the labeling process have explored how a label of deviance influences the behavior of an individual. This reflects the influence of Edwin Lemert's (1951, 1967) formulation of labeling theory, with an emphasis on secondary deviation produced by societal reaction and the internalization of cultural stereotypes surrounding the labeled behavior. Labeling theorists contend that labeling helps to create and reinforce deviance. In addition, they contend that labels encourage offenders to view themselves as deviant and, therefore, act in deviant ways.

The labeling theory proposes that sanctions against deviance can inadvertently contribute to continued deviant behavior (Ulmer, 1994). Early statements of labeling theory emphasized two important themes. First, formal and informal sanctions against deviant behavior may hinder opportunities for employment and relationships (Lemert, 1951; Schwartz & Skolnick, 1962). Second, recurrent labeling as deviant may lead to deviant self-concepts (Becker, 1963; Lofland, 1969). This idea has been prominent in labeling theory since its earliest statements and has received empirical support (Ageton & Elliott, 1974; Schmid & Jones, 1991; Stager, Chassin, & Young, 1983).

Robert Stebbins' (1971) *Commitment to Deviance* investigated how formal and informal penalties intended to punish or deter deviance can actually foster it. The study demonstrates how convicted felons experience penalties as they attempt to reenter conventional life, and tend to become further committed to criminal behavior as a result. Giordano, Cernovich, and Pugh (1986) noted that sanctions on deviant behavior could give individuals access to networks of deviant individuals (Lofland, 1969) and thus foster the development of friendships with other deviant individuals. Placement in deviant identities mobilizes negative expectations and stereotypes, resulting in the exclusion from mainstream society of individuals who have been labeled deviant (Lemert, 1951; Matza, 1969).

The proposition that labeling causes deviant behavior has been harshly criticized (Gove, 1975). Aside from this proposition, labeling may have ramifications and lead to labeling on other areas of the individual's life. Research by Link and his colleagues (Link, 1987; Link,

Cullen, Struening, Shrout, & Dohrenwend, 1989) has shown that negative labels may have other powerful short-term and long-term outcomes.

Most of the research regarding labeling theory has focused on the relationship between criminal sanctions and recidivism, or criminal sanctions and self-concepts (Stager et al., 1983). Some have discussed how the organizational features of police departments and the court system affect the way in which criminal labels are imposed. The focus of labeling theory has been expanded to include a social constructionist approach to social problems and societal reaction (Schur, 1971).

Labeling theory also has promoted the following criticisms:

1. Social reaction theory pays insufficient attention to the causes of primary deviance (Gove, 1975).
2. Empirical evidence is lacking to support the idea that deviant labels produced continuity in deviant behavior (Gibbs, 1966).
3. Recidivism rates support the idea that formal sanctions act as a deterrent rather than a cause of further deviance.
4. Involvement in deviance fosters continuity (Gove, 1975).

Although the exact empirical implications of labeling perspectives are sometimes ambiguous (Gove, 1975), most observers interpret it to mean that sanctions lead to negative social labels, and that labeling leads to a deviant identity.

Labeling theory implies that labels and an altered identity intervene between primary deviance (norm violation independent of labeling) and secondary deviance (norm violation resulting from labeling). When an individual is labeled deviant, a process of identity transformation is presumably set in motion. Once a person develops a sense of self as a deviant, that person is likely to engage in the deviant behavior implied by that identity to maintain consistency and to provide social reaction to confirm the new identity.

Ward and Tittle (1993) conducted research and, in contrast to the ambiguous findings in most other research, found evidence supportive of at least one of the two contending arguments. Their findings appear to be consistent with other recent research supporting labeling. Hagan and Palloni (1990) stated that until more methodologically sound research is conducted:

> Sanctions and peer labeling for deviant behavior help to produce a deviant identity that increases the probability of recidivism . . . however, recidivism of deviance also results from other factors, so that at best one can conclude

only that labeling may be one among a number of processes through which sanctions may influence recidivism. (p. 61)

Perhaps the greatest effect of labeling may be the selective reinforcement of an individual's deviant behavior by significant others in the individual's environment, resulting in an increased frequency of subsequent deviant behavior, corresponding shaping of other behaviors, and psychological socialization in terms of self-concept (Lynch, Norem-Hebeisen, & Gergen, 1981; Wahler, Winkel, Peterson, & Morrison, 1965; Watson, 1982). This process denies the individual the opportunity to acquire the academic and social skills necessary to participate in the social and economic environment. For example, inaccurate labeling by a teacher might be related to the teacher's expectations of children's achievement in the classroom setting. Thus, if a child is labeled as deviant, the teacher may develop the expectation that the child may not be able to perform on academic tasks as well as other children (Braun, 1976; Rosenthal, 1966; Rosenthal & Jacobson, 1968; Rosenthal & Rosnow, 1969). The child, therefore, may be denied the opportunity to acquire necessary academic and social skills for participation in the job market. Likewise, when professional change agents label a child as antisocial, deviant, violent, disruptive, or unsocialized, expectations for behavioral change are elicited that usually indicate that little change can be expected to occur in the child.

Rosenbaum and Prinsky (1991) studied the juvenile justice system in California within the context of labeling theory and concluded that labeling minors as juvenile delinquents or mentally ill because of their dress and tastes in music may have the effect of pushing them into a deviant role. They argue that without the negative label, the offending adolescent might simply grow up.

Labeling theories have relevance for the field of human services and the helping professions because they presumably contribute to accurate processing of clients who exhibit deviant behavior. Many dysfunctional aspects of labeling processes remain, and rigorous empirical investigation of variables that contribute to these aspects of the labeling processes are needed so that social work practitioners may develop procedures to decrease the occurrence of inaccurate labeling of clients.

## ESSENTIAL COMPONENTS: LABELING AND BEHAVIORS

Perhaps the most important variable that should be conceptualized, isolated, and delineated for accurate identification of deviancy is the behavior itself. This behavior must be defined by the individuals and institutions that comprise the social system, such as client peer groups and significant others, which include spouses and employers. In addition, the measurement process or processes used to secure relevant data must be clearly stated. Thus, the phenomenon depends on who defines it, the context of the behavior, and the measurement process (Balch, 1975; Conger & Coie, 1975; Elion & Megargee, 1975; Emerson, 1969; Erikson, 1962; Lundman, 1976).

All psychological measures involve someone's perception of the observed phenomena. Such measures include rating scales, direct observations, clinical interviews, and structured psychological tests. Since people's perceptions may differ, best practice dictates use of multiple methods and sources of information.

Other crucial variables involved in defining deviant behavior include: the frequency of the act; the seriousness of the act (e.g., the labeler's perception of how violent it is); the duration of the act; how consistently the act occurs; the intensity of the act; how visible the act is; the social power of the individual; social distance between the individual and agents of social control; and the tolerance level of the community for norm violation (Gibbs, 1966; Moos & Clemes, 1967; Platt, 1969; Schur, 1971). Future research must delineate how all these variables interact to produce a behavior that the labeler designates as deviant, thus initiating the process of referring the labelee to a social service agency.

The next crucial question pertains to how an individual labeler selects the human behavior to be labeled; that is, what are the parameters of such a process? Recent evidence suggests the following factors enter into the labeling of client behaviors: clients' age, sex, attitude, educational background, physical attractiveness, social power (e.g., lack of resources to resist the application of the label), race, socioeconomic class, appearance (dress, grooming), and demeanor (respectful or fearful). In addition, clients who act in certain ways, fail to show the proper degree of personal control, and have prior records of deviance are also labeled similarly (Cicourel, 1967; Dion, 1972; Levitin, 1975; Schur, 1971; Sigall & Landy, 1973; Sigall & Ostrove, 1975; Thornberry, 1973). There is little evidence to date showing that characteristics of an individual interact with the behavior exhibited to determine whether the behavior will be labeled as deviant.

Another essential component in the labeling process consists of the characteristics of the individuals who inaccurately label (e.g., number of years as a behavioral change agent, theoretical background, professional training, discriminability, authoritarianism, cognitive complexity, cognitive dimensionality, and Machiavellianism; Adomo, 1950; Bieri et al., 1966; Case & Lingerfelt, 1974; Christie & Geis, 1970; Cline, 1955; Hostorf, Schneider, & Polelka, 1970; Sarbin et al., 1960; Simmons, 1965; Solley & Murphey, 1960; Stuart, 1970). Important questions are: What essential variables are involved in developing a deviant self-concept that in turn leads to an individual's exhibiting residual or secondary deviance? and, Does this concept develop in different stages (Rogers & Buffalo, 1974)? If so, what are the essential variables involved in each stage? An excellent example of preliminary research delineating these variables is the investigation conducted by Ageton and Elliott (1974), which examined how legal processing affects development of the self-concept of delinquent orientations in male and female children from the 9th through the 12th grades. In this study each contact with a criminal justice agency increased the child's development of a delinquent orientation.

All these variables must be delineated if labeling theory is to accurately predict the incidence of deviant behavior. At this point we merely have a series of statements that relate a series of behaviors to a series of characteristics of the labeler and labelee. These inferences do not allow for accurate prediction of defiant behavior (e.g., high-risk clients). Further, it does not help to identify the critical point at which the individual's behavior is processed as deviant and in need of remedial services, or when the client will internalize by developing a self-concept that is deviant. What factors are involved in the continuation and acceleration of the developmental process of the deviant self-concept? A serious, long-term evaluation of labeling theory should consider the specific contributions of each component (Derogatis, Yevzeroff, & Wittlesberger, 1975).

## INDEPENDENT AND DEPENDENT VARIABLES

One aspect of a sophisticated body of knowledge is its capability for specifying dependent and independent variables (i.e., detailing how variables are related to the phenomenon that clinicians are interested in). Such capability produces a very potent experimental methodology on which to empirically base relationships among variables being studied. A critical conceptual question for social work researchers who are studying the labeling of human behavior is: "What are the relevant independent and dependent variables?" At present, much research in this area fails to specify those variables. Until such relationships are specified, however, research will remain descriptive and incapable of predicting relationships and crucial variables (Shearing, 1973; Siegel & Siegel, 1967). For the purposes of this chapter, independent variables consist of the characteristics of such individuals as teachers, social workers, psychologists, and psychiatrists who may label a behavior of a given client. Individuals chosen as the labelers may differ in the following characteristics: theoretical backgrounds, professional training, number of years as behavioral change agents, and cognitive complexity. At the same time, a standard unit of behavior that they will label is decided upon and becomes the dependent variable. The behaviors to be labeled may consist of a videotape of children interacting in group finger painting exercises, building model airplanes, or discussing topics of mutual interest (e.g., difficulties at school, with parents, with peers, drugs, or sex). These children would have formerly exhibited a constant incidence of antisocial behavior that had been empirically determined. In addition, characteristics such as age, sex, education, social background, and physical attractiveness of the children exhibiting the behaviors should be varied.

Few methodological studies such as this have been executed in the area of labeling theory, even though in order for labeling theory to be viable, the isolation of the essential components of labeling processes must occur. The Gingerich et al. (1976a, 1976b) experiment is a prototype of this type of study. This brings to awareness how services can be offered to children, utilizing different criteria in defining deviant behavior. This criteria can include: official and unofficial delinquencies; inventory data provided by children, parents, significant other adults or professionals; and globally defined behavioral categories, such as "antisocial behavior," "predelinquent" and "delinquent behavior," "deviant behavior," "asocial behavior," "aggressiveness," "illegal behavior," and "juvenile problems." However, such a diversity of measures leads to a problem of compatibility between theoretical concepts and research investigations and adds little to theory building.

## EXPECTATION THEORY: THE PROFESSIONAL'S CONTRIBUTION TO LABELING

Much of the support for labeling theory is derived from expectation theory. This body of knowledge seems to indicate that individuals tend to see what they want to see in other people. Zilber and Niven (1995) assert that important information is conveyed about a group based on the label placed upon them. For example, many individuals who have been labeled black prefer to be referred to as African Americans because they believe that this label more accurately describes who they are. Individuals who advocate the use of the term African American believe that this term conveys a sense of pride in their ethnicity, whereas being labeled as a black individual "connotes otherness" (p. 655).

Behavioral expectations of others influence the behavioral exchanges between them (e.g., professionals differentially respond to individuals to secure behavior that confirms their expectations; Goldstein, 1962; Rosenthal, 1966; Rosenthal & Rosnow, 1969; Shapiro, 1971). The communication of expectations can occur in the clinical situation in several ways that contribute to the labeling of the client. The first, and probably the most important, is that expectations can be communicated through verbal cues, such as association and clustering of words, duration of utterances, number of interruptions, questions, summary and interpretive statements, and length of silent periods. Nonverbal details, such as facial expressions, voice qualities, posture, gestures, eye contact, interpersonal distance, and touching are also important. In the clinical interactional context these behaviors may unintentionally communicate the clinician's expectations, which shape more deviant behavior in the client. In addition, clinicians may select those behavior cues that support these expectations and ignore others. An example of this phenomenon is the labeling of clients by social workers as resistant or unmotivated. Cohen (1985) states, "Most often, it is the social worker who decides to what degree the client is motivated. In this sense social workers create unmotivated as well as motivated clients" (p. 275). What Cohen seems to be inferring is that social workers may create positive or negative situations with clients, depending upon the labels that they attribute to clients.

According to Nisbett and Ross (1980), clinicians and other professionals are prone to a number of cognitive biases and errors. In processing large quantities of client information, they tend to invoke judgmental heuristics, or cognitive simplification strategies, which deviate from normative principles of statistics and probabilities (Dawes, 1986; Dumont & Lecomte, 1987; Faust, 1986). Though these cognitive shortcuts can result in accurate judgments, they also can impair the accuracy of clinical decision making, resulting in clinical bias (e.g., illusory correlation), and confirmatory bias (Strohmer, Shivey, & Chiodo, 1990). It has been noted that not all clinicians form biased clinical judgments all the time (Cline, 1985; Garb, 1984; Kleinmuntz, 1963; Rock, Bransford, Maisto, & Morey, 1987; Spengler, 1991).

Margolin (1992) conducted an analysis of official child abuse records in an attempt to determine the processes by which social workers labeled individuals as abusers. The analysis found that social workers frequently simplified the labeling process by omitting information about alleged perpetrators that may have absolved them of wrongdoing. One of the methods by which this was done was to simply omit interviews with alleged perpetrators, or by labeling them as noncredible or unreliable. Although it could be argued that simplifying the labeling process may be positive in that individuals thought to be dangerous to others are more swiftly dealt with, there are also very negative consequences for individuals who are inaccurately labeled as child abusers.

One way to protect against clinical judgment bias is to have clear guidelines for accepting a client for services and to have mechanisms that provide the clinician with a crosscheck on the labeling of a client (e.g., having other clinicians independently rate the client or having an independent professional from another agency validate the labeling process) to ensure that it is being consistently applied. Such a validation may be costly to the agency, but the social destructiveness of inaccurate labeling of a client justifies the costs. Thus, adequate reliability procedures are necessary in assessing the client's behavior. Moreover, reliability checks by independent clinicians are needed to ensure that treatment is being applied consistently, and not in such a manner as to confirm the expectation of the clinician. The clinician may develop an expectation of limited behavioral change and communicate this to the client. If the sessions are videotaped, the opportunity is provided to determine whether certain cues were given differentially to the client and to specify how they influenced the labeling process. Moreover, such tapes provide a rich basis for future research.

When human observation or interpretation is involved in clinical practice and experimental or evaluative research, biasing factors can affect the dependent variables unless adequate methodological procedures are used. Thus, although expectation biases tend to be unintentional, they often introduce extraneous factors into experiments, which could lead to unreliable data if left uncorrected. One possible avenue that may control such biasing effects is training clinicians to use global labels less often, and specifying more concretely the behavior with which they are going to work. In addition, practicing clinicians could be trained in time-sampling procedures to assist them in conducting more accurate assessments of behavior. This would reduce negative aspects as a result of inaccurate labeling due to inadequate sampling procedures.

In a vast majority of cases, intervention by mental health professionals begins (and often ends) with reports of deviant behavior by nonprofessionals (Baer, 1988; Witt, 1990). From a social labeling perspective, behavior is judged to be deviant based on an interaction of behavior, the tolerance of the observer, and the context in which the behavior occurred (Ullmann & Krasner, 1969).

Martens (1993) comments on a corollary of this social-labeling sequence that is particularly noteworthy. This corollary is that mental health professionals do not typically determine if behavior is deviant, but rather how best to classify and treat behavior that has been labeled deviant by another person. Interestingly, dire consequences have resulted when the labeling sequence was reversed. In the well-known case of Tarasoff versus Regents of the University of California (1974), a clinical psychologist working in the counseling clinic at the university judged the behavior of a student was deviant. The psychologist informed the campus police the student was dangerous and warranted being committed. The campus police then interviewed the student and determined he was not dangerous. Therefore, they did not commit him. Two months later, the student followed through on his threats to murder Tatiana Tarasoff (Stone, 1984).

## DIAGNOSTIC MANUALS

The *Diagnostic and Statistical Manual of Mental Disorders* (*DSM*) is the most frequently used publication in the field of mental health, and has often been referred to as the "Psychiatric Bible." Social workers have long supported the use of this diagnostic tool although remaining firm on the importance of including psychosocial stressors and other situational or environmental factors whenever possible. Today, social workers are the largest group of professionals in the field of mental health, and a survey of clinical social workers indicated that this manual is the publication used most often (Kutchins & Kirk, 1988). Carlton (1989) points out that although the professions may use the same diagnostic tools, there are essential differences in the purpose of psychiatry and the purpose of social work. Psychiatry is a medical specialty, and its focus is on pathology. The focus of social work in health care is on the ability of clients to manage their lives effectively under conditions of physical or mental illness and disability.

The first official *DSM* was published by the American Psychiatric Association (APA) in 1952 and reflected a psychobiological point of view. A second edition, *DSM–II*, was published in 1968 (APA, 1968) but, unlike its predecessor, it did not reflect a particular point of view. Both editions were highly criticized by many for being unscientific and for contributing to the negative labeling of those who suffered from mental health problems (Eysenck, Wakefield, & Friedman, 1983). The developers of a third edition, *DSM–III*, published in 1980 (APA, 1980), tried to calm the controversy by claiming that this new edition was unbiased and more scientific (Spitzer, 1980). Even though many of the earlier problems still persisted, they were overshadowed by an increasing demand for *DSM–III* diagnoses for clients to qualify for reimbursement from private insurance companies or from governmental programs.

A new debate erupted in 1983 over the alleged masculine bias of the system (Kaplan, 1983a, 1983b; Kass, Spitzer, & Williams, 1983; Williams & Spitzer, 1983). Before independent researchers could critically evaluate the *DSM–III* and test its reliability, the developers aborted the process by starting work on a revision of the manual. Reliability of the *DSM–III* was moot, and all attention was focused on the new revision. APA published this revision of the third edition, *DSM–III–R* in 1987, but this did not end the controversy. Despite data from field trials that the developers claimed validated the system on scientific grounds, serious questions were raised about its diagnostic reliability, its possible misuse, its potential for misdiagnosis, the ethics of its use, and other matters (Dumont, 1987; Kutchins & Kirk, 1986; Milich, 1986).

Kutchins and Kirk (1993) note that it is surprising that neither the developers nor independent investigators saw any immediate need to conduct reliability tests on the *DSM–III–R*. They go on to say that, although the new edition preserved the same structure and all of the innovations of the *DSM–III*, there were many changes in specific diagnoses. More than 100 categories were altered, some were dropped, and others were added. No one will ever know whether these changes improved or detracted from diagnostic reliability, because no effort was made to compare the reliability of the new manual with the old. Nor were any attempts made to test the overall reliability of the *DSM–III–R*, even after it was published. According to Kutchins and Kirk, our knowledge of the reliability of the manual is no greater today than it was almost two decades ago when the massive innovations were initiated.

Less than one year after the publication of the *DSM–III–R*, the APA initiated the next revision. *DSM–IV* was originally scheduled for publication in 1990. However, the date was repeatedly set back until finally it was published in May 1994. Some believed that this new edition would have the same disruptive impact on research on the overall reliability of *DSM–III–R* as its publication had on its predecessor (Zimmerman, 1988). This new addition of the *DSM–IV* was clearly based in research with over 500 field trials initiated to support the diagnostic categories outlined (American Psychiatric Association, 1994). And recently, the *DSM–IV–TR* adds additional supporting information to this research basis (American Psychiatric Association, 2000).

Based on a general dissatisfaction with the DSM multi-axis diagnostic system, the National Association of Social Workers (NASW) decided to construct its own diagnostic system (Karls & Wandrei, 1996), which was called Person in Environment (PIE). This system was not meant to be a substitute for *DSM–IV*, but rather would serve more as a complimentary alternative that was meant to evaluate the social environment and to impact the revisions of the DSM. The only noticeable influence that the PIE has had on the revisions of the DSM is that in *DSM–IV*, Axis IV is now called "psychosocial and environmental problems," which is a name change from "severity of psychosocial stressors."

Overall, even after the development of the PIE social workers have not actively pushed the initiation and development of the PIE as the exclusive classification and diagnostic system reflective of the field. Many social workers still tend to rely on psychiatric typologies. For a current description and comparison of the *DSM–IV* and the PIE see Dziegielewski (1998).

In 1966 Bieri and colleagues noted that this reliance among social workers was problematic because psychiatric typologies have been developed for classification of mental illness and, therefore, are not adequate for social work diagnoses.

> The categories are not psychosocial and do not define situations or units larger than the individual. When a caseworker classifies his cases within a typology of mental illness, he is reducing the problem these cases present to varieties of, mental illness. (p. 142)

The absence of an accepted system of classification and diagnosis for social work has been a burden for practitioners. Because insurance companies require a medical diagnosis before they will reimburse for services, social workers, along with psychologists and other mental health professionals, have waged a long and difficult fight to use *DSM* independently for third-party payment purposes. Carlton (1989) questions whether this largely successful fight has been fought on the right battleground. He questions whether social workers should have fought to be reimbursed for social work services based on a well-developed system of social work assessment.

> Any diagnostic scheme must be relevant to the practice of the professionals who develop and use it. That is, the diagnosis must direct practitioners' interventions. If it does not do so, the diagnosis is irrelevant. *DSM–III*, despite the contributions of one of its editors who is a social worker, remains essentially a psychiatric manual. How then can it direct social work interventions? (p. 85)

In closing, it appears that research findings suggest that many social workers may not use DSM to direct their interventions at all. Rather, they only use it for third-party reimbursement purposes, and further, when doing so they may select more or less severe diagnoses to qualify clients for services or to avoid stigmatizing them (Kutchins & Kirk, 1986).

## RESEARCH AND CLINICAL ISSUES

Several topics deserve high priority in future research on the accurate labeling of clients. Current research in this area is rudimentary, and at best suggestive. However, analysis of the following factors can help to substantially increase our knowledge and understanding of labeling theory, as well as lead to more accurate labeling of human service clients so that they may receive the necessary remedial services.

### Specification of Professional Training

One implication of the findings reviewed is that social work educators must be more specific about what professional training entails, and what effects they expect training to have on social workers' behaviors. Only when training can be defined in a reasonably specific manner and measured empirically can the social work profession then assess its effects on social worker behavior. With the contemporary emphasis of professional accountability, the effort to predict and document specific outcomes of professional training is timely.

The data also suggest that one way in which professional training can be further enhanced is through differential selection of specified treatment methods. Because different treatment methods are addressed to different causative variables (e.g., some emphasize such internal states as ego controls, whereas others focus on such overt acts as differentially reinforced behavior), the data indicate that social workers' attentions are directed to different kinds of stimuli in the course of assessing the client's behavior. The results are a differential tendency to use evaluative labels as defined by Case and Lingerfelt (1974). Perhaps more important, however, training in different treatment methods might also lead to different degrees of accuracy. This seems apparent among trained social workers. Hence, treatment method does seem to have an effect on social workers' behavioral assessments. Though we cannot be certain how to interpret this interaction, one plausible explanation is that traditional methods, which still comprise a great part of professional training in social work and emphasize dispositional diagnoses, may result in diminishing accuracy of behavior assessment (see Case & Lingerfelt; Stuart, 1970). These data, and those reported by Stuart, indicate that educators can improve the accuracy of client behavioral evaluations through the introduction of specific training in behavioral assessment. Clinical assessment, particularly when it emphasizes client behaviors, is a skill that can be transmitted (Dziegielewski & Leon, 2001). Therefore, accuracy is, at least in part, a function of specific training.

## THE LABELING OF DEVIANCE

One assumption of the labeling perspective is that individuals are identified or tagged as deviant for reasons other than, or in addition to, their own behavior (Becker, 1963; Lemert, 1967; Platt, 1969; Schrag, 1971; Schur, 1971). Although a fairly large number of studies have attempted to test this assumption empirically, the evidence is still probably best described as equivocal (Cohen, 1985; Dion, 1972; Gove, 1975; Schur, 1971; Shoemaker, South, & Lowe, 1973). This state of affairs may be due, in part, to several methodological features that have limited, and perhaps, biased many of the attempts to investigate labeling phenomena. First, labeling, when measured by official records, is usually treated as a dichotomous variable (e.g., as either present or absent). Second, the criteria of deviant behavior typically consist of self-reports that are subject to the well-known biases of self-perception, memory loss, and dishonesty. Third, the more serious deviant acts (e.g., nonstatus delinquencies and violent crimes) are usually the subject of prime interest despite the fact that they occur rarely, thus yielding relatively little variance to be investigated.

Perhaps a somewhat different approach to the study of labeling can yield more conclusive information regarding the extent and correlates of discrimination in the application of the deviant label. The research reported by Gingerich et al. (1976a, 1976b) represents a beginning attempt to remedy some of the methodological problems of previous studies. Specifically, we assume that individuals are more likely to vary in degree of behavioral deviance than in categorical type of deviance. Hence it would seem more appropriate to treat labeling as a continuous variable, rather than as a nominal or ordinal variable. The latter approaches have predominated in most research to date; yet few individuals are either deviant or nondeviant unless clearly defined and delineated behavioral criteria are consistently applied, as shown in certain well-formulated legal definitions of deviance. Furthermore, if criteria of deviant behavior were expanded, more variance could be generated, which in turn would permit more sophisticated methodological and theoretical analysis. In addition, the use of systematically observed behaviors rather than self-reports would likely increase the reliability and validity of the empirical criteria. Finally, most of the previous studies of the determinants of labeling have been unidimensional. Few have focused simultaneously upon features of the labeler and the labeling situation, or on characteristics of the labelee.

## Components of the Labeling Process

In general, no studies have attempted to isolate the effects of each of the several components of the labeling process. Because much of the data have shown significant effects when focused on limited facets of the labeling process, the audience does not know which of these are simply due to one or two components, and which depend on a combination or interaction of several components. Thus, the body of knowledge has not begun to delineate key relationships among variables. It is essential to isolate the effects of each component, the characteristics of the labeler and the labelee, and the behavior, to make labeling theory more powerful, to reduce its irrelevant facets, and to provide a rationale for interventions.

## Parameters of Deviant Behavior

What are the parameters involved in the definition of deviant behavior? Various parameters have been suggested here. However, the ways in which these parameters are blended so that an individual act is defined as deviant presently remains somewhat speculative. Perhaps the most important issue involves the conceptualization of deviant behavior, not as an all-or-none categorical behavior, but as a behavior that occurs at different intensities, frequencies, and duration. The use of such measurement techniques as different time-sampling methods derived from behavior analysis may alleviate the difficulties involved in specifying and measuring deviant behavior. The studies reviewed indicate that relatively small proportions of observed deviant behavior are usually associated with over attributions of that behavior by relevant others. In addition to its methodological implications, this finding has substantive significance. Another explanation of the overattribution of deviant behavior asserts that evaluations of others generally emphasize the negative, even apart from methodological constraints (Watson, 1982). Both interpretations suggest that evaluations of the proportion of deviant behavior engaged in by others may represent systematic overattributions, especially in low-frequency deviant behaviors. This illuminates the conceptual and methodological problems involved in measuring the accuracy or inaccuracy of social labeling.

Labels and concepts, such as codependent and dysfunctional family, have recently come under attack both in the professional literature (Walters, 1990) and in the national press because of their tendency to stigmatize and pathologize people. Such diagnoses have been criticized because of their tendency to blame the victim and ignore any social construction of behavior (Walters, 1990). Concepts, such as "good mother," are often discussed without making any reference to behavior (Rugel, 1992). Bentley, Harrison, and Hudson (1993) state that due to their trendiness and widespread use, terms such as codependent, dysfunctional family, borderline, and addiction have been referred to as designer diagnoses. These terms are used profusely despite the fact that many of these terms do not have clear meanings or definitions. The costs to individuals who are labeled with these terms may be great. One of the major problems regarding the use of designer diagnoses is that there is a tendency to blame the victim (often the individual who has been labeled).

Critics of labeling theory often assert that the relationship between labeling and its consequences is spurious, and is observed only because other relevant variables have been inadequately controlled. The question, as Link (1987, p. 108) sees it, becomes: "Is a supposed labeling effect real or is it simply a product of the failure to control adequately for the true cause—a patient's psychiatric condition?" The adequacy of controls rests on the reliability and validity of their measurement. Sobell and Sobell (1975) found that harsher penalties were recommended when a criminal suspect was labeled an alcoholic than when not so labeled. It also has been postulated that the stigma attached to being labeled an alcoholic can be a reason for drinkers' reluctance to enter treatment (Roizen, 1977). This assertion was supported in a 1992 study of people who had resolved an alcohol problem without treatment. Forty percent reported that they had not sought treatment because of the stigma attached to being labeled an alcoholic (Sobell, Sobell, & Toneatto, 1992). A study by Dean and Poremba (1983) found that 75% of the words used by respondents to describe an alcoholic reflected the image of a skid row bum. Drug addicts were also viewed negatively (Dean & Rud, 1984).

## Characteristics of Labelers

What are the critical characteristics of individuals in power positions who select a behavior to be labeled as deviant? The data suggest the advisability of including labeler-related predictors in future examinations of labeling discrepancies. Labelers cannot be treated as a constant in the labeling process. Studies that assume labelers, such as human service practitioners, judges, and policemen, are nonvariant in their judgmental processes and will not account for a sizable proportion of the variance in social labeling. Additionally, the data indicate that different categories of labelers are likely to differentially engage in the labeling process. Categories of labelers vary according to social relationships with the labelee (e.g., parent, teacher, peer, and police officer). The differences in labeler discrepancies clearly suggest that different categories of labelers view the same labelee differently and that, at least in part, labelers' views are a function of their particular social relationship with the individuals being assessed.

Martens (1993) addressed several issues of concern for school psychology practice. Research has shown that expectancy biases can influence the eligibility and placement decisions of school staffing teams (Ysseldyke & Algozzine, 1981), and that stigmatizing labels can adversely affect children's perceptions and interactions with their peers (Haring & Lovetti, 1992; Milich, McAninch, & Harris, 1992). As Martens pointed out, the first step in the social labeling process for children is usually a request for help from a parent or a teacher. These types of requests are usually initiated because the adult judges the child's behavior as deviant.

Children who have been labeled as learning disabled often are segregated from the mainstream school population with very little empirical evidence to support this decision. In addition, definitions of learning disability vary widely among different states. Unfortunately, it appears that children are often grouped by label rather than educational needs (Pfeiffer, 1980).

Clinical attributes investigated so far (i.e., age, gender, race, experience, expertness, confidence, profession, and theoretical orientation) have been criticized for inconsistent and contradictory results, as well as for lack of relevance to tasks associated with clinical decision making (Bieri et al., 1966; Faust, 1986; Rock et al., 1987). Spengler and Strohmer (1994) proposed that most of these variables do not reflect how clinicians' process information and more research is needed to determine how clinicians process information. This research could lead to empirically based recommendations for improving the accuracy of clinical judgment.

In client variable biases, one source of information is emphasized at the expense of minimizing another. In an extensive review of the literature on clinical judgment, Lopez (1989) observed that support for client variable biases is usually mixed. Of the many biases reviewed, only diagnostic overshadowing (Reiss, Levitan, & Szyski, 1982) received consistent support. Diagnostic overshadowing represents the underemphasis of a coexisting mental disorder when clients have mental retardation. In other words, a client who is mentally retarded is less likely to be diagnosed and treated for a coexisting mental disorder than would a nonmentally retarded client with the exact same symptoms (Levitan & Reiss, 1983; Reiss & Szyski, 1983).

In conclusion, it seems apparent that a behavioral approach toward social labeling may be more sensitive, valid, and reliable than the traditional official labeling approach. Such an approach serves to clarify conceptual inconsistencies regarding labeling and methodological deficiencies in measurement. The treatment specificity in conceptualization and measurement required by the behavioral approach may contribute to a more adequate understanding of this basic social phenomenon.

## Other Aspects of Labeling

The exact percentage of variance accounted for by various components will necessitate the utilization of factorial designs to investigate variables such as characteristics of the labeler, and characteristics and behavior of the labelee. Other variables to investigate in more sophisticated studies will involve the context of deviant behavior and the means by which it is measured. In addition, the social consequences of inaccurate labeling should be investigated more fully relative to self-concept formation and preparation for adulthood regarding education and social skills. An analysis of the ways in which clients are currently processed for treatment is necessary. Treatment according to client attributes, social worker attributes, techniques, and treatment context must be developed and empirically validated.

## SUMMARY

A major interest in this chapter relates to the importance of the experience or training and professional identification of the trained helping professional. Professional training is considered an important variable because of the assumption that training ensures consistency in assessment. Earlier studies of the relationship between professional training and clinical assessments have yielded contradictory information. Professional training, referred to in the aforementioned studies, represents a relatively nonspecific, global, and undefined variable. It usually means that the social worker has received a professional education or has had some experience as a professional social worker. However, the nature and content of the training or experience is undefined. In the field of social work, professional training customarily includes socialization to a set of values, the acquisition of a body of theoretical and applied knowledge, and student practice in performing the functions of a professional social worker (Bartlett, 1970; Pincus & Minahan, 1973). Beyond a general description, however, it is not possible to state the nature of the specific content of professional training or how it influences the accuracy of clinical assessment. Therefore, training could result in undue assessment of client pathology. Another hypothesis is that training increases acuity and preciseness and, therefore, sharpens clinical assessment. A third possibility is that a selection factor may operate that ensures that people, with more or less accuracy in person perception, differentially decide to seek professional training. Moreover, it is possible that several of these hypotheses, and perhaps still others, may together influence the accuracy of clinical assessment. This information gives insight into the reasons that research studies have been unable to show consistent effects of training on clinical assessment.

It is recommended that professional training in social work should include how to construct observable and reliable categories of behavior, with training in various systems of observation (e.g., the time-sampling method). The findings presented here should lead educators, not only to reevaluate the content of professional education, but also to question what educators want to train social workers to do. If students continue to be trained in traditional methods, one consequence is that accuracy in behavioral assessment could decrease. By any measure, such an outcome is manifestly undesirable for any form of contemporary professional education. If the relevant body of knowledge is to advance, descriptive and after-the-fact research must be replaced by experimental studies utilizing time-series and multivariate designs, as well as statistical procedures such as analysis of covariance and path analysis. Only then will labeling theory begin to test empirical relationships, and thus become a truly viable body of knowledge upon which clinical intervention can be accurately based.

## REFERENCES

Adomo, T. W. (1950). *The authoritarian personality.* New York: Harper & Row.

Ageton, S., & Elliott, D. C. (1974). The effects of legal processing on self-concept. *Social Problems, 22,* 87–100.

American Psychiatric Association. (1952). *Diagnostic and statistical manual of mental disorders.* Washington, DC: American Psychiatric Association.

American Psychiatric Association. (1968). *Diagnostic and statistical manual of mental disorders.* Washington, DC: American Psychiatric Association.

American Psychiatric Association. (1980). *Diagnostic and statistical manual of mental disorders* (3rd ed.). Washington, DC: American Psychiatric Association.

American Psychiatric Association. (1987). *Diagnostic and statistical manual of mental disorders* (3rd ed., rev.). Washington, DC: American Psychiatric Association.

American Psychiatric Association. (1994). *Diagnostic and statistical manual of mental disorders* (4th ed.). Washington, DC: American Psychiatric Association.

American Psychiatric Association. (2000). *Diagnostic and statistical manual of mental disorders: Text Revision* (4th ed.). Washington, DC: American Psychiatric Association.

Baer, D. M. (1988). If you know why you're changing a behavior, you'll know when you've changed it enough. *Behavioral Assessment, 10,* 219–223.

Balch, R. W. (1975). The medical model of delinquency—theoretical, practical and ethical implications. *Crime and Delinquency, 21,* 116–130.

Bartlett, H. M. (1970). *The common base of social work practice.* New York: National Association of Social Workers.

Becker, H. S. (1963). *Outsiders: Studies in the sociology of deviance.* New York: Free Press.

Bentley, K. J., Harrison, D. F., & Hudson, W. W. (1993). The impending demise of "designer diagnoses": Implications for the use of concepts in practice. *Research on Social Work Practice, 2* (4), 462–470.

Berleman, W. C., Seaberg, J., & Steinburn, T. W. (1972). The delinquency prevention experiment of the Seattle Atlantic Street Center: A final evaluation. *Social Service Review, 46,* 323–346.

Bieri, J. (1961). Complexity-simplicity as a personality variable in cognitive and preferential behavior. In D. Fiske & S. Maddi (Eds.), *Functions of varied experience.* Homewood, IL: Dorsey.

Bieri, J., Atkins, A. L., Briar, S., Leaman, R. L., Miller, H., & Tripodi, T. (1966). *Clinical and social judgment: The discrimination of behavioral information.* New York: Wiley.

Braun, C. (1976). Teacher expectation: Sociopsychological dynamics. *Review of Educational Research, 46* (2), 185–213.

Bruner, J. G. (1951). Personality dynamics and the process of perceiving. In R. Blake & G. Ramsey (Eds.), *Perceptions: An approach to personality.* New York: Ronald Press.

Bruner, J. G. (1957). On perceptual readiness. *Psychological Review, 64,* 123–152.

Carlton, T. O. (1989). Classification and diagnosis in social work in health care. *Health and Social Work,* 83–85.

Case, L. P., & Lingerfelt, N. B. (1974). Name-calling: The labeling process in the social work interview. *Social Service Review, 48,* 75–86.

Christie, R., & Geis, F. L. (1970). *Studies in Machiavellianism.* New York: Academic.

Cicourel, A. V. (1967). *The social organization of juvenile justice.* New York: Wiley.

Cline, T. (1985). Clinical judgment in context: A review of situational factors in person perception during clinical interviews. *Journal of Child Psychology and Psychiatry, 26,* 369–380.

Cline, V. B. (1955). Ability to judge personality assessed with a stress interview and soundfilm technique. *Journal of Abnormal and Social Psychology, 50,* 183–187.

Cohen, B. Z. (1985). Applying the "unmotivated" label to clients in social service agencies. *Journal of Sociology & Social Welfare, 12* (2), 274–286.

Conger, A. J., & Coie, D. J. (1975). Who's crazy in Manhattan: A re-examination of "treatment" of psychological disorder among urban children. *Journal of Consulting and Clinical Psychology, 43,* 179–182.

Crow, W. J. (1957). The effect of training upon accuracy and variability in interpersonal perception. *Journal of Abnormal and Social Psychology, 55,* 355–359.

Dawes, R. M. (1986). Representative thinking in clinical judgment. *Clinical Psychology Review, 6,* 425–441.

Dean, J. C., & Poremba, G. A. (1983). The alcoholic stigma and the disease concept. *International Journal on Addiction, 18,* 739–751.

Dean, J. C., & Rud, R. (1984). The drug addict and the stigma of addiction. *International Journal on Addiction, 19,* 859–869.

Derogatis, L. R., Yevzeroff, H., & Wittlesberger, B. (1975). Social class, psychological disorder and the nature of the psychopathologic indicator. *Journal of Consulting and Clinical Psychology, 43,* 183–191.

Dion, K. K. (1972). Physical attractiveness and evaluation of children's transgressions. *Journal of Personality and Social Psychology, 24,* 207–213.

Dumont, F., & Lecomte, C. (1987). Inferential processes in clinical work: Inquiry into logical errors that affect diagnostic judgments. *Professional Pathology: Research and Practice, 18,* 433–438.

Dumont, M. P. (1987). A diagnostic parable: First edition—Unrevised. *A Journal of Reviews and Commentary in Mental Health, 2,* 9–12.

Dziegielewski, S. F. (1998). *The changing face of health care practice: Professional practice in the era of managed care.* New York: Springer.

Dziegielewski, S. F., & Leon, A. M. (2001). *Social work practice and psychopharmacology.* New York: Springer.

Elion, V. H., & Megargee, E. I. (1975). Validation of the MMPI scale among black males. *Journal of Consulting and Clinical Psychology, 43,* 166–172.

Emerson, R. M. (1969). *Judging delinquents: Context and process in juvenile court.* Chicago: Aldine.

Erikson, K. T. (1962). Notes on the sociology of deviance. *Social Problems, 9,* 307–314.

Eysenck, H., Wakefield, J., & Friedman, A. (1983). Diagnosis and clinical assessment: The DSM–III. *Annual Review of Psychology, 34,* 167–193.

Faust, D. (1986). Research on human judgment and its application to clinical practice. *Professional Psychology: Research and Practice, 17,* 420–430.

Garb, H. N. (1984). The incremental validity of information used in personality assessment. *Clinical Psychology Review, 4,* 641–655.

Gibbs, J. P. (1966). Conceptions of deviant behavior: The old and the new. *Pacific Sociological Review, 9,* 9–14.

Gingerich, W., Feldman, R. A., & Wodarski, J. S. (1976a). Accurate and inaccurate attributions of anti-social behavior: A labeling perspective. *Sociological and Social Research, 61,* 204–222.

Gingerich, W., Feldman, R. A., & Wodarski, J. S. (1976b). Accuracy in assessment: Does training help? *Social Work, 2* (10), 40–48.

Giordano, P., Cernovich, S., & Pugh, M. D. (1986). Friendships and delinquency. *American Journal of Sociology, 91,* 1170–1202.

Goldstein, A. P. (1962). *Therapist-patient expectancies in psychotherapy.* New York: Pergamon.

Gould, L. C. (1969). Who defines delinquency: A comparison of self-reported and officially reported indices of delinquency for three racial groups. *Social Problems, 16,* 325–336.

Gove, W. W. (Ed.). (1975). *The labeling of deviance: Evaluating a perspective.* New York: Wiley.

Hagan, J., & Palloni, A. (1999). Sociological criminology and the mythology of Hispanic immigration and crime. *Social Problems, 46* (4), 617–632.

Haring, K. A., & Lovett, D. L. (1992). Labeling preschoolers as learning disabled: A cautionary position. *Topics in Early Childhood Special Education, 12* (2), 151–173.

Hostorf, A. H., Schneider, D. J., & Polelka, J. (1970). *Person perception.* Reading, MA: Addison-Wesley.

Kaplan, M. (1983a). The issue of sex bias in DSM–III: Comments on articles by Spitzer, Williams, & Kass. *American Psychologist, 38,* 802–803.

Kaplan, M. (1983b). A woman's view of DSM–III. *American Psychologist, 38,* 786–792.

Karls, J. M., & Wandrei, K. M. (Eds.). (1996). *Person-in-environment system: The PIE classification system for social functioning problems.* Washington, DC: NASW.

Kass, F., Spitzer, R. L., & Williams, J. B. W. (1983). An empirical study of the issue of sex bias in the diagnostic criteria of DSM–III Axis II personality disorders. *American Psychologist, 38,* 799–801.

Kleinmuntz, B. (1963). MMPI decision rules for the identification of college maladjustment: A digital computer approach. *Psychological Monographs, 77* (4), 577.

Kutchins, H., & Kirk, S. A. (1986). The reliability of DSM–III: A critical review. *Social Work Research & Abstracts, 22,* 3–12.

Kutchins, H., & Kirk, S. A. (1988). The business of diagnosis. *Social Work, 33,* 215–220.

Kutchins, H., & Kirk, S. A. (1993). DSM–IV and the hunt for gold: A review of the treasure map. *Research on Social Work Practice, 3* (2), 219–235.

Lemert, E. (1951). *Social pathology: A systematic approach to the theory of sociopathic behavior.* New York: McGraw-Hill.

Lemert, E. M. (1967). *Human deviance, social problems, and social control.* Englewood Cliffs, NJ: Prentice-Hall.

Levitan, G. W., & Reiss, S. (1983). Generality of diagnostic overshadowing across disciplines. *Applied Research in Mental Retardation, 4,* 59–64.

Levitin, T. E. (1975). Deviants as active participants in the labeling process: The visibly handicapped. *Social Problems, 22* (4), 548–557.

Link, B. (1987). Understanding labeling effects in the area of mental disorders: An assessment of the effects of expectations of rejection. *American Sociological Review, 52,* 96–112.

Link, B., Cullen, F., Struening, E., Shrout, P., & Dohrenwend, B. (1989). A modified labeling theory approach to mental disorders: An empirical assessment. *American Sociological Review, 54,* 400–423.

Lofland, J. (1969). *Deviance and identity.* Englewood Cliffs, NJ: Prentice-Hall.

Lopez, S. R. (1989). Patient variable biases in clinical judgment: Conceptual overview and methodological considerations. *Psychological Bulletin, 106* (184–203).

Lundman, R. J. (1976). Will diversion reduce recidivism? *Crime and Delinquency, 2* (4), 428–437.

Lynch, M. D., Norem-Hebeisen, A. A., & Gergen, K. J. (1981). *Self-concept: Advances in theory and research.* Cambridge, MA: Ballinger.

Margolin, L. (1992). Deviance on record: Techniques for labeling child abusers in official documents. *Social Problems, 3* (90), 58–70.

Martens, B. K. (1993). Social labeling precision of measurement, and problem solving: Key issues in the assessment of children's emotional problems. *School Psychology Review, 22* (2), 308–312.

Matza, D. (1969). *Becoming deviant.* Englewood Cliffs, NJ: Prentice-Hall.

Milich, R. (1986). Reliability of DSM–III [Letter to the editor]. *Archives of General Psychiatry, 37,* 1426–1427.

Milich, R., McAninch, C. B., & Harris, M. J. (1992). Effects of stigmatizing information on children's peer relations: Believing is seeing. *School Psychology Review, 21,* 400–409.

Moos, R. H., & Clemes, S. R. (1967). Multivariate study of the patient-therapist system. *Journal of Consulting Psychology, 31,* 119–130.

Nisbett, R., & Ross, L. (1980). *Human inference: Strategies and shortcomings of human judgment.* Englewood Cliffs, NJ: Prentice-Hall.

Pfeiffer, S. I. (1980). The influence of diagnostic labeling on special education placement decisions. *Psychology in the Schools, 1* (70), 346–350.

Pincus, A., & Minahan, A. (1973). *Social work practice: Model and method.* Itasca, IL: R. E. Peacock.

Platt, A. (1969). *The child savers: The invention of delinquency.* Chicago: University of Chicago Press.

Postman, L. (1951). Toward a general theory of cognition. In J. Rohrer & M. Sherif (Eds.), *Social psychology at the crossroads.* New York: Harper and Row.

Quicke, J., & Winter, C. (1994). A labeling and learning: An interactionist perspective. *Support for Learning, 9* (1), 16–21.

Reiss, S., Levitan, G. W., & Szyski, J. (1982). Emotional disturbance and mental retardation: Diagnostic overshadowing. *American Journal on Mental Deficiency, 86,* 567–574.

Reiss, S., & Szyski, J. (1983). Diagnostic overshadowing and professional experience with mentally retarded persons. *American Journal on Mental Deficiency, 87,* 396–402.

Rock, D. L., Bransford, J. D., Maisto, S. A., & Morey, L. (1987). The study of clinical judgment: An ecological approach. *Clinical Psychology Review, 7,* 645–661.

Rogers, J. W., & Buffalo, M. D. (1974). Fighting back: Nine models of adaptation to a deviant label. *Social Problems, 22,* 101–118.

Roizen, R. (1977). *Barriers to alcoholism treatment.* Berkeley, CA: Alcohol Research Group.

Rosenbaum, J., & Prinsky, L. (1991). The presumption of influence: Recent responses to popular music subcultures. *Crime & Delinquency, 17* (4), 528–535.

Rosenthal, R. (1966). *Experimenter effects in behavioral research.* New York: Appleton-Century-Crofts.

Rosenthal, R., & Jacobson, L. (1968). *Pygmalion in the classroom: Teacher expectation and pupils' intellectual development.* New York: Holt, Rinehart & Winston.

Rosenthal, R., & Rosnow, R. L. (Eds.). (1969). *Artifact in behavioral research.* New York: Academic.

Rugel, R. (1992). Self-esteem maintenance in "accepting-open" and "devaluing-closed" marital systems. *American Journal of Family Therapy, 20* (1), 36–51.

Sarbin, T. R., Taft, R., & Bailey, D. E. (1960). *Clinical inference and cognitive theory.* New York: Holt, Rinehart & Winston.

Schmid, T., & Jones, R. (1991). Suspected identity: Identity transformation in a maximum-security prison. *Symbolic Interaction, 1* (40), 415–432.

Schrag, C. (1971). *Crime and justice: American style.* Washington, DC: Center for Studies of Crime and Delinquency.

Schur, E. M. (1971). *Labeling client behavior: Its sociological implications.* New York: Harper & Row.

Schwartz, R., & Skolnick, J. (1962). Two studies of legal stigma. *Social Problems, 10* (2), 133–140.

Shapiro, A. K. (1971). Placebo effects in medicine, psychotherapy, and psychoanalysis. In A. Bergin & S. Garfield (Eds.), *Handbook of psychotherapy and behavior change: An empirical analysis.* New York: Wiley.

Shearing, C. D. (1973). How to make theories untestable: A guide to theorists. *American Sociologist, 8,* 33–37.

Siegel, L., & Siegel, L. C. (1967). A multivariate paradigm for educational research. *Psychological Bulletin, 8* (5), 306–326.

Sigall, H., & Landy, D. (1973). Radiating beauty: Effects of having a physically attractive partner on person perception. *Journal of Personality and Social Psychology, 28,* 218–224.

Sigall, H., & Ostrove, N. (1975). Beautiful but dangerous: Effects of offender attractiveness and nature of the crime of juridic judgment. *Journal of Personality and Social Psychology, 31,* 410–414.

Simmons, J. L. (1965). Public stereotypes of deviants. *Social Problems, 13* (2), 223–232.

Sobell, L. C., & Sobell, M. B. (1975). Drunkenness, a "special circumstance" in crimes of violence: Sometimes. *International Journal on Addiction, 10,* 869–882.

Sobell, L. C., Sobell, M. B., & Toneatto, T. (1992). Recovery from alcohol problems without treatment. *Self-control and addictive behaviors* (pp. 198–242). New York: MacMillan.

Solley, C. M., & Murphey, G. (1960). *Development of the perceptual world.* New York: Basic.

Spengler, P. M. (1991). *Counselors' preference for problem type and level of cognitive complexity as moderators of the diagnostic overshadowing bias.* Unpublished doctoral dissertation, University at Albany, State University of New York.

Spengler, P. M., & Strohmer, D. C. (1994). Clinical, judgmental biases: The moderating roles of counselor cognitive complexity and counselor client preferences. *Journal of Counseling Psychology, 41* (1), 8–17.

Spitzer, R. (1980). Introduction. *Diagnostic and statistical manual of mental disorders. Washington, DC: American Psychiatric Association.*

Stager, S., Chassin, L., & Young, R. (1983). Determinants of self-esteem among labeled adolescents. *Social Psychology Quarterly, 46,* 3–10.

Stebbins, R. (1971). *Commitment to deviance: The nonprofessional criminal in the community.* Westport, CT: Greenwood.

Stone, A. A. (1984). *Law, psychiatry, and morality: Essays and analysis.* Washington, DC: American Psychiatric Press.

Strohmer, D. C., Shivey, V. A., & Chiodo, A. L. (1990). Information processing strategies in counselor hypothesis testing: The role of selective memory and expectancy. *Journal of Counseling Psychology, 37,* 465–472.

Stuart, R. B. (1970). *Trick or treatment: How and when psychotherapy fails.* Champaign, IL: Research Press.

Thornberry, T. (1973). Race, socioeconomic status, and sentencing in the juvenile justice system. *Journal of Applied Behavior Analysis, 6,* 31–47.

Tripodi, T., & Miller, H. (1966). The clinical judgment process: A review of the literature. *Social Work, 11,* 63–69.

Ullmann, L. P., & Krasner, L. (1969). *A psychological approach to abnormal behavior.* Englewood Cliffs, NJ: Prentice-Hall.

Ulmer, J. T. (1994). Revisiting Stebbins: Labeling and commitment to deviance. *The Sociological Quarterly, 5* (1), 135–153.

Wahler, R. G., Winkel, G. H., Peterson, R. F., & Morrison, D. C. (1965). Mothers as behavior therapists for their own children. *Behavior Research and Therapy, 3,* 113–124.

Walters, M. (1990, July/August). The codependent Cinderella who loves too much . . . fights back. *Family Therapy Networker,* 53–57.

Ward, D. A., & Tittle, C. R. (1993). Deterrence or labeling: The effects of informal sanctions. *Deviant Behavior: An Interdisciplinary Journal, 14,* 43–64.

Watson, D. (1982). The actor and the observer: How are their perceptions of causality divergent? *Psychological Bulletin, 92* (3), 682–700.

Williams, J. B. W., & Spitzer, R. L. (1983). The issue of sex bias in DSM–III: A critique of "A woman's view of DSM–III" by Marcie Kaplan. *American Psychologist, 38,* 793–798.

Witt, J. C. (1990). Complaining, precopernican thought and the univariate linear mind: Questions for school-based behavioral consultation research. *School Psychology Review, 19,* 367–377.

Ysseldyke, J. E., & Algozzine, B. (1981). Diagnostic classification decisions as a function of referral information. *Journal of Special Education, 15,* 429–435.

Zilber, J., & Niven, D. (1995). Black versus African American: Are Whites' political attitudes influenced by the choice of racial labels? *Social-Science-Quarterly, 76* (3), 655–664.

Zimmerman, M. (1988). Why are we rushing to publish DSM–IV? *Archives of General Psychiatry, 45,* 1135–1138.

# PART II

# Mezzo and Macro Perspectives: Group Variables in Human Growth and Development

# Mezzo and Macro Perspectives: Group Variables in Human Growth and Development

Carolyn Hilarski, Sophia F. Dziegielewski, and John Wodarski

Part I gave an overview of the process of human growth and development and their interactions between the individual and the environment. In Part II, the authors stress the point that no one theory can stand alone, because individuals are social creatures who have infinite influences on their development and the resulting behaviors. The authors invite the reader to explore theoretical models that adopt a broader base for interpretation of group and policy variables. These approaches encompass and support the mezzo and macro aspects of social work practice. When looking at these broader-based theoretical models or environmental approaches, social workers attempt to explain and predict behavior based on learning and past experience. Therefore, in this section, the mezzo and macro areas (system, group, or social learning aspects) relative to human growth and development are explored. Environmental issues that relate directly to practice with families, small groups, and communities from a macro or larger scale intervention process will be addressed.

To facilitate this process, the authors provide a brief summary of different theoretical models that often fall into this area. Similar to Part I, the presentation of these theoretical models set the stage by providing background information with selected readings. The authors provide selected readings that are designed to: (a) provide a brief overview of the theoretical model; (b) discuss how empiricism can be applied to the model; and (c) discuss interventive strategies in measuring the concepts. Special attention is paid to the importance of linking each of the theoretical perspectives to how they can relate to empirically based practice strategy and effectiveness. The selected readings highlight learning theories, group variables, and the inclusion of macro concepts, which provide the reader with much greater depth in terms of understanding and application.

## MEZZO AND MACRO: GROUP- AND POLICY-BASED THEORETICAL MODELS: INTRODUCTORY CONCEPTS

### Ecological and System's Approaches

In the first 60 years of social work education, practice training was based on the medical model. In the medical model, the primary goal of client-worker interaction is to assess the client's problem and treat what is identified. In this approach the client's presenting problem was conceptualized as being caused by a combination of factors (e.g., genetic, metabolic, infectious, or internal conflict); and it appeared more humane when compared with previous approaches that often demonized, blamed, and persecuted the client. As social work practice approached the 1960s, however, the medical model did not seem adequate in explaining the extent of the client's circumstance, nor was it found to be effective in helping the client (Zastrow & Kirst-Ashman, 1990). Therefore, another approach began to gain in popularity with its emphasis on ecological constructs. One of the founders of this ecological perspective was William E. Gordon (1969). Gordon asserted that behavior was the result of a transaction that occurs when a person and an environment come together at what is called an *interface* (Brower, 1988). His basic premise being "person-in-environment." In this approach, the client is viewed as being influenced by many systems, through evolutionary and adaptive forces (Bartlett, 1970; Brower, 1988). For example, a family might be viewed as interacting with its environment, while at the same time, it is effected by its internal composition and transactions.

This model views coping behaviors as attempts by the individual or systems to interact with the environment (Wodarski, 1987) to find a "goodness of fit," a "niche," or "life space" for survival or homeostasis (Brower, 1988, pp. 412–413). Individuals and systems are seen as "active, goal seeking, and purposeful—they make decisions and choices, and take actions, guided by the memory of past experiences and by anticipating future possibilities" (Brower, p. 412). Stasis develops between the person and its environment through continuous interaction with a mutual goal of continuous adaptation (Dore, 1990; Gibson, 1991; Thyer & Myers, 1998; Wodarski, 1987). Based in the importance of the environment, system's theory is based on several important concepts that describe the family and its interactions. These concepts include: systems, homeostasis, boundaries, input, output, feedback, and entropy and negative entropy. (See Table 1 for concepts and terms most often related to system's theory.)

Therefore, models of practice that guide social work interventions from a mezzo perspective such as the ecological or systems perspective seek to understand individuals in relation to their environment. In these approaches, the interaction between the person and its environment create a client system where the importance of family, friends, and other support systems cannot be underestimated. Systems approaches propose that human development remains active, and are based on relationships that interact with the environment. Individuals and their families as a whole are affected by their environmental systems. For example, if mother becomes pregnant, the whole family is influenced by many environmental systems including (but not limited to): day care, health care, and living arrangements. In addition to negotiating a new place and physical space for a new member of the family, the entire family will experience a new or modified structure within the system that will require that family members adjust and adapt.

## Evaluation of Theory

Theoretical modalities that utilize these concepts are enticing to practitioners in that they understand that all behaviors are present within and between systems. Moreover, Thyer and Myers (1998) assert that the concept inherent in the ecological model is "the most widely adopted generic practice perspective in social work today . . . " (p. 34). Yet, often times these types of ecological models are seen as "too abstract to produce practice guidelines" (Brower, 1988, p. 413). Additionally, it does not " . . . offer [a] prescription for intervention . . . (and) . . . does not specify outcomes" (Thyer & Myers, 1998, p. 34). Furthermore, several social workers have suggested that until the *process* is more explicitly defined, it is seen as irrelevant to practice (Brower, 1988; Thyer & Myers, 1998).

**TABLE 1   Concepts and Definitions Relative to System's Theory**

A *system* is a nonrandom interrelated relationship of conditions that together perform a function and act as a whole (Zastrow & Kirst-Ashman, 1990, p. 118). Systems come in many forms. For instance, a community, school, or a family.

*Homeostasis* refers to the system's endeavor for balance. A family in equipoise is generally thriving and growing. Thus, the maintenance of homeostasis means the system must be able to change, negotiate, and bend with internal and external circumstances.

*Subsystems* consist of groups within the system. For example, mom and dad are a subsystem. The children can form many different sorts of dyads or triads and parents can form subgroups with children. In a family with substance abuse, the nonabusing parent will often form an alliance with a child or children against the abuser. These subgroups can be quite destructive to the system's balance and the behaviors are often generational.

*Boundaries* are "invisible barriers which surround individuals and subsystems, regulating the amount of contact with others" (Nichols, 1984, p. 474). Thus, boundaries define inclusion and exclusion. They may also characterize the subsystems of the family.

*Input and output* are elements of interaction. This involves communication and action between and within systems and is crucial to the maintenance of the system.

*Feedback* is "any kind of direct information from an outside source about the effects and/or results of one's behavior" (Wolman, 1973, p. 143). This positive or negative information can be offered, from within or from without, to any part or the system as a whole. An example might be a school report card or mom's raise at work.

*Entropy* relates to the scientific understanding that all systems proceed toward death. Change is inevitable and desirable. An unchanging family would not be in balance. Negative entropy is a system that is evolving and willing to adapt to the new internal and external circumstance it faces.

In contrast, when looking specifically at ecological theory, the work of Vicente and Wang's (1998) study of memory recalls enthusiastically the framework in several ways. First, they report that the ecological theory is applicable to perceptual motor behavior as well as to a cognitive phenomenon. Indeed, they propose that the ecology theory may encapsulate many micro theories of learning. Moreover, their conclusions sustain the ecological theories' basic premise of the necessity of understanding the environmental constraints on behavior (Vicente & Wang, 1998, p. 49).

Ecological research currently dominates the study of criminology and contributes to a deeper understanding of the relationships between community, crime, and social control (Klinger, 1997, p. 277). A recent study (see Klinger, 1997) of police behavior found that police tend to be more lenient in high-crime communities than their colleagues in lower-crime communities. The level of police action in a given circumstance is related to the seriousness of the perpetrating offense, the "group" rules about "vigor," the perception of deservedness of the perpetrator, the district workload, the officer's understanding of the district's deviance, as well as the level of district's deviance (Klinger, 1997, p. 298).

## Interventive Implications

Assessment is vital to any intervention effort and from a system's perspective; the first area of evaluation for understanding the individual and family system involves goals to achieve homeostasis. Of course, the authors understand that no family or individual is functioning perfectly at a given time; however, it is obvious that a perceived threat to a system's serenity or balance can cause great harm to all that interact within the system. For example, if a new baby is born into a family, the parents may be elated at the culmination of a long-awaited addition to their family. However, the *new baby*'s sibling might have very negative feelings about this unwanted intruder and consequently, *acting out* behavior might be seen in school or at home. The family system must now interact with other ecological systems (e.g., school, counseling, church) to gain a renewed or reorganized homeostasis.

A second area of possible threat to the system's homeostasis is the ratio of inputs to outputs. If a family is in need of utilizing more resources than it's receiving, then a threat to the system's economic vitality is at hand. For instance, a family in poverty may expend great energy in attempting to maintain its existence, while receiving little or no aid or support.

A third domain involves inherited family and cultural boundaries that can affect the ability to change within the environment. The resistance to change is a "systems" defense mechanism that is attempting to maintain a homeostatic integration of the group. The double-bind theory is descriptive of the outcome of a dysfunctional communication pattern that in effect creates "rubber boundaries," restricting the ability of the individual and family to move forward into positive change (Becvar & Becvar, 1988). The "no win" communication pattern is described in the paradoxical model. The social worker, in attempting to change negative behavior, provides a counter-paradoxical message that is designed to force the family to redefine its relationships and allow for new, positive growth (Becvar & Becvar, 1988).

The ecological and system's approaches focus the practice interventions and goals toward three domains: the client, the systems, and the interface between the client and systems (Henry, Stephenson, Hanson, & Hargett, 1993; Zastrow & Kirst-Ashman, 1990, p. 14) (see Figure 1).

A fundamental component of this paradigm postulates that individuals (micro systems), families (mezzo systems), and other groups (macro systems) often experience difficulties as they evolve through life stages. Thus, a thorough grasp of the inherent course of human development within the client's cultural boundaries, and an understanding of the common social issues, stresses, and crisis affecting specific life transitions is essential.

Individuals within families commonly experience critical life stages that can affect adaptation of its members. For example, this may occur when a child leaves home ("the empty nest"), with a recent marriage, or with the changes that come with retirement. A core concern for the professional social worker who incorporates the ecological model is that the social worker understands the presenting problem *in and between* the client's systems in order to facilitate the negotiation of goals that will benefit all. These goals might include insuring an exchange of activity between the individual and the environment. This can be accom-

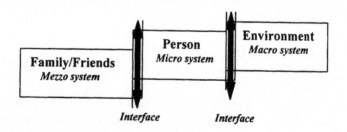

FIGURE 1    Ecology and system's approaches.

plished through interventions aimed at changing the coping behaviors of the individual and changing the interactions of environmental systems toward a more homeostatic match between *person in environment* (Wodarski, 1987). Brower (1988) cites several specific interventions, such as "helping the client understand their decision-making patterns and options, to allow more freedom of choice for responding to situations (cognitive restructuring), and to teach new responses (augment skill deficits for better problem solving) when appropriate" (p. 426). Germain and Gitterman (1980) suggest specific objectives, one of which involves cognitive restructuring of the irrational self and world perceptions that could lead to an increased understanding of positive environmental resources. In looking at a recent example, Thyer and Myers (1998) conducted a study that looked at parent education interventions from an ecological point of view. The research was interested in finding how parents (mothers 25–48 years old) and children (aged 5–7) interact, in an endeavor to help family therapists in their parent training efforts.

## RECOGNIZING THE IMPORTANCE OF CULTURE

Social work practitioners have precedence in promoting the importance of understanding culturally diverse populations. Every culture and every person within his or her culture has unique components of relating and interacting with the environment. Many theories have been discussed thus far; however, interactional theory presents a model that can serve the professional in the importance of recognizing the ramifications of daily social interactions to the way an individual or system responds. In this way, cultural diversity can be respected as the characteristics and beliefs of individuals and systems are directly attributable to social interactions and not necessarily a reaction to others. Coleman and Cressey (1984) assert that,

> People develop their outlook on life from participation in the symbolic universe that is their culture. They develop their conceptions of themselves, learn to talk, and even learn how to think as they interact early in life, with family and friends. However, unlike the Freudians, interactionists believe that an individual's personality continues to change throughout life in response to changing social environments. Young children blindly imitate the behavior of their parents, but eventually they learn to "take the role of the other," pretending to be "Mommy" or "Daddy." In addition, from such role-taking children learn to understand the interrelationships among different roles

and to see them selves as they imagine others see them. Eventually, . . .
dren begin to take the role of a generalized other. In doing so, they ad
a system of values and standards that reflect the expectations of people .
general, not just those in the immediate present. In this way, reference groups
as well as actual membership groups come to determine how the individual
behaves. (p. 21)

Lawrence Schulman (1991, 1993) attempted to adapt the interactional model to social work practice by focusing on the process of
interchange between worker and client. The interaction is conducted
with the intention of promoting genuine positive regard and helps
facilitate change in the client's negative self-identification. Schulman's
(1968) concepts also incorporate the *game model*, in which human behavior is seen as an interaction composed of the roles individuals take on
in a given situation and the rules that govern the interaction (Kelly &
Thibaut, 1978). Game analysis (see Berne, 1964) was developed by Eric
Berne and proposes that *games* are,

a set of transactions with a gimmick (that is, a hidden plan for attaining an
end). In a game, one or more participants are consciously or unconsciously
striving to achieve an ulterior outcome by using a hidden scheme. People
who are attempting to achieve a hidden outcome may or may not be aware
of their intentions—or aware of the gimmick they are using. (Zastrow & Kirst-
Ashman, 1990, p. 337)

Finally, Nelson (1997) reports that empowering individuals involves
attending to the person's need for connectiveness in an interchange.
Fostering genuine positive regard in a therapeutic environment can aid
to decrease a client's negative self-image or negative self-identification.
Thus, the interactional model supports and respects cultural diversity
because it can help to focus and develop the encouragement of connected power (p. 125). Pinderhughes (1997) elaborates on the subject
of power, roles, and interaction by asserting:

The dynamics of difference and power constitute an essential element in the
socio/cultural processes which affect people's behavior. Racial and other
differences between people make them vulnerable to anxiety and negative
responses when they interact with others. How African Americans and the
practitioners who work with them behave in relation to having and lacking
power as a result of these societal roles must be understood by all practitioners
who seek to empower African American clients. (p. 323)

# POLICY AND MACRO IMPLICATIONS REGARDING THEORY-DRIVEN PRACTICE

Theories of human behavior must include macro-level principles, as research increasingly suggests that a great portion of social bias is the result of cultural dynamics (Lyons, Wodarski, & Feit, 1998). Many of the theories discussed address change at the micro level. However, effective practice embraces social and political factors as well. Despite the fact that most social work is done individually, the whole environment must be considered. Therefore, Lyons et al. maintain:

> The prevailing ideology of demand for outcome effectiveness is likely to lead to a greater role of social work on the larger canvas. This will continue to manifest itself both in attempts to ameliorate the conditions leading to *unhealthy communities* as well as in efforts to create environments which make behavioral change more durable and transferable. (p. 12)

Social science endeavors to explicate cultural phenomena that appear in many of the theories and approaches presented in this text although many aspects of change appear strongest when utilizing a micro or mezzo perspective. After all, we are a practice-based profession and often macro changes require more time and connections outside the client system that must be changed. The changes needed may not show direct or immediate benefit to the client served and this may result in a decrease of efforts of this nature. Although the practice environment can make many of the aforementioned suppositions more attainable to *micro and mezzo* work, the importance of *macro* work cannot be underestimated. The attempts in this area, although they may appear more difficult, remain needed. Therefore, theories that accent a macro perspective generally tend to make sense of the behavior of large groups of people and the activities of entire societies and it is this large-scale observation that results in *macro*-level explanations. Assumptions most often used to explain macro level phenomena are the ecological, interactional, and functional models. In the following, the reader will be shown how we examine these behavioral models that may be very helpful in macro work.

## Theory, Social Issues, and Macro Practice

Ephross and Reisch (1982) maintain that client dilemma is caused by the social structures of society; for example, schools, welfare organizations, hospitals, and the norms of the culture. This belief contends that it is not the defective client but the inadequate societal structures that need to change. Hence, *macro-level change* in the social-psychological, sociological, economic, and political arenas of our society would alleviate client problems (Lyons et al., 1998; Mathis, 1975; Weinert, 1982).

## Macro Functional Model

The macro functional model encompasses both a micro and macro philosophy. The preceding pages presented a composition of micro and mezzo practice theories. From there the authors will now present a brief glimpse of a macro view that is offered before elaborating further on the implications of theoretical macro work offered in chapter 9.

Macro-level functionalism, developed by the French sociologist Emile Durkheim during the 1930s (Grigsby, 1995), is considered one of the most influential sociological theories. This model promotes the community as an interconnected and dependent *system* continually reaching for homeostasis through common norms and rules. Analogous to this is the human body, which comprises many parts or systems, each with its own function. When, however, one of these *systems* fails to perform, the body can become ill or break down. Functionalism asserts that, like the human body, society's systems are not always achieving optimum health or equilibrium. When a segment of the community fails to secure social essential endeavors for its members, the system is considered *dysfunctional* (Zastrow & Kirst-Ashman, 1990). Although a system change may be needed to regain homeostasis, systems have a tendency to oppose change. Certainly, history has shown that with change come unexpected events and change can be perceived as troubling or anxiety provoking. For example, birth control answered a social need to reduce unwanted pregnancy; yet, it is perceived by some to have increased another social problem of premarital or extramarital relationships. In the functional view, some societal functions are considered overt, while others are covert. For example, the legal system's overt function is to reduce crime; while a covert function might be the "labeling" (e.g., delinquent) of perpetrators, by law officers, which studies show (see Klinger, 1997) tends to increase crime.

Macro functionalism asserts that when society as a whole or in part becomes disorganized, social problems occur. Disorganization is the result of a lack of structure and goals—chaos reigns. Functionalists view the fundamental cause for disorganization as powerful social change. For example, technological advances are currently more rapid than at any other time in history, but our culture has failed to keep pace with the resulting state of affairs associated with these sweeping transformations (Zastrow & Kirst-Ashman, 1990). Consequently, issues such as medical advances that have prolonged life expectancy and increased population have become political, economical, and moral concerns (Zastrow & Kirst-Ashman, 1990).

Additionally, *macro functionalism* asserts that poverty is the result of an impaired economy. The examples given are "rapid industrialization . . . (and a) dysfunctional welfare system" (Zastrow & Kirst-Ashman, 1990, p. 403). It is apparent that industrial progress has negatively affected specific groups in our society. Particularly, those without an education, who are generally forced into low-wage positions and are the first to be replaced when mechanization arrives. Further, the social welfare system adds to the dilemma by failing to provide adequate and up-to-date job skills training.

Macro functionalists also believe that poverty is sustained because it provides a *functional* purpose to our society. For example, the poor are available to do disagreeable tasks; they provide a cheap labor force, absorb the cost of change, and provide mobility and the feeling of righteousness for "others" (Zastrow & Kirst-Ashman, 1990, p. 402). If our society were to eradicate poverty, it would mean that income would have to be redistributed. History has revealed the awkward political attempts at reducing poverty. The rich are generally opposed to any legislation that would effectively attend to the problem, such as guaranteed annual income programs (Gans, 1968, p. 133). Julian and Kornblum (1986) assert that, "Our government has the resources to eliminate poverty, but not the will" (p. 485).

*Interactionists* focus on the inherent characteristics of interchange between individuals and their environment. This model indicates that the poor can internalize the perceptions of themselves through the labeling and interactions, as well as cultural beliefs about poverty while living in a society that is success oriented. This can result in a negative self-perception, withdrawal and emotional difficulties, or worse, criminal behavior. Beckett (1994) has shown the enormous impact of labeling on certain segments of our culture. She contends that government and media labeling reinforce negative perceptions in our nation. Ryan (1976) maintains that "Blaming the poor for their circumstances is a convenient excuse" (p. 84). When society decides to stop labeling poverty because of culture, and offers hope through improved assistance and opportunity programs, interactions and self-identification will change.

Sadly, Zastrow and Kirst-Ashman (1990) report that, "No single theory provides a complete picture of why racial and ethnic discrimination occurs" (p. 528). It is suggested that different elements of multiple theories can explain this phenomenon; therefore, the macro strategies suggested by Zastrow and Kirst-Ashman to change discrimination incorporate many behavioral and or learning theory principles (e.g., civil rights legislation and community action).

Thyer and Myers (1998) maintain that,

> Behavioral principles have been applied in community settings to such topics as reducing unemployment, crime, employee absenteeism, school vandalism, and highway speeding, as well as promoting public health practices, industrial safety, and community-based recycling efforts. Most legislative action uses explicit contingencies, usually in the form of punitive fines or penal sentences. (pp. 46–47)

In addition, Thomas Szasz (1961) used the interactional model (the premises of labeling and daily interactions) to support his belief that mental illness is not a disease, but the result of client difficulties in interactions with others. For example, assignment of a diagnosis or *label* often affects the client's self-perception and other's perception of the client, which in turn affects interactions. Cooley's *looking glass self-concept* (1902) may help explain that, " . . . we develop our self-concept . . . in terms of how other people react to us. If someone is labeled mentally ill, other people are apt to react to him as if he were mentally ill, and that person may well define himself as being different, crazy, and begin playing that role" (Zastrow & Kirst-Ashman, 1990, p. 264). Moreover, the *labeling* of disease is seen as enabling the client to refuse accountability for personal difficulties. To illustrate, a client diagnosed with an incurable disease is *released* to await the cure rather than work on understanding the reasons for the client's presenting problems and any possible corrections that could be made.

Additionally, interactionalists attempt to explain the problem of alcohol and drug abuse. Interactional theory is often offered as a model for explaining this problem (Brook et al., 1998). Their hypotheses contend that alcohol abuse is learned from culturally acceptable drinking interactions with others, and illegal drug use occurs via the interactions with a drug-using subculture (Wodarski, 1996). To illustrate, Brook et al. (see Figure 3 on page 7 in work cited) interviewed 1,687 (45% female) South American youth, aged 9–18, regarding personality, family, peer, and ecological variables in relation to drug use. The study found that all the variables tested were found to connect through social interactions and the youth's choice to use drugs (Brook et al., 1998).

The ecological and system's perspectives strive to improve the interactions of people and their environments in order to facilitate desired goals at both levels. Inevitably, macro social work will be an important practice issue as the professional incorporates the client's environment into the treatment plan. The professional social worker uses the skills of brokering and advocacy when the environment fails to provide needed resources. Indeed, it is often found that the environmental system needs reforming to meet the needs of the client. When MacNair (1996) used the ecological model to analyze group cohesion in a community action project, he found that patterns of organizing, reduction of costs, specialization of function, and styles of intervention were essential components of group members engaging in community intervention. His findings support the understanding of how a community action group can improve the likelihood for positive mediation efforts on the part of the social worker. Likewise, Crittenden (1992) used the ecological model to analyze and improve services for maltreated children (p. 22). Finally, Emerson (1990) studied the effect of social welfare needs on the academic achievement of 153 disadvantaged undergraduates. The ecological paradigm helped to explain the negative effects that a lack of health, housing, and income had on academic achievement.

## SUMMARY

This overview has given the reader a summary of several of the most popular theories that look directly at the mezzo aspects (groups and systems) and the macro aspects (policy formulation) and implications these can have for social work practice. The following selected readings are provided to help further explain and expand on several of these selected theories.

Chapters 6 and 7 describe the contributions that result from the application of theories and learning principles for understanding human growth and development. Over the last 30 years these theories have gained in popularity along with the increased emphasis on professional accountability and practice effectiveness. Given both the pressures in the environment, as well as the established need for determining practice efficiency and effectiveness, social workers could benefit greatly from the knowledge of various learning theories and their applications to social work practice. Chapter 6 provides special attention to defining the theoretical premises of the "operant respondent" and "modeling" paradigms. The relevance of these models to social work practice is highlighted for the purpose of promoting a greater understanding of how the learning theories can contribute and provide intervention guidance. In chapter 7, social exchange theory is used to understand such topics as the exchanges between individuals, which can later lead to complex power relationships in organizations and communities. These authors are firm in their belief that the postulates of social exchange theory can easily be integrated with other theories, resulting in a wide range of applications and important implications for contributing to the understanding of human development and behavior.

Chapter 8 outlines the advantages of using group interventions as opposed to individual ones. The authors believe that recognizing the importance of group level variables can facilitate the development of desired goals and behaviors. Group participation enables individuals to be better prepared for participation in larger society. In addition, groups offer a forum for members to address and work collectively on issues. In this setting collective decision making and new behaviors are tested in a realistic atmosphere. In closing, this chapter presents the components of groups that the social worker can employ to facilitate the execution of relevant tasks.

Chapter 9 addresses macro-level variables that influence client behavior that cannot be addressed by individual (micro) and mezzo interventions. These macro-level variables are crucial to professional social workers in the understanding of the helping process and include broad-based organizational and societal interventions that can help address systemic problems. Chapter 9 also examines macro-level variables that can help individual clients get what they need, as well as support change efforts in the broader societal and political arenas. The historical foundations of macro-level practice are identified along with recommendations for future practice development in this area.

## REFERENCES

Bartlett, H. M. (1970). *The common base of social work practice.* New York: National Association of Social Workers.

Beckett, K. (1994). Setting the public agenda: "Street crime" and drug use in American politics. *Social Problems, 41* (3), 462–470.

Becvar, D. S., & Becvar, R. J. (1988). Toward a unified concept of reality for the social sciences. *Journal of Strategic and Systematic Therapies, 7* (4), 67–72.

Berne, E. (1964). *Games people play*. New York: Grove Press.

Brook, J. S., Brook, D. W., DeLaRosa, M., Duque, L. F., Rodriguez, E., Montoya, I. D., & Whiteman, M. (1998). Pathway to Marijuana use among adolescents: Cultural/ecological, family, peer, and personality influences. *Journal of the American Academy of Child and Adolescent Psychiatry, 37* (7), 759–766.

Brower, A. M. (1988). Can the ecological model guide social work practice? *Social Service Review, 62* (3), 411–429.

Clancy, J. (1995). Ecological school of social work: The reality and the vision. *Social Work in Education, 17* (1), 40–47.

Coleman, J. W., & Cressey, D. R. (1984). *Social problems* (2nd ed.). New York: Harper & Row.

Cooley, C. H. (1902). *Human nature and the social order*. New York: Scribner.

Crittenden, P. M. (1992). The social ecology of treatment: Case study of service system for maltreated children. *American Journal of Orthopsychiatry, 62* (1), 22–34.

Dore, M. M. (1990). Functional theory: Its history and influence on contemporary social work practice. *Social Service Review, 64* (3), 358–374.

Emerson, B. W. (1990). Academic interference: A study of social welfare needs as factors in the achievement of disadvantaged students in higher education. DSW Dissertation, Columbia University.

Ephross, P. H., & Reisch, M. (1982). The ideology of some social work texts. *Social Service Review, 56* (2), 273–291.

Gans, H. J. (1968). *More equality*. New York: Pantheon.

Germain, C. B., & Gitterman, A. (1980). *The life model of social work practice*. New York: Columbia University Press.

Gibson, E. J. (1991). *An odyssey in learning and perception*. Cambridge, MA: MIT Press.

Gordon, W. E. (1969). Basic constructs for an integrative and generative conception of social work. In G. Hearn (Ed.), *The general systems approach: Contributions toward an holistic conception of social work*. New York: Council on Social Work Education.

Grigsby, R. K. (1995). Determinism versus creativity: A response to Peile. *Social Work, 40* (5), 706–707.

Henry, C. S., Stephenson, A. L., Hanson, M. F., & Hargett, W. (1993). Adolescent suicide families: An ecological approach. *Adolescence, 28* (110), 292–308.

Julian, J., & Kornblum, W. (1986). *Social problems* (5th ed.). Englewood Cliffs, NJ: Prentice-Hall.

Kelly, H. H., & Thibaut, J. W. (1978). *Interpersonal relations: A theory of interdependence*. New York: Wiley.

Klinger, D. A. (1997). Negotiating order in patrol work: An ecological theory of police response to deviance. *Criminology, 35* (2), 277–304.

Lyons, P., Wodarski, J. S., & Feit, M. D. (1998). Human behavior theory: Emerging trends and issues. *Journal of Human Behavior in the Social Environment, 1* (1), 1–21.

MacNair, R. H. (1996). Theory for community practice in social work: The example of ecological community practice. *Journal of Community Practice, 3* (3/4), 181–202.

Mathis, T. P. (1975). Educating for black social development: The politics of social organization. *Journal of Education for Social Work, 11* (1), 105–112.

Nelson, M. L. (1997). An interactional model for empowering women in supervision. *Counselor Education and Supervision, 37* (2), 125–139.

Nichols, M. (1984). *Family therapy: Concepts and methods.* New York: Gardner Press.

Pinderhughes, E. B. (1997). The interaction of difference and power as a basic framework for understanding work with African Americans: Family theory, empowerment, and educational approaches. *Smith College Studies in Social Work, 67* (3), 323–347.

Ryan, W. (1976). *Blaming the victim.* New York: Vintage.

Schulman, L. A. (1968). A game model theory of interpersonal strategies. *Social Work, 13* (3), 16–22.

Schulman, L. A. (1991). *Interactional social work practice.* Itasca, IL: F. E. Peacock.

Schulman, L. A. (1993). Developing and testing a practice theory: An interactional perspective. *Social Work, 38* (1), 91–97.

Szasz, T. S. (1961). *The myth of mental illness.* New York: Hoeber-Harper.

Thyer, B. A., & Myers, L. L. (1998). Social learning theory: An empirically based approach to understanding human behavior in the social environment. *Journal of Human Behavior in the Social Environment, 1* (1), 33–52.

Vicente, K. J., & Wang, J. H. (1998). An ecological theory of expertise effects in memory recall. *Psychological Review, 105* (1), 33–57.

Weinert, B. A. (1982). A dialogue for change: Policy politics and advocacy. *Administration in Social Work, 6* (2/3), 125–137.

Wodarski, J. S. (1987). *Social work practice with children and adolescents.* Springfield, IL: Charles C Thomas.

Wodarski, J. S. (1996). Suicide and homicide among adolescents. *Social Work with Groups, 19* (1), 103–105.

Wolman, B. B. (1973). *Dictionary of behavioral science.* New York: Van Nostrand Reinhold.

Zastrow, C., & Kirst-Ashman, K. K. (1990). *Understanding human behavior and the social environment* (2nd ed.). Chicago: Nelson-Hall.

## CHAPTER 6

# Learning Theories: Their Application to Understanding Human Behavior

## Gerald Moote, Jr., David Skiba, and Jennifer Hall

To better understand human growth and development, the learning theories can be used to represent a diverse conceptual framework for understanding and changing human behavior. This chapter gives special attention to defining the theoretical premises of the "operant respondent" and "modeling" paradigms and their relevance to social work practice. The focus of this chapter is to help provide the reader with a general understanding of how the learning theories can contribute to understanding as well as provide guidance for intervention relating directly to social work. The chapter concludes with a call for increased attention to be given to the more valid, powerful, and relevant social work practice strategies for the future.

In social work education the learning theories have become increasingly popular paradigms with which to view human behavior. This increase is supported by the increased emphasis on professional accountability and practice effectiveness. Therefore, behaviorally based interventions conceptualized on various learning theories have received increased attention in the literature (Commons, Fantino, & Branch, 1993; Grinnell, 2001; Thyer, 1992; Thyer & Hudson, 1987; Thyer & Wodarski, 1990; Wodarski, 1983). Given the current political and economic conditions, social work methods emphasizing traditional theories and intrapsychic changes, which are often considered difficult if not impossible to measure, have come under increased scrutiny and criticism. Given both the pressures in the environment and the established need for determining practice efficiency and effectiveness through outcomes-based research (Thyer, 2000), social workers could benefit greatly from accessible knowledge of various learning theories and their applications to social work practice.

## OPERANT MODEL

Historically, the idea that human beings are motivated to seek pleasure and to avoid pain is central to the operant model, postulated before Christ, by the Greek philosophers Epicurus and Aristippus (Gergen, 1969). This principle formed the basis of the philosophical doctrines of hedonism and utilitarianism, and became an integral part of Freud's psychoanalytic theory regarding the pleasure-pain principle. Thorndike, an early twentieth century psychologist, engaged in a series of investigations that resulted in his postulation of the *law of effect* (Kimble, 1961). This law specified that responses followed by satisfying events are more likely to recur and conversely, responses followed by unsatisfying events are less likely to recur.

B. F. Skinner presented a modern version of the law of effect in his formulation of the law of the operant, demonstrating that the types of consequences following a behavior determine the probability of that behavior occurring in the future. Hence, positively evaluated consequences more often induce certain behaviors than negatively evaluated consequences (Skinner, 1953, 1966, 1969, 1971). Additionally, Skinner's findings opened the way to rapid conditioning, strengthened by intermittent reinforcement, which made behavioral change applicable in a variety of contexts (Iverson, 1992).

### Philosophy

The basic concepts of the operant model involve the probabilities of behaviors occurring and the events controlling the rate of occurrence. The central focus is on changing the rates of behavior. Therefore, the model is concerned with gaining knowledge of the antecedent events (i.e., the events in the client's environment occurring just prior to the behavior) and consequences (i.e., events in the client's environment occurring just after the behavior), which control the rate of certain behaviors. Depending upon the situation, either one or both of these concepts are utilized in the alteration of behavior. The goal is to develop descriptive statements about events that affect rates of behavior. Thus, whatever behaviors are to be changed must be observable and countable (Kazdin, 1975; Skinner, 1966).

Proponents of the operant model believe that it lends itself to a precise and reproducible account of why behaviors change. Therapeutic processes are operationalized concretely, as opposed to other models for social work practice that focus on the inner psychic processes that precede behavioral change. An example of the use of operant learning might be of a social worker utilizing the principles of the framework to help a child with antisocial tendencies. The social worker should specify those behaviors the child should decrease, such as fighting or verbal aggression. Next, those behaviors the child wished to increase, such as academic and social behaviors, ability to concentrate on a given task, appropriate verbal statements, and self-care behaviors would be identified. After determining desirable behaviors to replace undesirable behaviors, the worker would proceed to determine the antecedent events and consequences controlling such behaviors. Following the isolation of these events, the worker could employ a variety of techniques to modify the client's behavior, such as eliminating stimuli that bring on a particular behavior, reducing available reinforcement for deviant behavior, and reinforcing pro-social behaviors.

Widespread application of operant learning has also included the treatment of obese children, the obsessive-compulsive nature of adult obesity, distorted body image in adults, and the use of pharmacological interventions for both obesity and bulimia nervosa (Craighead & Agras, 1991; Mount, Neziroglu, & Taylor, 1990; Rosen, Orosan, & Reiter, 1995).

Many professionals in the field of social work often emphasize the importance of the determination of environmental events and their functional relationship in controlling or changing a person's behavior, and the manipulation of these relationships to achieve desired effects. Primarily, within the last two decades, learning theorists have placed an increased emphasis on the cognitive aspects of behavior (i.e., what clients are saying to themselves) while helping clients gain cognitive control over their behavior (Cautela, 1971; Fox & McEvoy, 1993; Mahoney, 1977; Smith, Siegel, O'Connor, & Thomas, 1994; Wong, Woolsey, & Gallegos, 1987; Zirpoli & Melloy, 1993).

Meichenbaum (1993), a clinical psychologist, in reviewing cognitive-behavioral modification, discusses three major metaphors existing within this discipline: conditioning, information processing, and constructive narratives. Although cognitive-behavioral treatments (CBTs) have demonstrated a wide applicability to both anxiety and depressive disorders (Butler, Fennell, Robin, & Gelder, 1991; Jacobson et al., 1996), substantial empirical evidence is necessary to determine the effective ingredients of these CBT with respect to particular groups, such as children for example (Durlak, Fuhrman, & Lampman, 1991). Cognitive-behavioral approaches involve helping clients learn how to control their behavior through many techniques. Two common techniques are structuring cognitive consequences for appropriate behaviors and eliminating or controlling the antecedent conditions, which cause behaviors. Analogous development has been evident in social work with the shift between individual and environmental factors. Richmond (1965) placed considerable emphasis on the environment as a treatment vehicle in her explication of social diagnosis. Actually, her social diagnosis could have been considered a forerunner of the operant analysis of behavior. Her ideas are compatible with the relationship postulated by the operant model, showing that change in an environmental event leads to a change in the client's behavior.

A social worker might determine that a couple should engage in more positive behaviors, like exchanging compliments, practicing active listening, and engaging in more pleasurable activities. Both partners can be taught to exhibit more reinforcing behaviors, resulting in increased frequency of positive behaviors toward each other (Bagarozzi & Wodarski, 1978; Wodarski, 1997).

An integration of social work's historic emphasis on an individual's personality and environmental events at different time periods was accomplished in Hollis' *Casework, a Psycho-Social Therapy* (1972). Her conceptualization of diagnosis and treatment, which emphasizes that people must be considered in the total stimulus environment in which they are operating, encompasses the assumptions of other theorists. A parallel is made in the development of human behavior theory that looks at assessing an individual's internal as well as external environment. The study of genetic influences on family environments and the subsequent role played in personality development has also applied this concept (Chipuer, Plomin, Pederson, McClearn, & Nesselroade, 1993; Traunt, 1995). Walker, Freeman, and Christensen (1994) applied a derivative of this theory in their use of Restricting Environmental Stimulation (REST) as a catalyst for improving the cognitive behavioral treatment of individuals who suffer from an obsessive-compulsive disorder.

## Model Components

The three basic elements of the operant model are discriminative stimuli (Sd), the operant (B), and the consequences (C) that follow the operant. The equation for the analysis of behavior is Sd > B > C. When the theory of operant learning is applied to practice situations, the social worker may wish to examine these three elements in order to facilitate client change. Actually, this conceptual framework is similar to Hollis' conceptualization of behaviors that result from the forces inside the individual (stresses), and influences of the environment (presses), as well as the interaction that takes place between them.

Depending on a client's life situation, stresses and presses can be regarded as either discriminative stimuli or consequences. *Discriminative stimuli* (i.e., antecedent events that occur in the individuals' environment before the behavior) indicate to individuals what conditions of reinforcement exist within their contexts; that is, they indicate what the probability is for receiving reinforcement as a result of exhibiting particular behavior(s) for that setting. These stimuli gain a controlling function over an individual's behaviors, since past experiences have taught the client that certain behaviors will be reinforced (in the presence of particular stimuli), and that other stimuli (neutral, negative, or aversive) will be received. The number of reinforcing stimuli can be extensive, such as the 89 individually rated items that make up the Adolescent Reinforcement Survey Schedule (Holmes, Cautela, & Sakano, 1996).

The operant is synonymous with the particular verbal, physical, and cognitive behaviors that an individual exhibits. Consequences are the events that either increase or decrease the probability of an operant behavior occurring in the future. Thus social workers, in analyzing why a particular couple quarrels, should know what antecedent events, such as negative commands, disapproval, or teasing, occur before the quarreling. Also needed are consequences, such as acquiring a reinforcer, terminating an aversive event, and so forth, that occurs afterward. This represents a significant departure from traditional diagnostic frameworks that focus primarily on the antecedent determinants of behavior.

In social work practice the caseworker serves as a discriminative stimulus for the client and vice versa. Clients present certain behaviors, such as stating problems and exhibiting anxiety through verbal and nonverbal channels, which serve as discriminative stimuli for the caseworker. These cues indicate to caseworkers that they should be warm, accepting, and reassuring; convey confidence and encouragement—exhibit trust, interest, and sympathetic listening; and convey concern for the client's well-being while gathering information about the antecedents and consequences that control such behaviors. Likewise, disruptive behaviors exhibited in the therapeutic context indicate that the caseworker should set limits. Actually, one function of graduate social work education is to train social workers to respond accurately to different discriminative stimuli presented by clients, and not to reinforce undesired behaviors, directly or indirectly.

After a number of sessions, a therapist's behaviors become signals for clients to exhibit certain types of behaviors via their interaction with the therapist. Examples of these behaviors might be talking about problematic areas such as sex, drugs, school performance, or relationships with others, or providing data on the frequencies of certain behavior. Time, day of week, length of session, physical aspects of the therapeutic context, type of agency, and office furnishings also serve as discriminative stimuli for the social worker and client behaviors (Dinges & Oetting, 1972; Guerin, 1992; Kazdin, 1975; Lauver, Kelly, & Froehle, 1971).

All verbal, cognitive, and physical behaviors have operative components. *Operant behaviors* and their rate of occurrence are altered by the antecedent events occurring before the behavior, and the consequences occurring after the behavior. Social work practice focuses primarily on verbal behavior, though verbal behaviors are often combined with physical behaviors to accomplish change. Such change, however, is debated, concerning visual versus auditory stimulus acting as factors in determining differences in outcomes (Mauro & Mace, 1996). The most relevant operant model literature indicates that verbalizations in the therapeutic interview are increased by techniques easily available to social workers. Examples of these techniques are positive reinforcers such as (a) a smile or a nod of the head; (b) various expressions of the face, hands, and body; (c) positive body position (leaning forward, maintaining a comfortable, distance); (d) eye contact; and (e) standard statements of a positive nature occurring after verbalizations (e.g., "please elaborate," or "tell me more about that"). Likewise, certain consequences such as interruptions, lack of appropriate inflection in speech, inadequate interpersonal distance, negative body position, and so forth tend to decrease verbalization.

For example, clients who suffer from multiple problems such as failure to keep a job, marital discord, and inability to manage their children, might be encouraged through positive statements of praise. Difficulties in these areas, when discussed, could increase the resolution of these difficulties. The question that social work practitioners must ask is whether this type of verbal conditioning is beneficial and does what is learned in the session(s) carry over into contexts outside the helping process (Verplank, 1955).

Several authors have suggested that behaviors modified through verbal conditioning be maintained beyond the interview setting (Herbert, Nelson-Gray, & Herbert, 1992; Miller & Berman, 1983; Naug, 1985). A related study by Strathman, Gleicher, Boninger, and Edwards (1994), examined the effects to which individuals are influenced by persuasive communication. Findings indicated, using data collected across seven samples of college students, that *consideration of future consequences* (CFC), was a predictor of health and environmental behaviors better than other related constructs.

Behavior is controlled not only by discriminative stimuli but also by environmental events, or consequences, occurring after the behavior. A central assumption of the operant model is that consequences affect the probability of the behavior occurring in the future. *Consequences* may be viewed as either the addition of a new stimulus or the removal of a stimulus already present within the environment (Cooper, Heron, & Heward, 1987). Consequences are defined relative to their reinforcing properties, which either increase or decrease the future probability of a behavior. Positive reinforcers increase the probability of the behavior occurring later and are usually considered to be of three types: primary, secondary, and generalized (Keller, 1954). Factors influencing reinforcement patterns include immediacy of the response, the combined verbal praise with the reinforcer, and the schedule, type, quality, quantity, the provider, and consistency of the reinforcer (Zirpoli & Melloy, 1993).

The primary positive reinforcers of food, water, and sexual activities are reinforcing because of their biological basis. Their reinforcing power is intensified as deprivation increases. For example, candy (a primary reinforcer) is often used with autistic children to establish eye contact and to increase social and linguistic behaviors (Hamblin, Buckholdt, Ferritor, Kozloff, & Blackwell, 1971). Even though their use in social work practice is often not intentional, primary positive reinforcers are used and have many indirect effects. A general mode of operation for social work practitioners is to make themselves more attractive by dispensing reinforcers. Think of the times you have taken a child out to get a soda, helped a mother with a task, or helped a client with a difficulty in securing employment. It is through such reinforcing operations and through the dispensation of primary reinforcers that we make ourselves acquire secondary reinforcing properties.

Secondary reinforcers acquire reinforcing properties through repeated association with a stimulus having positive properties. Secondary reinforcement occurs when a teacher dispenses candy bars to children for working mathematics problems toward a certain level of performance and then pairs this distribution of the candy bars with a verbal expression such as "good." After a number of associations the children will work for the expression of "good" because, through the pairing, it has acquired reinforcing properties (Hamblin et al., 1971).

Social workers utilize various types of reinforcers in clinical interviews. During the first interview, the social worker goes through a series of anxiety-reducing operations, which probably account for the client's decision to return for subsequent interviews (Berscheid & Walster, 1969; Houston, 1974). The entire process of defining the problem and discussing means of rectifying it, that is, the process of structuring, leads to the reduction of anxiety. The procedure is reinforcing for the client and thus leads to the social worker's acquisition of reinforcing properties. Reinforcing clients for their participation by smiling, nodding the head, and using positive verbal statements throughout the process helps to assure their continued participation. Positive reinforcing statements, such as "you did well" when they report back that they attained the goal, increase the probability that they will carry out other treatment objectives, adding to the attractiveness of the practice context.

A stimulus that both follows a behavior and enables the individual to secure other reinforcers is called a generalized reinforcer (Ayllon & Azrin, 1968). In certain treatment milieus "tokens" or *token reinforcement* have been used as generalized reinforcers. In these in-patient settings tokens are usually exchangeable for valued items such as cigarettes, food, or possible passes home. In everyday life resources such as money, prestige, and social status are common generalized reinforcers because they can be exchanged readily for other desired items. Today, however, social workers do not utilize these reinforcers extensively with clients despite the efficacy shown in behavioral medicine (e.g., where fixed-interval and fixed-ratio schedules have produced dramatic behavioral responses; DeLuca & Holburn, 1990).

Yet, social workers can enable clients to more readily secure generalized reinforcers. For example, a caseworker may help children to secure social skills such as getting dressed without help, making their bed, developing proper eating habits, and increasing conversational competence. Then the child not only gains self-worth but, through exhibition of these behaviors, also secures additional reinforcers such as social approval from peers and significant adults. Thus, each time these events occur they increase the value of positive behavior and decrease the value of negative behavior. Generalizations can also be enhanced when incorporating the role of self-instruction. Here, subjects who developed self-generated rules show a greater likelihood of having schedule-typical behaviors, compared with subjects without such rules.

## Interventions to Decrease Undesirable Behaviors

There are six types of interventions that can be utilized in social work practice to decrease behavior: punishment, avoidance conditioning, escape conditioning, time-out, extinction, and stimulus control (Bandura, 1969). These procedures are discussed individually for the purpose of conceptual clarity and to illustrate how they may operate in practice. However, these techniques should always be paired with procedures that increase the frequency of pro-social behavior to be exhibited by a client. These interventions, used solely to decrease undesirable behaviors, increase the likelihood that the client will evaluate the treatment context as negative, increasing the probability that the client will terminate treatment prematurely. These interventions may decrease behavior temporarily, but unless clients develop appropriate behaviors, which are reinforced by their environment, the behavior is likely to return to its former level and frequency (Wodarski, Feldman, & Flax, 1974).

*Punishment* applies to an aversive stimulus occurring after a behavior that decreases the probability of that behavior occurring in the future. When clients introduce certain topics, the social worker may punish them by not attending to that subject, changing to another topic, pointing out deficiencies in their behavior, probing an area before they are ready, or not providing the appropriate positive reinforcer for the accomplishment of a behavioral task. *Response cost* is the withdrawal of a certain amount of a reinforcer. An example of response cost would be paying a fine (withdrawal of money) for receiving a speeding ticket. This serves to discourage future speeding behavior. More important, there are a number of instances when the social worker may want to decrease certain behaviors, such as inability to address oneself to a discussion of a certain area, the commitment of antisocial acts, or the failure to carry out treatment objectives (Campbell & Church, 1969).

In escape conditioning, an aversive stimulus occurs and the client terminates the stimulus by exhibiting an undesired behavior. Typically, a welfare worker may threaten to remove a child from an inadequate home if the parents do not improve the care of the child. Hence, the parent(s) may terminate the aversive stimulus (threatened removal of the children) by improving their child-rearing habits. Spouses may nag in order to secure a desired item and their partners may provide the item to reduce the nagging. Contingent escape has been utilized to decrease disruptive behaviors in children (Allen, Loiben, Allen, & Stanley, 1992), showing reduced rates of aberrant behaviors, while at the same time increasing task completion (Lalli, Casey, & Kates, 1995).

Avoidance conditioning involves exhibiting some behavior that prevents an aversive stimulus from occurring. It is different from escape conditioning in that it requires an "anticipatory response" to prevent the aversive stimulus from occurring (Kaplan & Saddock, 1988, p. 87). During interviews, clients may avoid probing questions and topics of conversation they evaluate as negative. Clients who characteristically choose to withhold information that is necessary to work on difficulties may be asked a number of probing questions. After a period of time the client learns that by giving the social worker desired information the aversive stimulus of probing questions such as "Why can't you talk about your father?" can be avoided. This avoidant behavior typifies the antisocial child who is referred by the court for casework and avoids the stimulus of incarceration by going to the treatment context as the judge has ordered.

The procedure called *time-out* involves removing the person from a reinforcing situation for a period of time to decrease a behavior. When social workers terminate an interview prematurely because they feel the client is not participating adequately, time-out is being employed. The social worker may indicate to the client that an interview will be rescheduled for a later date, hoping clients will use the time beneficially to reevaluate their part in the helping process. Similarly, when clients fail to return for interviews this can serve as a "time-out," allowing the social worker to modify interviewing behaviors. Time-out is a technique utilized by educators and parents to encourage the use of appropriate social behavior with children and has worked well in situations that are highly reinforcing to the individual (Mash & Barkley, 1989).

Withholding reinforcers when a client exhibits a certain behavior is designated as *extinction*. In social work practice certain types of verbal responses are extinguished through withholding reinforcement when the client exhibits these behaviors. Thus, if the goal of interviews is to discuss how to refuse drugs, and young clients spend a large portion of this time talking about how disagreeable their parents are, caseworkers might choose to ignore this behavior by (a) breaks in eye contact, (b) silence, or (c) increasing the distance between themselves and the child. Ducharme and Van Houten (1994) discuss the use of extinction procedures in the treatment of severe maladaptive behavior in humans. Extinction is an effective technique with various populations (Barrett, Deitz, Gaydos, & Quinn, 1987; Higgins, Morris, & Johnson, 1989), and is gaining popularity particularly with the use of extinction in the field of interpersonal communication.

*Stimulus control* refers to the removal of stimulus that elicits certain undesirable behaviors. For example, if the behavior to be changed is the consumption of alcohol, the worker should help the client remove the stimuli that elicit the negative behavior from the environment. The social worker should encourage clients to remove the alcohol from their dwelling. Furthermore, the client will be encouraged to reduce interactions with individuals who also abuse alcohol, and avoid frequenting the places where the consumption of alcohol is promoted. Since research suggests that alcoholics respond differently than nonalcoholics when exposed to alcohol-related stimulus cues (Abrams & Niaura, 1987; Monti et al., 1987), various interventions for addressing smoking, drinking, and substance abuse behaviors need to utilize a "cue" reactivity framework that can predict, identify, and avoid behaviors that could lead to relapse (Grabowski & O'Brien, 1981; Hodgson, 1991; Niaura et al., 1988).

The foregoing intervention techniques should be used in conjunction with positive reinforcement for pro-social behavior. This combination of techniques provides social workers with a very potent means of changing behavior. However, if these techniques are used without positive reinforcement, the following negative consequences can occur: (a) client avoidance of the social worker, (b) undesirable side effects as an emotional response, (c) termination of treatment by the client, and (d) negative reactions generalizing to positive behavior. Follow-up results using family support with behavioral techniques have been shown effective for reduction of drug use and in maintaining effect over time (Azrin et al., 1996).

*Shaping* is another useful technique involving reinforcement, whereby progressive changes are highly orchestrated in pursuit of the desired behavior. For example, a social worker might wish to shape problem-solving attempts. Initially, the social worker would reinforce elementary attempts at problem solving, gradually reinforcing more elaborate problem-solving attempts until the terminal behavior is reached. The key to successful utilization is stating a goal that is achieved readily by the client at the onset of treatment. Likewise, once the terminal behavioral goal is reached, the behavior should be placed on a schedule of reinforcement that maintains the desired behavior and the possibility of the behavior generalizing to other contexts (Kazdin, 1989; Snell & Zirpoli, 1987). The frequency of reinforcement should be reduced once the appropriate rate is established (Ducharme & Van Houten, 1994; Wodarski, 1980). The reader is also referred to Wodarski and Bagarozzi (1979, chap. 2) for an extensive discussion of the effects of schedule on the maintenance of behavior.

Analogous to the concept of shaping is *sequence of responses* training, which involves learning a series of behaviors required for completion of a complex task, such as securing employment. In this type of behavior sequencing, clients are made aware of how to best present themselves for fulfillment of such tasks (Azrin & Besalel, 1980).

## RESPONDENT MODEL

Historically, the theoretical rationale for three techniques often utilized in social work intervention (*progressive relaxation, systematic desensitization, assertiveness training*) is derived from classical conditioning theory. Classical conditioning, often referred to as Pavlovian conditioning, was discovered in the course of a series of studies conducted by the eminent Russian physiologist I. P. Pavlov in the early 1890s, focusing on the physiology of digestion and preparatory reflexes of the stomach.

Pavlov discovered that if a previously neutral stimulus occurs just before food is placed in a dog's mouth, the neutral stimulus itself gradually could elicit salivation. In Pavlovian terms, food in the mouth is an unconditioned stimulus, eliciting the unconditioned response of salivation. With repeatedly paired unconditional stimulus, the previously neutral stimulus acquires the eliciting powers of the unconditioned stimulus, and hence is called the conditioned stimulus. In Pavlov's original conditioning experiment he rang a bell (a neutral stimulus) just prior to placing food (unconditioned stimulus) in a dog's mouth. The unconditioned food stimulus elicited salivation (unconditioned response) and, after repeatedly pairing the neutral bell stimulus with the unconditioned food stimulus, the neutral stimulus by itself gained the power of eliciting the salivation. Thus, in conditioning theory, this has become a conditioned stimulus.

Although Pavlov first demonstrated the classical conditioning process using laboratory animals, other researchers explored this concept further. For example, Watson and Rayner (1920) worked with a baby less than a year old, named Albert, who was conditioned to fear a rat. Each time the child was in the presence of the rat, a piece of metal was struck that produced a loud noise near the child. Soon the child began to cry when only the rat was present. The following schematic diagram and narrative illustrates the classical conditioning paradigm used to condition Albert's crying at the mere sight of the rat.

UCS (loud noise) → elicits response without pairing → UCR (fear)
CS (white rat) → elicits response with pairing → CR (fear)

The loud noise (unconditioned stimulus; UCS) produced by vigorously striking a steel bar placed directly behind the infant's head elicited a fear response (unconditioned response; UCR). A white rate (neutral stimulus) was repeatedly paired with the loud noise until by itself the white rat (now a conditioned stimulus; CS) was able to elicit a fear response (conditioned response; CR).

These conditioned stimuli, however, did extend beyond what was originally expected to happen. For example, not only did Albert, in the Watson and Rayner study, respond with fear to the conditioned white rat stimulus, but also his fear generalized to other stimuli such as a rabbit, dog, cat, or a simple ball of wool that resembled the rat. Second, the principle of extinction states that the conditioned stimulus loses its elicitation power unless periodically paired with the unconditioned stimulus. Therefore, if the white rat was continuously presented to Albert without being intermittently paired with the loud noise, the fear response would eventually extinguish. The neutral stimuli, by being paired a number of times with an eliciting stimulus, acquires properties similar to the unconditioned stimulus. After the neutral stimulus acquires such properties it must be paired occasionally with the original stimulus to maintain them. For instance, a client can develop a fear of airplane travel through the pairing of the travel with bad weather, unpleasant reasons (family illness or death), and so forth. This fear is maintained through avoiding the learning situation and the occasional pairing of the airplane travel with aversive stimuli.

## Techniques for Behavioral Change

The maintenance of anxiety, fears, and nonassertive behavior is based on the assumption that individuals do not place themselves in learning situations that enable them to acquire new responses to stimuli that currently elicit these behaviors. Progressive relaxation training, systematic desensitization, and assertiveness training are all based on the assumption that these procedures facilitate the establishment of responses that are incompatible with anxieties and fears. Various explanations have been proposed as to why these techniques change behavior; theories include: expectations (Brown, 1973; Kazdin & Krouse, 1983; Wilkins, 1971); reciprocal inhibition theory (Yates, 1975); counter-conditioning (Davison, 1968; Osterhouse, 1976); operant shaping (Kazdin & Wilcoxon, 1976); relationship factors such as warmth (Andrews, 1966; Goldstein, 1980; Krapfl & Nawas, 1969; Woldwitz, 1975); cognitive factors (Borkovec, 1973; Davison & Valins, 1969; Lott & Murray, 1975; Rosen, 1976); modeling (see Kazdin & Wilcoxon); and muscular activities (Craighead, 1973; Farmer & Wright, 1971). A review of the literature, however, does not support any one of these explanations over another and seems to indicate that all factors are operative to some extent.

As a clinical example of the use of the techniques of relaxation therapy, a therapist would educate clients, explaining to them the role of tension in the total problem situation, and indicate that from a social learning point of view tension or anxiety is a learned behavior. Clients learn that they have been exposed to experiences that originally resulted in anxiety and fear. These repeated exposures teach the client to associate the anxiety response with a variety of stimuli similar to the original precipitating event(s). These stimuli in themselves should no longer elicit the anxiety response; however, because of the laws of learning, the anxious behavior continues as clients encounter stimuli of this sort.

Contemporary research suggests the continued utilization of many interventions premised on this theoretical framework. This framework supports behaviorally based techniques and methods such as systematic desensitization, progressive relaxation, mental imagery, and stress inoculation in the treatment of various violent behaviors, phobias, anxiety, post-traumatic stress disorder (PTSD), and alcoholism (Ball, 1993; Hall, Bemoties, & Schmidt, 1995; Horne, Vatmanidis, & Careri, 1994; King, 1993; Schneider & Nevid, 1993; Seidel, Gusman, & Abueg, 1994; Strumpf & Fodor, 1993).

Eye-movement desensitization and reprocessing (EMDR) is a relatively new treatment approach for addressing trauma-related anxiety (Shapiro, 1989a, 1989b). The technique involves both imaginal exposure to the traumatic event and eye movement. In case studies using five hospitalized Vietnam combat veterans, Lipke and Botkin (1992) confirmed Shapiro's findings, although to a lesser degree, showing a rapid decrease in distress associated with PTSD symptoms. Given the paucity of empirically sound studies from a psychophysiologic perspective, many questions regarding the effectiveness of EMDR remain unanswered (Aciemo, Hersen, Van Hasselt, Tremont, & Meuser, 1994; Lohr, Kleinknecht, Tolin, & Barrett, 1995).

## MODELING PARADIGM

Thus far the basic principles of operant and respondent learning have been reviewed, explaining the acquisition of behaviors, their maintenance, and the modification of unwanted behaviors. A third type of learning, the *observational* or *modeling paradigm*, was postulated by the social learning school of human behavior (e.g., Bandura, 1969, 1971a, 1971b, 1977a, 1977b, 1986; Bandura, Adams, & Beyer, 1977; Bandura & Walters, 1963; Rosenthal, 1976). This modeling paradigm of human learning differs significantly from the respondent and operant models because from this perspective a person's learning not only comes through direct experience it also comes from observing the behaviors exhibited by others. That is, learning can take place without an individual exhibiting the desired behavior or being reinforced for it.

The following list shows that virtually all learning that results from direct experience can occur vicariously through observing the performances of social models (Bandura, 1969; Bandura & Walters, 1963; Edelstein & Eisler, 1976; Kazdin, 1989; Ladoucer, 1983):

1. Intricate and complex behaviors such as cooperative, moral assertive, aggressive, and linguistic and emotional reactions such as anxiety, fears, and phobias may be acquired by observing the behaviors of others.
2. Fear and avoidance responses may be extinguished, altered, or acquired vicariously through observational processes.
3. Behaviors that already exist in a person's repertoire may be inhibited from further expression depending upon the consequences

experienced by the model, that is, whether the observer witnesses a model being rewarded or punished for exhibiting a particular behavior or sequence of behavioral responses.

4.  The performance of behaviors that have been acquired previously may be enhanced and altered by the observation of competent models.

Vicarious consequences may be either reinforcing or punishing. Vicarious reinforcers convey information about appropriate behaviors, arouse pleasurable or satisfying emotions in the observer, and can generate incentive-motivational effects. An example of a vicarious reinforcer would be viewing a high-status actor (model) endorsing a product on a television commercial. Vicarious punishment typically conveys information about inappropriate behaviors, which has a restraining effect on the observer and devalues the model's status. An example of vicarious punishment would be viewing a high-status athlete (model) apprehended and convicted of a high-profile crime.

## Explaining Human Growth and Development

During the early part of this century, the attribution of *instinctual forces,* such as life and death instincts accounted for human behavior, received both popular and scientific support. Modeling or copying of another's behavior also was attributed to the innate propensities of humans (McDougall, 1908; Morgan, 1896; Trade, 1903). Individuals exhibited a particular behavior because their tendencies were inherited and, when the environment gave the proper cues, the behavior would appear. As the value of such explanations came into question, behavioral scientists discarded instinctual theories in favor of respondent and operant learning explanations of modeling.

Learning theorists from classical schools have postulated *respondent explanations* such as copying behavior occur because stimuli associated with the modeled performance of behaviors also become cues for observers' subsequent performances (i.e., copying behavior occurs when original cues are presented to the observer; Allport, 1924). However, this explanation is incomplete by social learning standards (Bandura, 1969, 1971a, 1971b) because it does not explain how previously learned behaviors might be elicited by the original stimulus cues. Therefore, it does not explain: (a) why observational learning is controlled by social stimuli such as the physical characteristics of the model; (b) how new responses are learned; and (c) how an individual learns a behavior without practice and reinforcement, or the psychological mechanisms underlying the acquisition of novel responses.

According to *operant explanations* of this viewpoint, observational learning takes place because modeled behavior is reinforced. Members of the operant school do not abandon the assumption that learning occurs through association, but they stress the importance of reinforcement in determining which responses will be copied. The following list contains essential elements of the modeling process as conceptualized by operant theorists (e.g., Baer & Sherman, 1964; Gewirtz & Stingle, 1968; Lundin, 1974; Miller & Dollard, 1941; Skinner, 1953):

1. The observer must be motivated to acquire the desired behavior. This motivation is believed to stem from the observer's anticipation of receiving reinforcements for exhibiting modeled responses.
2. Modeling cues for the target behavior, that is, accurate and detailed presentations of the behavior to be acquired, must be available. Modeling cues, in this respect, serve as discriminative stimuli to which observers must attend if they are to copy faithfully the modeled behavior. These cues guide the performance of the observer to facilitate the acquisition of the modeled behavior.
3. Observers must perform matching responses. The observer must attempt to reproduce the modeled behavior by exhibiting differential responses that resemble those exhibited by the model.
4. Matching behaviors must be reinforced. Inaccurate, irrelevant, or inappropriate responses are either not reinforced or are punished.

Bandura (1969, 1971a, 1971b) and Bandura and Walters (1963) were highly critical of the operant explanation of the modeling paradigm. They argued that this perspective fails to explain how learning takes place without overt performance of the model's responses during the acquisition phase and without direct reinforcement being received by the model or the observer. Furthermore, it does not explain why the appearance of the acquired responses may be delayed for long periods of time after initial exposure. According to Bandura (1969, 1971a, 1971b), the operant paradigm fails to explain how new behaviors are acquired without the organism practicing the behaviors and receiving reinforcement for them.

The operant procedure of shaping responses through the process of successive approximations is seen by social learning theorists as insufficient to account for the acquisition of all novel (original) responses. This procedure assumes that the organism learns a particular behavior, and that behavior has to be performed in a random course, which accidentally matches the modeled behaviors. A positive reinforcement then has to occur immediately after the performance for its acquisition to be ensured. Social learning theorists question whether many of the complex behavioral patterns exhibited by most members of society would ever be acquired if social training took place solely through this lengthy process of shaping. This is believed to be true of behaviors for which no reliable eliciting stimuli are present apart from the cues, such as verbal statements and physical mannerisms. From this perspective, even when other stimulus cues exist, social learning theorists believe the process of acquiring novel responses can be shortened when a social model provides detailed instructions on the responses that are to be acquired (Bandura & McDonald, 1963).

Mowrer (1960) posited another explanation of modeling phenomena related to *affective feedback* as he argued that when a model exhibits a particular response and rewards the observer for performing the behavior, the observer would imitate the model's behaviors. This concept becomes highly valued when associated with positive reinforcements. Thus, the repeated association of the modeled response and rewards acquire secondary reinforcing properties. Through stimulus generalization, the observer learns to reproduce self-rewarding experiences by performing the model's behaviors. It is also assumed that the observer experiences, vicariously, the affective consequences (reinforcing or punishing) that models enjoy as a result of their performance. The observer, through vicarious conditioning, becomes predisposed to reproduce the modeled behavior to gain the attendant pleasurable effects. Svartdal (1995), using feedback contingencies to examine the interdependency of observed behaviors, found that contingency adaptation was not dependent on verbalizations alone, suggesting that vicarious learning was indeed underway.

While Mowrer (1960) explains the acquisition of emotional responses, he does not adequately account for the acquisition of a model's specific behavioral performances that occur without reinforcement. Therefore, Bandura (1971a) believed that relying on feedback as a primary means for learning new behaviors was limited, because human functioning would be highly inflexible and unadaptive if such processes controlled acquisition of behavior. Looking at the highly discriminative character of social responsiveness, it becomes highly improbable that a substantial proportion of behaviors are controlled by secondary reinforcing properties inherent in the behaviors themselves. Bandura (1971a) argued the importance of considering the social context relative to the target behavior. He believed that situational cues were essential to accurately predict which modeled responses were critical for understanding human behavior.

In *Contiguity-Mediation theory*, postulated by Albert Bandura, extensive research on modeling phenomena has been explored (Bandura, 1965, 1969, 1977b). This is a multiprocess theory of observational learning that entails symbolic coding and central organization of modeling stimuli, the representation of stimuli in memory, verbal (word) and imaginal (picture) codes, and the stimuli's subsequent transformation from symbolic forms to motor equivalents. When individuals observe a model's behavior, but otherwise perform no overt responses, they can acquire the modeled responses through coding the behavior in a cognitive, representational form. Any learning under these conditions occurs purely on an observational or covert basis. This mode of responses acquisition has been designated as "no trial" learning because the observer does not engage in overt responding trials, although the observer may require multiple observational attempts to reproduce accurately modeled stimuli.

After modeling stimuli have been coded into words or images for memory representation, they function as mediators for subsequent acquisition, integration, facilitation, inhibition, and retrieval of responses reproduction. Later, reinstatement of these representational mediators, in conjunction with appropriate environmental cues, guides behavioral reproduction of matching responses. For example, in a study testing the stated intentions of two groups of work site employees and their follow-through with a prescribed exercise program, findings revealed a twofold increase in the frequency and intensity of exercise for the experimental group who received educational training, and who expressed structured statements outlining their intentions to change their behavior (Huddy, Hyner, Hebert, & Johnson, 1995). Performance of observationally learned responses is regulated largely by outcomes that are externally applied, self-administered, or experienced vicariously.

Several interrelated subprocesses such as attentional processes, retention processes, and incentive and motivational processes control modeling phenomena. The absence of modeling effects in any given case may result either from failures in sensory registration because of inadequate attention of relevant social cues, deficient symbolic coding of modeled events into functional mediators of overt behavior, retention decrements, motor deficiencies, or unfavorable conditions of reinforcement.

There are three major differences between the contiguity-mediation theory (Bandura, 1969, 1971a, 1971b; Bandura & Walters, 1963) and other learning explanations of the modeling process (Allport, 1924; Baer & Sherman, 1964; Gewirtz & Stingle, 1968; Holt, 1931; Lundin, 1974; McDougall, 1908; Miller & Dollard, 1941; Morgan, 1896; Mowrer, 1960; Skinner, 1953; Trade, 1903). First, learning takes place even though an individual is not reinforced for reproducing the model's responses at the same time the behavior is being observed. However, the likelihood of observers imitating a model's behavior increases if learners are rewarded for producing matching responses or observes a model being reinforced for their performance. Even if the behaviors are punished or ignored it can still become part of the learner's repertoire. These responses may be reproduced long after the observer's initial exposure to the model. According to the contiguity-mediation viewpoint, reinforcement is facilitative rather than essential for observational learning to occur.

Second, *cognitive mediational processes* have a central role in contiguity-mediation theory in explaining the learning process. Symbolic coding, organization, storage, and representation of modeling stimuli in both verbal and imaginal forms are believed to take place before modeling stimuli are reproduced motorically (Bandura, 1977a, 1977b; Bandura et al., 1977). After modeling stimuli have become coded they function as mediators for subsequent response retrieval. The performance of observationally acquired response patterns is believed to be regulated by reinforcing outcomes, which may take the form of external rewards that may be (a) dispensed by others, (b) obtained instrumentally by the individual, (c) self-administered overtly or covertly, and (d) experienced vicariously.

Third, exposure to modeled behavior does not result in simple mimicry of specified behavioral responses that have been observed previously. When the observer witnesses the performance of a variety of models, novel patterns of behavior are exhibited. New response patterns are created and generalized to new and different settings and situational contexts (Bandura & Mischel, 1965; Bandura, Ross, & Ross, 1963a). Bandura (1986) addressed this issue and felt that comparing modeling to response mimicry "has left a legacy that minimizes the power of modeling and has limited the scope of research for many years" (p. 48).

## Factors Influencing Observational Learning

For the child growing up, most professionals agree, simple exposure to the models does not automatically guarantee that behaviors witnessed by the observer will be learned. A variety of factors are known to influence the extent to which learning will take place by observing the behavior of others. With attentional processes, for instance, observers are more likely to acquire response patterns that accurately match those exhibited by a model if they are able to discriminate specific stimulus cues. These include appropriate eye contact, body language, and conversational characteristics such as sentence construction and voice qualities. Individuals will model the behavior of persons who hold their interest, that is, persons to whom they are attracted. Generally, physical, social, educational, and attitudinal attributes affect attractiveness, thus influencing the relevance of a model for any individual. Attentional processes may play a role in autism, because an autistic child employs attentional focus with a limited amount of available social cues (Bandura, 1986, p. 87). Other disorders such as Attention Deficit Hyperactivity Disorder (ATHD) also appear to involve complications in attentional processes.

Contiguity-mediation theorists assert that, in order for an individual to reproduce observed behaviors when the modeling cues are no longer present, the observer must be capable of certain *retention processes*. In this type of learning the original observational inputs are retained symbolically for verbal symbols, vivid images, or words. Combining memory and learning concepts into conditioning theory can expand our understanding and applications of cognitive-behavioral treatments. Overt practice and covert rehearsal (symbolic role-playing) can facilitate the retention of learned behaviors because repeated rehearsal enables the learner to code and organize elements allowing for behavioral reproduction. If the model's behavioral performance is presented over a prolonged period of time, the chances of the observer forgetting what has been learned are reduced.

The rate and amount of observational learning can be governed partially by the availability to the learner of essential *motor reproduction responses*. Obviously, learning will proceed more rapidly if observers can actually construct new performance patterns by utilizing behavioral responses they already possesses. On the other hand, if the observer does not possess the necessary component responses, the modeled behavior may be learned incompletely or reproduced inaccurately. In such cases, a graduated modeling procedure in an individually paced and graduated step-wise fashion can facilitate more complex and intricate performance sequences.

Accurate behavioral reproduction can be quite difficult if governed by responses that cannot be observed or easily discernible. Behavior practice along with the provision of necessary informative feedback will facilitate the achievement of desired performances.

*Administering incentive rewards* to the observer for imitating the behaviors exhibited by a model increase the probability of reproduced modeled responses. This likelihood of an observer reproducing the behavior of a model is increased if the model is rewarded rather than punished for the performance. According to Bandura (1986) the immediate sensory and social effects of an individual's actions can motivate infants and young children, and as experience and development increase so do the range and complexity of motivational processes (p. 91). Reinforcement influences what the individual attends to and affects how accurately the information is perceived and rehearsed. However, the behavior exhibited by a model who has been punished can still be acquired and stored symbolically by the observer, and may be reproduced at a later time when the threat of punishment is no longer present.

The extent to which modeled behavior is learned and reproduced is influenced by a variety of *observer characteristics*. For example, highly dependent individuals (Jakubczak & Walters, 1959; Kagan & Mussen, 1956; Ross, 1966); persons with low self esteem (De Charms & Rosenbaum, 1960; Gelfand, 1962); persons with low levels of competence (Kanareff & Lanzetta, 1960); persons with low intelligence (Bandura, 1971a); and individuals who have been frequently rewarded for imitative responses (Miller & Dollard, 1941; Schein, 1954), are especially prone to adopt the behaviors of successful models. Additionally, confident, talented, and motivated persons select models that possess valued skills that they wish to emulate (Bandura, 1986).

Models who are highly competent, expert, and famous or can confer symbols of status have been shown to be more influential than models that do not possess these qualities (Gelfand, 1962; Hovland, Janis, & Kelly, 1953; Mausner, 1953, 1954a, 1954b; Mausner & Bloch, 1957; Rosenbaum & Tucker, 1962). Models who are liked and physically attractive and who possess prized characteristics such as social power (Bandura & Huston, 1961; Bandura, Ross, & Ross, 1963b) are more likely to be imitated. Similarities between the models and observers in age (Bandura & Kupers, 1964; Hicks, 1965; Jakubczak & Walters, 1959), sex (Bandura et al., 1963a; Maccoby & Wilson, 1957; Rosenblith, 1959,

1961), ethnic status (Epstein, 1966), race, and socioeconomic status (Boyer & May, 1968) also influence the degree to which modeled responses are adopted. Warm and nurturing individuals elicit more spontaneous imitative behavior than models that do not posses these qualities (Bandura & Huston, 1961; Hetherington & Frankie, 1967; Mussen & Parker, 1965).

## Modeling As a Clinical Tool

Modeling has been shown to be an extremely powerful clinical technique that can be useful in modifying fears, increasing social skills and assertion, and modifying autistic and sexual behaviors (Bandura, 1969, 1971b). This section describes how modeling procedures have been applied successfully to the treatment of a variety of behavior problems, in a variety of environmental settings. To familiarize the reader with the ways in which modeling principles can be used to modify behavioral responses in clients, the following summary is offered.

Observational processes play a central role in personality formation. Numerous studies have shown that modeling cues may facilitate the exhibition of previously learned responses that are not deviant or maladaptive. Behaviors elicited from observers in responses to behavioral performances of models are among a variety of altruistic acts (Blake, Rosenbaum, & Duryea, 1955; Bryan & Test, 1967; Harris, 1968; Rosenhan & White, 1967). Some of these behaviors involve volunteering one's services (Rosenbaum, 1956; Rosenbaum & Blake, 1955), pledging to follow a specific course of action (Blake, Mouton, & Hain, 1956; Helson, Blake, Mouton, & Olmstead, 1956), and assisting persons in distress (see Bryan & Test). In addition, modeling can influence information seeking (Krumboltz & Thoreson, 1964; Krumboltz, Varenhorst, & Thoreson, 1967); the choice of specific items from among various selections, such as foods, activities, and toys (Bandura et al., 1963b; Barnwell, 1966; Duncker, 1963; Gelfand, 1962; Madsen, 1968); and decisions on moral issues (Bandura & McDonald, 1963). Therefore, modeling processes are key to the acquisition of socially redeeming behaviors.

Similarly, techniques based on modeling theory have been utilized in the education and training of social work students including (a) interactive computer video systems, for skill development of crisis counselors (Seabury, 1993); and (b) computer-assisted instruction, to teach graduate social work students the appropriate use of the *DSM* (Patterson & Yaffe, 1993) and to improve the interviewing skills of under-graduate social work students (Poulin & Walter, 1990).

The reduction of overly aggressive and domineering behaviors and the subsequent increase of socially acceptable behaviors such as sharing and cooperation in school children can be increased. In this process children observe a series of interaction sequences in which puppets modeled prosocial behaviors and cooperative solutions to interpersonal problems (Bandura & Walters, 1963; Chittenden, 1942). Aggressive responses to frustrating situations were reduced substantially in older children who were taught alternative responses through observation of models, behavioral enactment, and role playing (Gittelman, 1965). Filmed models of peers who exhibited approach behaviors to other children were used to reduce social isolation and withdrawal in pre-school children (O'Connor, 1969). Videotaped self-modeling has helped to increase cooperative classroom behaviors of elementary schoolchildren (Lonnecker, Brady, McPherson, & Hawkins, 1994), and videotaped peer modeling has been utilized to train students' job-related social skills (Sundel, 1994). Recent research has supported the use of multiple peer exemplars (models) to enhance the generalization of play skills of children with autism (Belchic & Harris, 1994). A combi-nation of modeling and verbal praise has also increased self-initiated social and work skills with autistic students (Rigsby-Eldredge & McLaug-hlin, 1992). Additionally, video simulation has been used in the treat-ment of adolescent enuresis (Ronen & Schecter, 1991). If modeling procedures are ineffective in modifying behaviors that are instrumen-tally rewarded, other behavioral techniques may be introduced.

Although many of our emotional responses are acquired by means of direct respondent conditioning, the learning of specific emotional responses to certain stimulus cues can also occur through vicarious conditioning. The same processes (laws of associative learning) govern vicarious conditioning as direct classical conditioning. The main differ-ence is that in direct classical conditioning the learner experiences the painful or pleasurable stimulation, whereas in vicarious conditioning the learner observes someone else experiencing the stimulation. Af-fective behaviors exhibited by the model serve as an arousal stimulus for the observer. The vicarious conditioning process requires the activa-tion of emotional responses in the observer and close temporal pairing of these behaviors with environmental stimuli, from which subsequent behaviors are controlled.

An example of vicarious conditioning is seen in the development of phobic behaviors. Phobias often arise from direct experience with the feared object, a result of observing the actions of others that show fear reactions. Avoidance behaviors or the experience of painful physical consequences result from their interactions with particular objects such as snakes, dogs, rats, heights, elevators, and examinations (Bandura, Blanchard, & Ritter, 1969; Bandura & Menlove, 1968).

The extinction of fears and deviant behavioral patterns through vicarious conditioning takes place in a similar fashion. Persons are presented with models that perform the fear-provoking behavior without experiencing anticipated adverse consequences. After gradual and repeated exposure, the impact of threatening stimulus to produce fear is reduced or neutralized, thus enhancing future approach behavior. In talking about the client's fears, in conjunction with modeling by the social worker of normal, nonanxious behavior, the fear-producing properties of the stimuli are reduced. Likewise, observing the model repeatedly exhibiting fearless behavior with the absence of unfavorable consequences, and making direct personal contact with the threatening object and experiencing no aversive results, may account for the changes seen in observational learning procedures. Once the client gains mastery over the feared situation or object, gains can be generalized across settings and into other areas of the client's life (Bandura, 1986, pp. 258–259).

Detailed procedures for eliminating phobic behaviors, and their accompanying affective responses, can be found in the classic studies undertaken to extinguish snake phobias, acrophobia, and fear of water, spiders, darkness, height, and dogs (Bandura et al., 1969; Bandura, Grusec, & Menlove, 1967; Bandura & Menlove, 1968; Blanchard, 1969; Leitenberg & Callahan, 1973; Lewis, 1974; Ritter, 1968).

The successful application of covert modeling techniques in the treatment of phobic behaviors has been reported (Cautela, 1971; Kazdin, 1976), and shown to be as effective as overt modeling in reducing phobic responses (Cautela, Flannery, & Hanley, 1974). The procedure of covert modeling consists of the therapist presenting a verbal stimulus to the client, who is then instructed to vividly imagine the behavior suggested by the therapist. This process is similar to systematic desensitization except that deep muscle relaxation is not employed and the model is imagined is not the client. In this procedure a stimuli is imagined. The utilization of cognitive behavior modification techniques is discussed in detail by several authors (Hughes, 1988; Manning, 1991).

The use of a variety of behavioral procedures in conjunction with modeling practices has been successful in helping clients acquire assertive behaviors and other social skills (Asher & Hymel, 1986; Eisler, Hersen, & Miller, 1973; Kazdin, 1976; Lazarus, 1966; McFall & Twentyman, 1973; O'Connor, 1972; Rathus, 1973). Published studies show that the effects of modeling can be strengthened when used in conjunction with other learning techniques such as behavioral rehearsal, practice, and guided instruction (Eisler et al., 1973; Lewis, 1974; Nay, 1975). This type of training via modeling of assertive behaviors involves the inhibition nonassertive responses, as well as learning new assertive behaviors, such as the ability to say "no," to express positive and negative feelings, to make requests, and to initiate and carry on social conversations.

Presented thus far is how novel behaviors are acquired and facilitated by the performance of previously acquired behaviors, which improves through repeated observation. Mechanisms through which emotional reactions are acquired vicariously by observers also have been outlined. In this section the role of vicarious punishment and reinforcement is discussed.

A number of studies have demonstrated that behavioral performance can be deterred if the observer witnesses models who are punished or experience negative consequences as a result of their behaviors (Bandura, 1965; Bandura, Grusec, & Menlove, 1967; Bandura & Kupers, 1964; Benton, 1967; Rosenkrans & Hartup, 1967; Wilson, Robertson, Herlong, & Haynes, 1979). A complicating factor involves the fact that both vicarious and direct reinforcement occurs together in many instances, making it difficult to determine the effect of each individually. Negative sanctions can provide a quick and simple means of eliminating deviant behavioral responses in clients. Yet, this notion is not altogether accurate because vicarious conditioning through the use of aversive control may result in variety of undesirable consequences. For example:

1. The inhibitory effects produced through punishment may only be temporary if the aversive consequences are not of sufficient strength to override the effects of other maintaining conditions or if more effective competing responses are not developed at the same time.
2. The effects of punishment may generalize to behaviors other than those that are punished. When this occurs, socially approved responses that are associated with the punishing behavior may also be suppressed.
3. The use of punishment may result in avoidance, escape, and discrimination learning. Here the client may learn to avoid or

flee from those situations in which punishment is received while continuing to exhibit the behavior in situations where no aversive consequences occur.

4. The negative emotional responses that inevitably accompany punishment may generalize to both the therapist and the therapeutic relationship.

Because the effects of punishment are not completely understood, and the risks of undesirable side effects are substantial, it is recommended that therapists refrain from utilizing such aversive techniques to modify deviant client behaviors. Furthermore, behavioral inhibitions can be established through vicarious punishment, previously suppressed or inhibited responses are also discouraged. Discouragement occurs as a result of observing models that are either not punished (Bandura, 1965), or are rewarded for exhibiting antisocial behaviors that previously had been punished (Bandura et al., 1963b; Epstein, 1966; Wheeler, 1966).

## THEORETICAL ISSUES

Learning models require that we thoroughly delineate and specify variables. For example, when the operant model is employed in the animal laboratory it is a simple matter to define a discriminative stimuli, behavior, and consequences. However, when the same concepts are used to analyze behaviors of concern to practitioners, ambiguities develop. Specifically, what are the dimensions of a discriminative stimulus? How does it differ from behavior? How does behavior differ from reinforcement?

As a result of their experience in trying to apply this model in group practice, Feldman and Wodarski (1975) struggled to isolate the discriminative stimuli and the consequences that control the antisocial behaviors of children in a group context. They found that problems stemmed from the numerous behavioral exchanges taking place in any practice situation, which increased the complexity of specifying behavioral concepts and interventive strategies. For example, when a social worker reinforces a child for exhibiting a pro-social behavior, does this reinforcing behavior of the worker also serve as a discriminative stimulus for the child, indicating that if additional reinforcers are desired, continuation of the pro-social behavior is needed? Likewise, the social worker's statement, "don't do that or punishment will occur," could reinforce certain behaviors or serve as a discriminative stimulus. Thus, behavioral concepts in clinical practice need greater delineation. Though there are proven benefits for utilizing an operant model, more development is needed directly relating it to social work. The exchange model presented later in this book provides a more powerful theoretical framework for capturing the comprehensive nature of the learning process in human interactional sequencing.

Certain reinforcers such as praise, candy, and money seem to be very effective with most individuals. Factors that can limit the reinforcement potential include: when deprivation occurs highlighting the extent of time that the individual has been without the reinforcer; the number of times the individual has received reinforcement in the past; the amount of the reinforcer others possess; and, other environmental factors that may remain unrecognized in the process. Since there appears to be little systematic knowledge of which reinforcers are most effective for a certain client, additional study in this area is needed. As an example, it would be beneficial to have an inventory of reinforcers that could be easily utilized by therapists working with children, clients in mental hospitals, and outpatient clients. Obviously, creation of a classification of reinforcers remains a formidable task because there will be differences in preferences among various populations. Nonetheless, the delineation of appropriate reinforcers in the operant learning process can create effective theory building and practice applications.

Most interventions based on learning theory models utilized in the past have occurred on a one-to-one basis with a specific focus on modifying the individual's behavior. This procedure, if continued, may allow for few transfer effects to the client's general environment (Koegel & Rincover, 1977; Wahler, 1969; Wodarski, 1980). By modifying the social system, prosocial behaviors can be encouraged and maintained. Thus, the question to be resolved is, how can social workers help individuals learn how to modify the system? Psychiatric hospitals, prisons, and institutions for persons with mental retardation represent systems that in many instances maintain the behaviors that they are structured to modify, and in addition, teach other maladaptive behaviors to clients (Wodarski & Bagarozzi, 1979).

Another issue raised by concerned colleagues is the application of the learning theory models in an *open setting*. Open settings do not readily provide the controls necessary to implement techniques based on learning theory. Difficulties are encountered in monitoring the clients' behaviors and having them carry out aspects of their treatment plans. This can be particularly troublesome when implementing treatments that need to consider stages of change, as with addictive behaviors (Prochaska, DiClemente, & Norcross, 1992). However, these concerns are characteristic of most treatment processes. To alleviate these difficulties clients must learn how to keep daily charts and to record what happened before and after problematic behaviors occur. In addition, adequate monitoring systems implemented by significant persons in the client's environment will place greater importance on the family in the role of being cotherapist to a client's change process (Wodarski, 1976, 1980). Finally, if treatment is taking place in a closed environment, education of certain staff members in the basic treatment plan is essential.

The role of expectations in learning theory models deserves consideration. There is substantial research indicating that one of the most crucial variables in the achievement of therapeutic change is therapist-to-client communications (Braun, 1976; Goldstein, 1962). Further research must clarify the role of expectations in the model and determine how expectations are therefore communicated.

This chapter has focused attention on those elements of observational learning that are the most pertinent for clinical practitioners, that is, the role of modeling in acquiring prosocial, nonsocial, and antisocial behavior. Application of learning theories to practice situations has been explicated, hopefully showing the pervasiveness of these concepts and behavioral techniques to social work intervention. Clinicians also should be aware of the influence that they have when interacting with clients. Knowing this, each clinician should consider the possible effects that conduct and personal appearance, as well as behaviors of mastery, competency, openness, warmth, have upon the therapist-client relationship.

Data on the uses of modeling in clinical training suggest that social work educators and practitioners can facilitate the transfer of clinical skills by well-designed videotaped, or audiotaped and live presentations by effective practitioners. Moreover, video modeling can be employed to illustrate to clients what kinds of behaviors they should exhibit to facilitate the therapeutic process and what behaviors they can expect from the social worker (Goldstein, 1973).

Therapeutic modeling has been translated to clients in the following conditions: pretherapy instructions, repeated modeling experiences, progressive increases in the complexity and fear-arousing properties of the modeled behaviors, use of multiple models and individuals that resemble the observers, and allowing models to describe their progress. Modeling is also facilitated by practice by the observer. Practice effects are in turn facilitated by repeated practice; guidance (verbal or physical); reinforcement and feedback (during and after practice); and favorable, nonthreatening conditions for practice. This will lead to an arrangement for sufficient reinforcement of the new behavior to assure performance; but the new behavior should be placed under general social reinforcement or self-reinforcement as soon as possible (Bandura, 1977b).

In the future more research is needed on the following issues:

1. Do models that provide verbalized or physical guidance or reinforcement facilitate modeling?
2. Are individuals who serve as models observed in the act of overcoming their own fears and acquiring mastery more effective than those who have already mastered their fears?
3. Is the use of live models more influential than videotaped models?
4. What is the role of repeated practice and repeated exposure to models?
5. How does use of multiple models and multiple fear-producing stimuli affect the modeling process?
6. What is the necessary number of successful exposures to the model and the total time needed for successful exposure to the model?

When these research issues are resolved the applicability of this sophisticated technology to social work practice will be facilitated.

## SUMMARY

This chapter has discussed various learning models presented as practice tools for social workers. Techniques based on operant, respondent, and modeling paradigms have an accumulated database, which potently illustrate application to social work practice situations. The aim is to give the practitioner a clear conceptualization of the models and issues involved in their use. The relevance of these models to social work practice has steadily increased in recent years, prompted in part by the multilevel problems clients present that respond favorably with the integration of learning theory components. Moreover, the influence of learning theory variables on behavioral exchanges between worker and client cannot be underestimated.

More theoretical development is needed to account for why the techniques work and to provide a rationale for their implementation. These techniques will become more powerful when more stringent criteria are developed regarding their application, what client behaviors may benefit from which techniques, and who is best prepared to apply these techniques effectively. Moreover, criteria should be developed for how long the techniques should be implemented, by whom, and where. Impinging in any theoretical application ultimately includes an accurate assessment of clients. Peterson and Sobell (1994) outline seven areas critical to an effective evaluation of behavioral intervention, which include: (a) initial diagnosis; (b) assessment of treatment context; (c) client's internal resources; (d) assessment as part of treatment planning; (e) assessment as a method of monitoring treatment progress; (f) assessment as a method of making treatment decisions; and (g) checking on maintenance of treatment gains.

Even though most of the treatment techniques reviewed in this chapter represent global intervention packages, more research is needed to streamline the packages and evaluate the effective components of each. As these components become isolated we can offer clients the most cost-effective procedures. Concepts discussed here were grouped under the various models: respondent, operant, and modeling. However, as research has shown, all models have common learning aspects. In the future we will witness the implementation of critical investigations, supplying data that will buttress a more formal theoretical framework and explaining the processes underlying effective and efficient behavior change.

## REFERENCES

Abrams, D. B., & Niaura, R. S. (1987). Social learning theory. In H. T. Blane & K. E. Leonard (Eds.), *Psychological theories of drinking and alcoholism* (pp. 131–178). New York: Guilford.

Aciemo, R., Hersen, M., Van Hasselt, V. B., Tremont, G., & Meuser, K. T. (1994). Review of the validation and dissemination of eye-movement desensitization and reprocessing: A scientific and ethical dilemma. *Clinical Psychology Review, 14* (4), 287–299.

Allen, K. D., Loiben, T., Allen, S. J., & Stanley, R. T. (1992). Dentist-implemented contingent escape for management of disruptive child behavior. *Journal of Applied Behavior Analysis, 25* (3), 629–636.

Allport, F. H. (1924). *Social psychology.* Cambridge, MA: Riverside.

Andrews, J. D. (1966). Psychotherapy of phobias. *Psychological Bulletin, 66,* 455–480.

Asher, S. R., & Hymel, S. (1986). Coaching in social skills for children who lack friends in school. *Social Work in Education, 8* (4), 205–218.

Ayllon, T., & Azrin, N. (1968). *A token economy: A motivational system for behavior rehabilitation.* New York: Appleton-Century-Crofts.

Azrin, N. H., & Besalel, V. A. (1980). *Job club counselor's manual: A behavioral approach to vocational counseling.* Austin: PRO-ED.

Azrin, N. H., Aciemo, R., Kogan, E. S., Donohue, B., Besalel, V. A., & McMahon, P. T. (1996). Follow-up results of supportive versus behavioral therapy for illicit drug use. *Behavior Research and Therapy, 34* (1), 41–46.

Baer, D. M., & Sherman, J. A. (1964). Reinforcement control of generalized imitation by reinforcing behavioral similarity to a model. *Journal of Experimental Child Psychology, 1,* 37–49.

Bagarozzi, D. A., & Wodarski, J. S. (1978). Behavioral treatment of marital discord. *Clinical Social Work Journal, 6* (2), 135–154.

Ball, G. G. (1993). Modifying the behavior of the violent patient. Special issue: Fifth Annual New York State Office of Mental Health Research Conference. *Psychiatric Quarterly, 64* (4), 359–369.

Bandura, A. (1965). Influence of models' reinforcement contingencies on the acquisition of imitative responses. *Journal of Personality and Social Psychology, 1,* 589–595.

Bandura, A. (1969). *Principles of behavior modification.* New York: Holt, Rinehart & Winston.

Bandura, A. (1971a). *Psychological modeling, Conflicting theories.* New York: Aldine-Atherton.

Bandura, A. (1971b). *Social learning theory.* Morristown, NJ: General Learning.

Bandura, A. (1977a). Self-efficacy: Toward a unifying theory of behavioral change. *Psychological Review, 84,* 191–215.

Bandura, A. (1977b). *Social learning theory.* Englewood Cliffs, NJ: Prentice-Hall.

Bandura, A. (1986). *Social foundations of thought and action.* Englewood Cliffs, NJ: Prentice-Hall.

Bandura, A., Adams, N. E., & Beyer, J. (1977). Cognitive processes mediating behavioral change. *Journal of Personality and Social Psychology, 3* (5), 125–139.

Bandura, A., Blanchard, E. B., & Ritter, B. (1969). The relative efficacy of desensitization and modeling approaches for inducing behavioral, affective, and attitudinal changes. *Journal of Personality and Social Psychology, 13,* 173–199.

Bandura, A., Grusec, J. E., & Menlove, F. L. (1967). Vicarious extinction of avoidance behavior. *Journal of Personality and Social Psychology, 5,* 16–23.

Bandura, A., & Huston, A. C. (1961). Identification as a process of incidental learning. *Journal of Abnormal and Social Psychology, 63* (3), 11–18.

Bandura, A., & Kupers, C. J. (1964). Transmission of patterns of self-reinforcement through modeling. *Journal of Abnormal and Social Psychology, 69,* 1–9.

Bandura, A., & McDonald, F. J. (1963). The influence of social behavior of models in shaping children's moral judgments. *Journal of Abnormal and Social Psychology, 67*, 274–281.

Bandura, A., & Menlove, F. L. (1968). Factors determining vicarious extinction of avoidance behavior through symbolic modeling. *Journal of Personality and Social Psychology, 8*, 99–108.

Bandura, A., & Mischel, W. (1965). Modification of self-imposed delay of reward through exposure to live and symbolic models. *Journal of Personality and Social Psychology, 2*, 698–705.

Bandura, A., Ross, D., & Ross, S. A. (1963a). Imitation of film-mediated aggressive models. *Journal of Abnormal and Social Psychology, 66*, 3–11.

Bandura, A., Ross, D., & Ross, S. A. (1963b). A comparative test of status envy, social power, and secondary reinforcement theories of identificatory learning. *Journal of Abnormal and Social Psychology, 67*, 527–534.

Bandura, A., & Walters, R. H. (1963). *Social learning and personality development*. New York: Holt, Rinehart & Winston.

Barnwell, A. K. (1966). Potency of modeling cues in imitation of vicarious reinforcement situations. *Dissertation Abstracts, 26*, 7444.

Barrett, D. H., Deitz, S. M., Gaydos, G. R., & Quinn, P. C. (1987). The effects of programmed contingencies and social conditions on response stereotype with human subjects. *Psychological Record, 37*, 489–505.

Belchic, J. K., & Harris, S. L. (1994). The use of multiple peer exemplars to enhance the generalization of play skills to the siblings of children with autism. *Child & Family Behavior.*

Benton, A. A. (1967). Effects of the timing of negative response consequences of the observational learning of resistance to temptation in children. *Dissertation Abstracts, 27*, 2153–2154.

Berscheid, A., & Walster, E. H. (1969). *Interpersonal attraction*. Reading, MA: Addison-Wesley.

Blake, R. R., Mouton, J. S., & Hain, J. D. (1956). Social forces in petition signing. *Southwestern Social Science Quarterly, 36*, 385–390.

Blake, R. R., Rosenbaum, M., & Duryea, R. (1955). Gift-giving as a function of group standards. *Human Relations, 8*, 61–73.

Blanchard, E. B. (1969). *The relative contributions of modeling, informational influences, and physical contact in the extinction of phobic behavior*. Unpublished doctoral thesis, Stanford University.

Borkovec, T. D. (1973). The role of expectancy and physiological feedback in fear research: A review with special reference to subject characteristics. *Behavior Therapy, 4*, 449–505.

Boyer, N. L., & May, J. G., Jr. (1968). *The effects of race and socioeconomic status on imitative behavior in children using white male and female models*. Unpublished manuscript, Florida State University.

Braun, C. (1976). Teacher expectation: Sociopsychological dynamics. *Review of Educational Research, 46* (2), 185–213.

Brown, H. A. (1973). Role of expectancy manipulation in systematic desensitization. *Journal of Consulting and Clinical Psychology, 41*, 405–411.

Bryan, J. H., & Test, M. A. (1967). Models and helping: Naturalistic studies in aiding behavior. *Journal of Personality and Social Psychology, 6,* 400–407.

Butler, G., Fennell, M., Robin, P., & Gelder, M. (1991). Comparison of behavior therapy and cognitive behavior therapy in the treatment of generalized anxiety disorder. *Journal of Consulting and Clinical Psychology, 59* (1), 167–175.

Campbell, B. A., & Church, R. M. (Eds.). (1969). *Punishment and aversive behavior.* New York: Appleton-Century-Crofts.

Cautela, J. R. (1971). Covert extinction. *Behavior Therapy, 2,* 181–200.

Cautela, J. R., Flannery, R. B., & Hanley, S. (1974). Covert modeling: An experimental test. *Behavior Therapy, 5,* 494–502.

Chipuer, H. M., Plomin, R., Pederson, N. L., McClearn, G., & Nesselroade, J. R. (1993). Genetic influence on family environment: The role of personality. *Developmental Psychology, 29* (1), 110–118.

Chittenden, G. E. (1942). An experimental study in measuring and modifying assertive behavior in young children. *Monographs of the Society for Research in Child Development, 7* (1), Serial No. 31.

Commons, M., Fantino, E., & Branch, M. N. (1993). Editorial. *Journal of the Experimental Analysis of Behavior, 60,* 1–2.

Cooper, J. O., Heron, T. E., & Heward, W. L. (1987). *Applied behavior analysis.* Columbus, OH: Merrill/Macmillan.

Craighead, L. W., & Agras, S. W. (1991). Mechanisms of action in cognitive-behavioral and pharmacological interventions for obesity and bulimia nervosa. *Journal of Consulting and Clinical Psychology, 59* (1), 115–125.

Craighead, W. E. (1973). The role of muscular relaxation in systematic desensitization. In R. Rubin (Ed.), *Advances in behavior therapy* (Vol. 1). New York: Academic.

Davison, G. C. (1968). Systematic desensitization as a counter-conditioning process. *Journal of Abnormal Psychology, 73,* 91–99.

Davison, G. C., & Valins, S. (1969). Maintenance of self-attributed behavior change. *Journal of Personality and Social Psychology, 11,* 25–33.

De Charms, R., & Rosenbaum, M. E. (1960). Status variables and matching behavior. *Journal of Personality, 28,* 492–502.

DeLuca, R. V., & Holburn, S. W. (1990). Effects of fixed-interval and fixed-ratio schedules of token reinforcement on exercise with obese and non-obese boys. *The Psychological Record, 40,* 67–82.

Dinges, N. G., & Oetting, E. R. (1972). Interaction distance anxiety in the counseling dyad. *Journal of Counseling Psychology, 19,* 146–149.

Ducharme, J. M., & Van Houten, R. (1994). Operant extinction in the treatment of severe maladaptive behavior: Adapting research to practice. *Behavior Modification, 18* (2), 139–170.

Duncker, K. (1963). Experimental modification of children's food preferences through social suggestion. *Journal of Abnormal and Social Psychology, 33,* 489–507.

Durlak, J. A., Fuhrman, T., & Lampman, C. (1991). Effectiveness of cognitive-behavior therapy for maladapting children: A meta-analysis. *Psychological Bulletin, 110* (2), 204–214.

Edelstein, B., & Eisler, R. (1976). Effects of modeling and modeling with instructions and feedback on the behavioral components of social skills. *Behavior Therapy, 7,* 382–389.

Eisler, R. M., Hersen, M., & Miller, P. M. (1973). Effects of modeling on components of assertive behavior. *Journal of Behavior Therapy and Experimental Psychiatry, 4* (1), 1–6.

Epstein, R. (1966). Aggression toward out-groups as a function of authoritarianism and imitation of aggressive models. *Journal of Personality and Social Psychology, 3,* 574–579.

Farmer, R. G., & Wright, J. M. C. (1971). Muscular reactivity and systematic desensitization. *Behavior Therapy, 2* (3), 1–10.

Feldman, R. A., & Wodarski, J. S. (1975). *Contemporary approaches to group treatment.* San Francisco: Jossey-Bass.

Fox, J. F., & McEvoy, M. A. (1993). Assessing and enhancing generalization and social validity of social skills interventions with children and adolescents. *Behavior Modification, 17* (3), 339–366.

Gelfand, D. M. (1962). The influence of self-esteem on rate of verbal conditioning and social matching behavior. *Journal of Abnormal and Social Psychology, 65,* 259–265.

Gergen, K. J. (1969). *The psychology of behavior change.* Reading, MA: Addison-Wesley.

Gewirtz, J. L., & Stingle, K. C. (1968). The learning of generalized imitation as the basis for identification. *Psychological Review, 75,* 374–397.

Gittelman, M. (1965). Behavior rehearsal as a technique in child treatment. *Journal of Child Psychology and Child Psychiatry, 6,* 251–255.

Goldstein, A. P. (1962). *Therapist-patient expectancies in psychotherapy.* New York: Pergamon.

Goldstein, A. P. (1973). *Structured learning therapy.* New York: Academic.

Goldstein, A. P. (1980). Relationship-enhancement methods. In F. H. Kanfer & A. P. Goldstein (Eds.), *Helping people change* (pp. 18–57). New York: Pergamon.

Grabowski, J., & O'Brien, C. P. (1981). Conditioning factors in opiate use. In N. K. Mello (Ed.), *Advances in substance abuse* (pp. 69–121). Greenwich, CT: JAI Press.

Grinnell, R. M. (2001). *Social work research and evaluation: Quantitative and qualitative approaches* (6th ed.). Itasca, IL: F. E. Peacock.

Guerin, B. (1992). Social behavior as discriminative stimulus and consequence in social anthropology. *Behavior Analyst, 15* (1), 31–41.

Hall, C., Bemoties, L., & Schmidt, D. (1995). Interference effects of mental imagery on a motor task. *British Journal of Psychology, 86,* 181–190.

Hamblin, R. L., Buckholdt, D. R., Ferritor, D., Kozloff, M. A., & Blackwell, L. J. (1971). *The humanization process: A social behavioral analysis of children's problems.* New York: Wiley.

Harris, M. B. (1968). *Some determinants of sharing in children.* Unpublished doctoral dissertation, Stanford University.

Helson, H., Blake, R. R., Mouton, J. S., & Olmstead, J. A. (1956). Attitudes as adjustments to stimulus, background, and residual factors. *Journal of Abnormal and Social Psychology, 52,* 314–322.

Herbert, J. D., Nelson-Gray, R. O., & Herbert, D. L. (1992). The effects of feedback on the behavior of depressed inpatients in two structured interactions. *Behavior Modification, 1* (60), 82–102.

Hetherington, E. M., & Frankie, G. (1967). Effects of parental dominance, warmth and conflict on imitation in children. *Journal of Personality and Social Psychology, 6,* 119–125.

Hicks, D. J. (1965). Imitation and retention of film mediated aggressive peer and adult models. *Journal of Personality and Social Psychology, 2,* 97–100.

Higgins, S. T., Morris, E. K., & Johnson, L. M. (1989). Social transmission of superstitious behavior in preschool children. *Psychological Record, 39,* 307–323.

Hodgson, R. J. (1991). Substance misuse. Special issue: The changing face of behavioral psychotherapy. *Behavioral Psychotherapy, 19* (1), 80–87.

Hollis, R. (1972). *Casework: A psycho-social therapy* (2nd ed.). New York: Random House.

Holmes, G. R., Cautela, J., & Sakano, Y. (1996). Adolescent reinforcement survey schedule: Summary of research and future directions. *Psychological Reports, 78,* 76–78.

Holt, E. B. (1931). *Animal drive and the learning process* (Vol. 1). New York: Holt.

Horne, D. J., Vatmanidis, P., & Careri, A. (1994). Preparing patients for invasive medical and surgical procedures: Using psychological interventions with adults and children. *Behavioral Medicine, 20* (1), 15–21.

Houston, T. (1974). *Foundations of interpersonal attraction.* New York: Academic.

Hovland, C. I., Janis, I. L., & Kelly, H. H. (1953). *Communication and persuasion.* New Haven, CT: Yale University Press.

Huddy, C. D., Hyner, G. C., Hebert, J. I., & Johnson, R. L. (1995). Facilitating changes in exercise behavior: Effect of structured statements of intention on perceived barriers to action. *Psychological Reports, 76* (1), 867–875.

Hughes, J. N. (1988). *Cognitive behavioral therapy with children in schools.* New York: Pergamon.

Iverson, I. H. (1992). Skinner's early research: From reflexology to operant conditioning. *American Psychologist, 47* (11), 1318–1328.

Jacobson, N. S., Dobson, K. S., Truax, P. A., Addis, M. E., Koerner, K., Gollan, J. K., Gortner, E., & Prince, S. E. (1996). A component analysis of cognitive-behavioral treatment for depression. *Journal of Consulting and Clinical Psychology, 64* (2), 295–304.

Jakubczak, L. F., & Walters, R. H. (1959). Suggestibility as dependency behavior. *Journal of Abnormal and Social Psychology, 59,* 102–107.

Kagan, J., & Mussen, P. H. (1956). Dependency themes on the TAT and group conformity. *Journal of Consulting Psychology, 20,* 29–32.

Kanareff, V. T., & Lanzetta, J. T. (1960). Effects of task definition and probability of reinforcement upon the acquisition and extinction of imitative responses. *Journal of Experimental Psychology, 60,* 340–348.

Kaplan, H. I., & Saddock, B. J. (1988). *Synopsis of psychiatry: Behavioral sciences clinical psychiatry* (5th ed.). Baltimore: Williams & Wilkins.

Kazdin, A. E. (1975). *Behavior modification in applied settings.* Homewood, IL: Dorsey.

Kazdin, A. E. (1976). Effects of covert modeling, multiple models, and model reinforcement on assertive behavior. *Behavior Therapy, 7,* 211–212.

Kazdin, A. E. (1989). *Behavior modification in applied settings* (4th ed.). Pacific Grove, CA: Brooks/Cole.

Kazdin, A. E., & Krouse, R. (1983).The impact of variations in treatment rationales on expectancies for therapeutic change. *Behavior Therapy, 14,* 657–671.

Kazdin, A. E., & Wilcoxon, L. (1976). Systematic desensitization and nonspecific treatment effects: A methodological evaluation. *Psychological Bulletin, 83,* 729–758.

Keller, F. S. (1954). *Learning: Reinforcement theory.* New York: Random House.

Kimble, G. A. (1961). *Hilgard and Marquis' conditioning and learning* (2nd ed.). New York: Appleton-Century-Crofts.

King, N. I. (1993). Simple and social phobias. *Advances in Clinical Child Psychology, 15,* 305–341.

Koegel, R. L., & Rincover, A. (1977). Research on the difference between generalization and maintenance in extra-therapy responding. *Journal of Applied Behavior Analysis, 10,* 1–12.

Krapfl, J. E., & Nawas, M. M. (1969). Client-therapist relationship factor in systematic desensitization. *Journal of Consulting and Clinical Psychology, 33,* 435–439.

Krumboltz, J. D., & Thoresen, C. E. (1964). The effects of behavioral counseling in group and individual settings on information seeking behavior. *Journal of Counseling Psychology, 11,* 324–333.

Krumboltz, J. D., Varenhorst, B. B., & Thoresen, C. E. (1967). Nonverbal factors in the effectiveness of models in counseling. *Journal of Counseling Psychology, 14,* 412–418.

Ladoucer, R. (1983). Participant modeling with or without cognitive treatment for phobias. *Journal of Consulting and Clinical Psychology, 51,* 930–932.

Lalli, J. S., Casey, S., & Kates, K. (1995). Reducing escape behavior and increasing task completion with functional communication training, extinction and response chaining. *Journal of Applied Behavioral Analysis, 28,* 261–268.

Lauver, P. J., Kelly, S. D., & Froehle, T. C. (1971). Client reaction time and counselor verbal behavior in an interview setting. *Journal of Counseling Psychology, 18,* 26–30.

Lazarus, A. A. (1966). Behavior rehearsal vs. nondirective therapy, vs. advice in effecting behavior change. *Behavior Research and Therapy, 4,* 209–212.

Leitenberg, H., & Callahan, E. J. (1973). Reinforced practice and reduction of different kinds of fears in adults and children. *Behavior Research and Therapy, 11,* 19–30.

Lewis, S. A. (1974). A comparison of behavior therapy techniques in the reduction of fearful avoidance behavior. *Behavior Therapy, 5,* 648–655.

Lipke, H. J., & Botkin, A. L. (1992). Case studies of eye desensitization and reprocessing (EMDR) with chronic post-traumatic stress disorder. *Psychotherapy, 29* (4), 591–602.

Lohr, J. M., Kleinknecht, R. A., Tolin, D. F., & Barrett, R. H. (1995). The empirical status of the clinical applications of eye movement desensitization and reprocessing. *Journal of Therapy and Experimental Psychiatry, 26* (4), 285–302.

Lonnecker, C., Brady, M. P., McPherson, R., & Hawkins, J. (1994). Video self-modeling and cooperative classroom behavior in children with learning and behavior problems: Training and generalization effects. *Behavioral Disorders, 20* (1), 24–34.

Lott, D. R., & Murray, E. J. (1975). The effect of expectancy manipulation on outcomes in systematic desensitization. *Psychotherapy, 12,* 28–32.

Lundin, R. W. (1974). *Personality: A behavioral analysis* (2nd ed.). New York: Macmillan.

Maccoby, E. E., & Wilson, W. C. (1957). Identification and observational learning from films. *Journal of Abnormal and Social Psychology, 55,* 76–87.

Madsen, C., Jr. (1968). Nurturance and modeling in preschoolers. *Child Development, 39,* 221–236.

Mahoney, M. M. (1977). Reflection on the cognitive-learning trend in psychotherapy. *American Psychologist, 32* (1), 5–13.

Manning, B. H. (1991). *Cognitive self-instruction for classroom processes.* Albany: State University of New York Press.

Mash, E. J., & Barkley, R. A. (Eds.). (1989). *Treatment of childhood disorders.* New York: Guilford.

Mauro, B. C., & Mace, C. F. (1996). Differences in the effects of Pavlovian contingencies upon behavioral momentum using auditory versus visual stimuli. *Journal of the Experimental Analysis of Behavior, 65,* 289–399.

Mausner, B. (1953). Studies in social interaction: III. Effects of variation in one partner's prestige on the interaction of observer pairs. *Journal of Applied Psychology, 37,* 391–393.

Mausner, B. (1954a). The effects of one partner's success in a relevant task on the interaction of observer pairs. *Journal of Abnormal and Social Psychology, 49,* 557–560.

Mausner, B. (1954b). The effects of prior reinforcement on the interaction of observer pairs. *Journal of Abnormal and Social Psychology, 49,* 65–68.

Mausner, B., & Bloch, B. L. A. (1957). A study of the additivity of variables affecting social interaction. *Journal of Abnormal and Social Psychology, 54,* 250–256.

McDougall, W. (1908). *An introduction to social psychology.* London: Methuen.

McFall, R. M., & Twentyman, C. T. (1973). Four experiments on the relative contribution of rehearsal, modeling, and coaching to assertion training. *Journal of Abnormal Psychology, 8L,* 199–218.

Meichenbaum, D. (1993). Changing conceptions of cognitive-behavior modification: Retrospect and prospect. *Journal of Consulting and Clinical Psychology, 61* (2), 202–204.

Miller, R. C., & Berman, J. S. (1983). The efficacy of cognitive behavioral therapies: A quantitative review of the research evidence. *Psychological Bulletin, 94,* 39–53.

Miller, R. E., & Dollard, I. (1941). *Social learning and imitation.* New Haven, CT: Yale University Press.

Monti, P. M., Binkoff, I. A., Zwick, W. R., Abrams, D. B., Nirenberg, T. D., & Liepman, M. R. (1987). Reactivity of alcoholics and non-alcoholics to drinking cues. *Journal of Abnormal Psychology, 96* (2), 122–126.

Morgan, C. L. (1896). *Habit and instinct.* London: Edward Arnold.

Mount, R., Neziroglu, F., & Taylor, C. J. (1990). An obsessive-compulsive view of obesity and its treatment. *Journal of Clinical Psychology, 46* (1), 68–78.

Mowrer, O. H. (1960). *Learning theory and the symbolic processes.* New York: Wiley.

Mussen, P. H., & Parker, A. L. (1965). Mother nurturance and girls' incidental imitative learning. *Journal of Personality and Social Psychology, 2,* 94–97.

Naug, R. N. (1985). Rapid treatment of hiccups by operant conditioning method. *Journal of Personality and Clinical Studies, 1* (1–2), 69–71.

Nay, W. R. (1975). A systematic comparison of instructional techniques for parents. *Behavior Therapy, 6* (1), 14–21.

Niaura, R. S., Rohsenow, D. J., Binkoff, J. A., Monti, P. M., Pedraza, M., & Abrams, D. (1988). Relevance of cue reactivity to understanding alcohol and smoking relapse. *Journal of Abnormal Psychology, 97* (2), 133–152.

O'Connor, R. D. (1969). Modification of social withdrawal through symbolic modeling. *Journal of Applied Behavior Analysis, 2,* 15–22.

O'Connor, R. D. (1972). Relative efficacy of modeling, shaping and the combined procedure for modification of social withdrawal. *Journal of Abnormal Psychology, 79,* 327–334.

Osterhouse, R. A. (1976). Group systematic desensitization of test anxiety. In J. D. Krumboltz & C. E. Thoreson (Eds.), *Counseling methods* (pp. 269–279). New York: Holt, Rinehart and Winston.

Patterson, D. A., & Yaffe, J. (1993). Using computer-assisted instruction to teach Axis II of the DSM–III–R to social work students. Special issue: Empirical advances in social work assessment. *Research on Social Work Practice, 3* (3), 343–357.

Peterson, L., & Sobell, L. C. (1994). Introduction to the state-of-the-art review series: Research contributions to clinical assessment. *Behavior Therapy, 25,* 523–531.

Poulin, J. E., & Walter, C. A. (1990). Interviewing skills and computer assisted instruction: BSW student perceptions. *Computers in Human Services, 7* (3–4), 179–197.

Prochaska, J. O., DiClemente, C. C., & Norcross, J. C. (1992). In search of how people change: Applications to addictive behaviors. *American Psychologist, 47* (9), 1102–1114.

Rathus, S. A. (1973). Instigation of assertive behavior through videotape mediated assertive models and directed practice. *Behavior Research and Therapy, 11,* 57–65.

Richmond, M. E. (1965). *Social diagnosis.* New York: Free Press.

Rigsby-Eldredge, M., & McLaughlin, T. F. (1992). The effects of modeling and praise on self-initiated behavior across settings with two adolescent students with autism. *Journal of Developmental & Physical Disabilities, 4* (3), 205–218.

Ritter, B. (1968). The group treatment of children's snake phobias using vicarious and contact desensitization procedures. *Behavior Research and Therapy, 6,* 1–6.

Ronen, T., & Schecter, Y. (1991). The use of video simulation as a therapeutic tool in cognitive behavioral intervention for the treatment of enuresis: A case study. *Psychotherapy in Private Practice, 9* (3), 67–78.

Rosen, G. M. (1976). Subject's initial therapeutic expectancies and subject's awareness of therapeutic goals in systematic desensitization: A review. *Behavior Therapy, 7* (1), 14–27.

Rosen, J. C., Orosan, P., & Reiter, J. (1995). Cognitive behavior therapy for negative body image in obese women. *Behavior Therapy, 26* (1), 25–42.

Rosenbaum, M. E. (1956). The effects of stimulus and background factors on the volunteering response. *Journal of Abnormal and Social Psychology, 53,* 188–121.

Rosenbaum, M. E., & Blake, R. R. (1955). Volunteering as a function of field structure. *Journal of Abnormal and Social Psychology, 50,* 193–196.

Rosenbaum, M. E., & Tucker, I. F. (1962). The competence of the model and the learning of imitation and non-imitation. *Journal of Experimental Psychology, 63,* 183–190.

Rosenblith, J. R. (1959). Learning by imitation in kindergarten children. *Child Development, 30,* 60–80.

Rosenblith, J. R. (1961). Imitative color choices in kindergarten children. *Child Development, 32,* 211–223.

Rosenhan, D., & White, G. A. (1967). Observation and rehearsal as determinants of prosocial behavior. *Journal of Personality and Social Psychology, 5,* 424–431.

Rosenkrans, M. A., & Hartup, W. W. (1967). Imitative influences of consistent and inconsistent response consequences to a model on aggressive behavior in children. *Journal of Personality and Social Psychology, 7,* 429–434.

Rosenthal, T. L. (1976). Modeling therapies. In M. Hersen, R. M. Eisler, & P. M. Miller (Eds.), *Progress in behavior modification* (Vol. 2). New York: Academic.

Ross, D. (1966). Relationship between dependency, intentional learning, and incidental learning in preschool children. *Journal of Personality and Social Psychology, 4,* 374–381.

Schein, E. H. (1954). The effect of reward on adult imitative behavior. *Journal of Abnormal and Social Psychology, 49,* 389–395.

Schneider, W. J., & Nevid, J. S. (1993). Overcoming math anxiety: A comparison of stress inoculation training and systematic desensitization. *Journal of College Student Development, 34* (4), 283–288.

Seabury, B. A. (1993). Interactive video programs: Crisis counseling and organizational assessment. *Computers in Human Services, 9* (3–4), 301–310.

Seidel, R. W., Gusman, F. D., & Abueg, J. (1994). Theoretical and practical foundations of an inpatient post-traumatic stress disorder and alcoholism treatment program. *Psychotherapy, 11* (1), 67–78.

Shapiro, F. (1989a). Eye movement desensitization: A new treatment for post-traumatic stress disorder. *Journal of Behavior Therapy and Experimental Psychiatry, 20,* 211–217.

Shapiro, F. (1989b). Efficacy of the eye movement desensitization procedure in the treatment of traumatic memories. *Journal of Traumatic Stress, 23,* 199–223.

Skinner, B. F. (1953). *Science and human behavior.* New York: Macmillan.

Skinner, B. F. (1966). Contingencies of reinforcement in the design of a culture. *Behavioral Science, 11,* 159–166.

Skinner, B. F. (1969). *Contingencies of reinforcement.* New York: Appleton-Century-Crofts.

Skinner, B. F. (1971). *Beyond freedom and dignity.* New York: Bantam Books.

Smith, S. W., Siegel, E. M., O'Connor, A. M., & Thomas, S. B. (1994). Effects of cognitive behavioral training on angry behavior and aggression of three elementary-aged students. *Behavioral Disorders, 19* (2), 126–135.

Snell, M. E., & Zirpoli, T. J. (1987). Intervention strategies. In M. E. Snell (Ed.), *Systematic instruction of persons with severe handicaps.* Columbus, OH: Merrill/Macmillan.

Strathman, A., Gleicher, F., Boninger, D. S., & Edwards, C. S. (1994). The consideration of future consequences: Weighing immediate and distant outcomes of behavior. *Journal of Personality and Social Psychology, 66* (4), 742–752.

Strumpf, J. A., & Fodor, I. (1993). The treatment of test anxiety in elementary school-age children: Review and recommendations. *Child & Family Behavior Therapy, 15* (4), 19–42.

Sundel, S. S. (1994). Videotaped training of job-related social skills using peer modeling: An evaluation of social validity. *Research on Social Work Practice, 4* (1), 40–52.

Svartdal, F. (1995). When feedback contingencies and rules compete: Testing a boundary condition of instrumental performance. *Learning and Motivation, 26,* 221–238.

Thyer, B. A. (1992). A behavioral perspective on human development. In M. Bloom (Ed.), *Changing lives: Studies in human development and professional helping* (pp. 410–418). Columbia, SC: University of South Carolina Press.

Thyer, B. A. (2000). Editorial: Social work research at the turn of the millennium: Progress and challenges. *Research on Social Work Practice, 10* (1), 9–14.

Thyer, B. A., & Hudson, W. W. (1987). Progress in behavioral social work: An introduction. *Journal of Social Service Research, 10* (2/3/4), 1–6.

Thyer, B. A., & Wodarski, J. S. (1990). Social learning theory: Toward a comprehensive conceptual framework for social work education. *Social Service Review, 64* (1), 144–152.

Trade, G. (1903). *The laws of imitation.* New York: Holt.

Traunt, G. S. (1995). Therapeutic models of psychopathology. Part III: The influence of activators, biological factors, and the childhood environment on the psychological organization. *American Journal of Psychotherapy, 49* (1), 19–27.

Verplank, W. S. (1955). The control and content of conversation: Reinforcement of statement of opinion. *Journal of Abnormal and Social Psychology, 51,* 668–676.

Wahler, R. G. (1969). Selling generality: Some specific and general effects of child behavior therapy. *Journal of Applied Behavior Analysis, 2,* 239–248.

Walker, W. R., Freeman, R. F., & Christensen, D. K. (1994). Restricting Environmental Stimulation (REST) to enhance cognitive behavioral treatment for obsessive-compulsive disorder with schizotypal personality disorder. *Behavior Therapy, 25,* 709–719.

Watson, J. B., & Rayner, R. (1920). Conditioned emotional reaction. *Journal of Experimental Psychology, 3,* 1–14.

Wheeler, L. (1966). Toward a theory of behavioral contagion. *Psychological Review, 73,* 179–192.

Wilkins, W. (1971). Desensitization: Social and cognitive factors underlying the effectiveness of Wolfe's procedure. *Psychological Bulletin, 76,* 311–317.

Wilson, C. C., Robertson, S. J., Herlong, L. H., & Haynes, S. N. (1979). Vicarious effects of time-out in the modification of aggression in the classroom. *Behavior Modification, 3,* 97–111.

Wodarski, J. S. (1976). Procedural steps in the implementation of behavior modification programs in open settings. *Journal of Behavior Therapy and Experimental Psychiatry, 7,* 133–136.

Wodarski, J. S. (1980). Procedures for the maintenance and generalization of achieved behavioral change. *Journal of Sociology and Social Welfare, 7* (2), 298–311.

Wodarski, J. S. (1983). Clinical practice and the social learning paradigm. *Social Work, 28* (2), 152–160.

Wodarski, J. S. (1997). *Research methods for clinical social workers.* New York: Springer.

Wodarski, J. S., & Bagarozzi, D. A. (1979). *Behavioral social work.* New York: Human Sciences.

Wodarski, J. S., Feldman, R. A., & Flax, N. (1974). Group therapy and anti-social children: A social learning theory perspective. *Small Group Behavior, 5* (2), 182–210.

Woldwitz, H. M. (1975). Therapist warmth: Necessary or sufficient conditions invivo desensitization. *Journal of Counseling and Clinical Psychology, 43,* 584–586.

Wong, S. E., Woolsey, I. E., & Gallegos, E. (1987). Behavioral treatment of chronic psychiatric patients. *Progress in Behavioral Social Work, 10* (2/3/4), 7–35.

Yates, A. J. (1975). *Theory and practice in behavior therapy.* New York: Wiley.

Zirpoli, T. J., & Melloy, K. I. (1993). *Behavior management: Applications for teachers and parents.* New York: Merrill/Macmillan.

## CHAPTER 7

# Social Exchange Theory in Understanding Human Growth and Development

## Lisa Rapp-Paglicci

As individuals grow and develop most professionals agree that much of what occurs can be explained from a conceptual framework that emphasizes the occurrence of social exchanges. Traditionally, social exchange theory has been used to understand topics as diverse as the exchanges between individuals that can lead to divorce, to the complex power relationships in organizations and communities. In general when looking directly at the social work literature, it becomes clear that social exchange theory has been underutilized and possibly ill applied. There may be many reasons for this limited usage; however, it appears that regardless of the reasons the lack of utility within the field of social work ultimately questions theoretical usefulness for direct application. For some social workers this resistance toward utility may be related to misunderstandings or possibly genuine disagreements with what the theory postulates. These authors, however, stress the need for reexamination of this issue, particularly the behavioral basis of social exchange theory. Studies have shown that the postulates of social exchange theory can easily be integrated with other theories, resulting in a wide range of applications and important implications for contributing to the understanding of human development and behavior (Lawler & Thye, 1999).

The editors would like to thank Eileen Lysaught for earlier contributions to this chapter.

# LEARNING THEORY

Since social exchange theory is composed of different theories and approaches toward learning, it is essential that the reader have a rudimentary understanding of three basic approaches: (a) classical conditioning, (b) operant learning, and (c) social learning theory.

The classical conditioning or respondent paradigm suggested by Glaser (1971) postulated that two events, which occur close together in time, could have similar effects on the response of the organism. This was highlighted in Pavlov's experiments in the early 1900s and lead to the recognition and foundation of the classical conditioning paradigm (Kimble, 1961). In his work, meat powder—the unconditioned stimulus, and a bell—a neutral stimulus, were paired closely in time to stimulate salivation. After repeated trials, the bell became a sufficient conditioned stimulus that alone could cause salivation. This was termed the conditioned response. In this way respondent conditioning can explain the relationship between seemingly nonrelated events. Conditioning or modifying an individual, group, or community's behavior is clearly important in the therapeutic process and is a critical part of exchange theory.

Operant or instrumental learning is based on B. F. Skinner's classic animal experiments (1938), and focuses on those discriminative stimuli preceding an event and the consequences that follow (Guttman, 1977). This learning paradigm (also called trial and error) asserts that learners behave in their environment and receive consequences for their actions. The basic types of consequences are positive and negative reinforcement and punishments. Reinforcements increase the probability of behavior occurring, while nonrewarding and punishing consequences decrease the probability of the behavior occurring (Long, Hammack, May, & Campbell, 1958; Salzinger, 1969). The frequency and regularity of punishments and reinforcements are known as "schedules of reinforcement" (Long et al., 1958; Salzinger, 1969).

## The Use of Reinforcement Schedules and Punishment

Since social exchange theory is predicated on basic behavioral theories, the importance of reinforcement schedules must be emphasized and delineated. Schedules of reinforcement determine how, and with what frequency, various behaviors will be reinforced. When appropriately designed, schedules of reinforcement elicit desired behaviors and help to maintain those behaviors at desired rates. The five basic schedules of reinforcement are: (a) continuous, (b) fixed-interval, (c) fixed ratio, (d) variable-ratio, and (e) variable-interval.

When individuals are reinforced every time they exhibit a desired behavior, then an individual is on a *continuous* reinforcement schedule. This is the simplest of all the schedules and usually results in a high rate of the desired behavior for a limited time period (Elkind, 1971). Caution, however, should be utilized when the reinforcement of every desired response is met to avoid satiation or a reduction in the power of the reward.

A *fixed-interval* reinforcement schedule rewards desired behaviors only after a fixed period of time. This schedule reduces desired behaviors when the next reinforcement interval is not soon and increases desired behaviors when the next reinforcement interval is approaching (Bachrach, 1962). In other words, individuals exhibit desired behaviors only when reinforcement is proximal. An individual on a *variable-interval* schedule receives reinforcement after time periods that are randomly selected. This schedule has been more effective than the fixed-interval schedule, especially with children (Long et al., 1958).

A *fixed-ratio* schedule reinforces individuals each time they produce a certain number of desired responses, and the number of desired responses necessary to receive a reward usually increase overtime. Individuals perform at a high rate on this schedule until the number of expected responses becomes so high that the rewards no longer outweigh the costs.

The *variable-ratio* schedule reinforces individuals after a number of appropriate behaviors have been emitted. The difference between this and the fixed ratio schedule is that the number of responses necessary to secure a reward is varied. This schedule is effective in producing the desired behavior in children (Orlando & Bijou, 1960).

These reinforcement schedules may be used singly or in different combinations to reinforce or discourage behaviors. Multiple schedules of reinforcement are probably at work, even when behavior appears simple. Acknowledging these complexly interacting schedules can bring new insight into social exchanges.

Punishment is usually part of any discussion involving the behavioral theories. Although punishment can be of use in reducing undesirable behaviors, its use should be infrequent. Research has consistently indicated that punishment is much less effective than reinforcement in reducing undesirable behaviors (Azoulay, 1999; Miller & Rollnick, 1991). Consequently, positive or negative reinforcement should be preferred over punishment.

## Learning Through Modeling

The basic postulate of the modeling paradigm, commonly known as social learning theory, is that individuals learn to mimic or replicate common behaviors within their social environment (Bandura, 1977, 1986). Social learning theory emphasizes the influence of cognitive processes in controlling, acquiring, and maintaining behavior. The leading social learning theorist, Albert Bandura, contends that traditional theories of learning generally depict behavior as a product of directly experienced behavioral consequences (Bandura, 1977). However, he states that much of learning can occur through observations of other people's behavior and its consequences. Social learning theory places a greater emphasis on cognitive variables than do the respondent and operant models, in that the individual learns overt behavior as well as covert thoughts, attitudes, and ideas from others (Parke, 1972). In other words, an individual may observe and learn the technique of smoking marijuana, in addition to the attitudes, beliefs, and opinions about the behavior. For example, "it's not a hard-core drug" or "I'm not hurting anyone." Although reinforcement is not mandatory for social learning to occur, it does increase the probability that the individual will perform the behavior.

In summary, the three paradigms are learning theories that are often used in social exchange theory: (a) the respondent paradigm focuses on the association between events, (b) the operant emphasizes the antecedents and (c) consequences and their relationships in controlling behavior, and modeling delineates cognitive processes and their role in learning new behaviors (Lysaught, Rapp, Wodarski, & Feit, 1999).

## SOCIAL EXCHANGE THEORY

When described in its most simple form, social exchange theory, in essence, is a conceptualization about relationships or social interactions among two or more people. All human beings feel the need to have and develop relationships, yet, while in these relationships individuals strive to maximize their rewards while minimizing their costs (Cate, 1981). Rewards can be defined broadly and can include an extensive range of commodities, resources, and skills that may or may not be tangible. For example, rewards may be money, material goods, information, praise, positive regard, gratitude, or anything else that satisfies human needs or desires. Social exchange theory suggests that social interactions be patterned by the knowledge that all human beings can control and disburse rewards (LaValle, 1999). To obtain rewards, however, an individual must provide something in exchange. This interactional process is viewed as a series of behavioral, material, and social exchanges occurring among two or more parties (Lysaught et al., 1999; Specht, 1986). Each individual evaluates the costs and rewards associated with interaction, and determines if the rewards are greater than the costs. In most cases it becomes obvious how most individuals choose to interact in more rewarding relationships and tend to avoid the less profitable exchanges. Some proponents of social exchange theory see such calculations as normal and natural for social development and therefore they are viewed as primary determinants of relational behavior. Though the emphasis may vary on how much emphasis should be placed on these exchanges, most professionals agree that recognition of social exchange behaviors remain important variables for assessment in human growth and behavior, which can lead to a richer understanding of the complex dynamics that surround human relationships.

## Power Exchanges

The mutual dependence of individuals on one another for rewards or reinforcers provides the primary basis for power relations (Molm, Quist, & Wisely, 1994). Power is an attribute of any relationship and is measured by A's dependence on B, and B's dependence on A. If both parties are equally dependent on each other their power is balanced. Unequal dependence produces imbalanced power. The greater the power imbalance in an exchange relationship, the more unequal the exchange will be (Markovsky, Willer, & Patton, 1988). The individual with the power advantage may receive more resources at a smaller cost, while the individual with the power disadvantage may receive fewer resources at a greater cost.

Although the use of punishment is not recommended in exchange relationships where equality and balance are favored, punishment still occurs. Molm et al. (1994) state that individuals' capacities to provide negative outcomes for another is called their punishment power. This power is separate from their reinforcement power, or capacity to provide rewards. For instance, a social worker may hold reinforcement power (interventions for the problem, verbal praise, etc.) as well as punishment power (the ability to call child protective services) over the client. The manner in which individuals use their reinforcement and punishment power determines the type of exchange and subsequently the type of relationship they will have.

Social workers tend to have more reinforcement and punishment power than their clients do. Most of this power is assigned to social workers simply because of their perceived authority. Authority is power, and is viewed by most of society as valid and legitimate (Martin, 1981). Typical examples of legitimate authority are: teacher-student, physician-patient, and social worker–client. Martin alleges that a professional-client relationship is, by its very nature, a power relationship. This must be addressed immediately upon initiation of the client–social worker relationship. The social worker's power must be mediated so that clients perceive their own power to be as equal to the social worker's as possible.

## SOCIAL EXCHANGE THEORY AND SOCIAL WORK PRACTICE

The knowledge and benefit that can be gained from understanding the relationship between human behavior and social exchange theory is pronounced, though it is infrequently discussed as part of the knowledge base for the field of social work. These authors believe that the social exchange theory is actually an essential theory for all levels of social work practice. Some of the applications of social exchange theory to social work practice are discussed next.

### Micro-Level Practice

Social exchange theory provides a useful conceptualization of the development and maintenance of the relationship between the social worker and the client. Research has indicated that the most effective tool for provoking change in clients is the therapeutic relationship (Beutler, Machado, & Neufeldt, 1994). Actually, for social workers the development of a therapeutic relationship is not very different from the development of interpersonal relationships (Altman & Taylor, 1973; Levinger & Snoek, 1972). Basically, it is believed that the decision to form a therapeutic relationship is based on the client's belief that the client will receive more rewards than punishments from the interaction (Molm et al., 1994; Tracy, 1995). The client should see the relationship as a mutually cooperative endeavor characterized by increased intimacy, self-disclosure, open communications, empathic understanding, and mutual satisfaction. When clients feel the exchanges are rewarding, or at least equitable, they will perceive their rewards as proportional to their investment in the therapeutic process, and this sense of satisfaction will support the advancement of the therapeutic process. When therapy is conceptualized in this fashion, each step in the process is seen as being preceded by a decision to continue or to terminate the association. If costs appear to outweigh benefits, termination of the relationship is likely. The use of punishment in social exchanges must be utilized prudently because it may eliminate future exchange completely if one party is threatened or perceives the other as aversive.

Social workers are able to provide multiple rewards for their clients. They can provide support, empathy, eye contact, verbal encouragement, effective interventions, and ultimately improvement on the presenting problem. In return, clients can provide verbal interaction, motivation for improvement, appreciation, follow-through on their treatment plan, and finally an improvement on their presenting problem. Social exchanges work to reinforce and encourage the client to initiate and continue in the counseling process. For instance, the social worker may utilize positive, supportive verbal comments to reinforce clients' discussions of their problems. In turn, clients may show an appreciation of the social worker's nonjudgmental attitude toward them. This reinforces the social worker to continue the desired behavior. This cycle is the process of social exchange.

The first few exchanges within a counseling situation are crucial, because these determine the client's sense of whether the counseling situation and this relationship in particular will provide more rewards than punishments. In general, the client's evaluation of the social worker's behavior is usually more critical than the social worker's evaluation of the client's behavior. That is because the social worker has been trained to expect fewer reinforcements from the client than the client expects to receive from the social worker. Thus, in the initial interactions, the social worker should provide a continuous schedule of reinforcement along with little or no punishment, and have an expectation of few rewards for themselves.

As the therapeutic relationship continues, expectations about long-term benefits will be established, and reinforcement will no longer need to occur on a continuous basis. Instead, reinforcement can be exchanged on a ratio or interval basis, with both client and social worker being satisfied that reinforcement will occur in the future. For example, the client may not need to have strong, positive verbal reinforcement from the social worker throughout the entire session, as long as this type of reinforcement is provided at the end of the session. The social worker who uses the principles of social exchange theory at the beginning of the therapeutic encounter will have established a pattern of exchange and an expectation in the client that reinforcement will be provided even if it is not instantaneous. Some reinforcing aspects of the relationship, however, would need to be more or less continuously present, such as attentive listening, eye contact, and empathy.

Power is a very significant variable within the relationship. Most therapeutic relationships tend to be unequal because social workers generally have more resources at their disposal and therefore have more power. It is important that the client does not believe that the social worker can control *all* of the reinforcements. Clients should feel that they also have rewards to exchange. Clinicians should attempt to reduce the power differential between themselves and the client by encouraging client participation in the therapeutic relationship and by encouraging and implementing the client's choices about treatment (Makoba, 1993; Miller & Rollnick, 1991; Tracy, 1995).

## Mezzo-Level Practice

Whether the social worker is working with an individual, family, or group, social exchange elements will be utilized to develop a therapeutic relationship. When working with mezzo systems such as groups or families, this task becomes more complex because multiple relationships are being developed and nurtured at the same time. In these situations, the social worker must develop a positive relationship with each member of the group or family, and each member must develop or strengthen their relationship with the others. As stated previously, relationships develop through reciprocal exchanges, and these exchanges require time, resources, and energy that may then take away from exchanges with others. In other words, when the social worker is developing a therapeutic relationship with one client, the social worker may be unable to develop another relationship with an additional person at the same time. The social worker may also not have enough resources to exchange with another person, or may not have the energy left to interact. Furthermore, social exchange interactions between two people may inhibit other exchanges. For instance, a member may feel jealous or angry about the social worker's interactions with others. This can be a serious problem in maintaining a group, since undesirable exchanges may induce group members to leave the group or provoke family members to refrain from therapy.

In addition to handling exchanges between themselves and each client, social workers must interact with the entire group or family. The group or family as a system must interact reciprocally with the social worker. The social worker's objective is to make sure the benefits of this interaction outweigh the costs so members do not leave the therapeutic situation prematurely.

Blau (1974) suggests that to become a part of a group, a potential member must be attracted to the group as well as be attractive to the other members. In other words, the potential reinforcement power that a member has to offer must be displayed and then examined by the group members. Group members must determine if these rewards will be worth the costs involved. Negative qualities, flaws, or inept skills are usually, initially concealed from the group (Early, 1992). Likewise, group members must exhibit the potential reinforcement power that the group can offer a member. The individual must evaluate these potential rewards and determine if they are worth the costs of membership in the group.

Most clients in group therapy have had difficulty with social interaction in prior relations. Clients bring a history of unprofitable social exchanges with relatives, friends, coworkers, and so forth into the therapeutic situation. Social exchange theory offers social workers a means of teaching clients new social skills. Social workers may use social exchange principles to teach clients about the theory of social exchange. In so doing, social workers model appropriate social interactions with others, highlighting the costs and benefits of each interaction. The social worker also mediates and facilitates the social interactions of clients with one another.

Family members are more complex to work with than group members are, since families bring their history of negative social interactions with them into the office. Again an important goal for the social worker is to assist clients in modifying their ineffectual social exchanges. Sometimes these negative exchanges have been developed and reinforced for years and appear to be beneficial for the family members (Call, Finch, Huck, & Kane, 1999; Ruben, 1998). Upon closer examination, however, these exchanges are not rewarding for all the members and therefore must be modified.

A marital dyad can be considered similar in structure and function to a group. Marital partners constantly assess the costs and benefits of their relationship. However, the benefits and costs in a marriage include more than just the social interaction. For instance, household goods, religious values, economic status, and children are all perceived as resources for a couple. When interactional costs outweigh benefits, couples usually dissolve their relationship (Donovan & Jackson, 1990). Power equity is very important between couples. Too much power held by one individual creates a power disparity that allows one person to leave the relationship more easily than the other. The social worker's tasks include equaling power and assisting the couple in learning more profitable exchanges.

Mezzo practice, similar to micro practice, requires social workers to mediate power differentials between themselves and the group or family members. The group or family therapy situation, however, may not provide the social worker with as much reinforcement power as micro practice. The group or family members actually hold a large amount of power or rewards. For example, the social worker is not the only one who can provide verbal praise to an individual client; other group or family members are capable of providing this reinforcer and may be seen as more significant and influential to the individual than the social worker.

Power differentials may also need to be mediated among clients. Change takes time to occur and, before clients have mastered profitable social interaction, negative or unequal social exchanges may take place within the group. The social worker is expected to assist clients in avoiding the repetition of negative interactions and to help them change those interactions into profitable ones. This cannot be done if clients continue interactions with one another in ways that are not effective and equitable. Social workers in mezzo practice must focus not only on social exchanges with individual clients, but also on interactions between themselves and the client system and on clients' interactions with one another. System's theory is a useful addition to social exchange theory in struggling with these complexities. In addition, power differentials must always be reconciled.

## Macro-Level Practice (Communities and Organizations)

As the client system becomes larger the number and complexity of social exchanges is amplified. The social worker again may use social exchange theories to initially develop positive, reciprocal relationships with large groups in communities and organizations. As in mezzo practice, social exchanges occur between the social worker and each individual group member as well as between the entire group and the social worker. The group also participates in social exchanges with the macro system.

The macro system itself is made up of smaller systems. For instance, within a community there are educational, health care, political, economic, and legal systems. Within an organization there are marketing, advertising, finance, and accounting departments (Emerson, 1976). These smaller systems are based on social exchanges. For example, the health care system is made up of hospitals, HMOs, clinics, and pharmacies; these organizations exchange needed resources to keep the system and each subsystem functioning.

The individual subsystems also maintain social exchange relationships with other subsystems. For instance, in most communities the educational system and the economic system exchange needed resources, as do the accounting and the marketing departments of an organization. These subsystems rely on this exchange and interdependence with others (Levine & White, 1961).

As social workers join the system and attempt to make changes, they must work within the systems' rules and boundaries. Social exchange assessment should focus on the exchanges that occur within and between subsystems or organizational departments (Emerson, 1976). Before this information is understood little progress can be made. The social worker must develop a relationship with the system and may utilize social exchange theorems to do so effectively.

Groups (i.e., citizens support groups, task-related groups) who are interested in modifying systems can be aided by an awareness of social exchange theory and its implications for systems and organizations. For these groups, understanding the environment and the relationships that will have to develop with each system before interventions can be initiated is a necessary practice skill (MacNair, 1981). Intervention into these systems require the development of exchanges that are more effective, efficient, and equitable. Groups must remember that a system probably will not develop a new social exchange relationship if the new relationship does not provide more benefits than the previous relationship. MacNair found that groups must also recognize that in most instances the community system or the organization will have more power than they have. This power must be mediated. In fact, power must be close to equitable or fairly balanced for the group to have any influence on the macro system. Otherwise, the community or organization will be able to ignore the interests of the group. When power is not equitable and social exchange relationships are not developed, conflict will often result (see MacNair; Maypole & Wright, 1979). Conflictual and competitive relationships are rarely profitable for either party, and macro change is rarely achieved in such circumstances, according to Maypole and Wright.

Work with communities and organizations can be quite complex because social exchanges within and between systems-departments must be constantly assessed and modified. Social workers can educate social action groups about social exchange theory and system's theory. These theories can then guide the assessment and intervention process. Reciprocal relationships must be developed within the change group, as well as between the group and the intended target systems. Without positive relationships, little progress can be made. The vision of a new social exchange relationship can motivate and facilitate systems change. As stated previously, no system will change unless there is a benefit to the change.

## CHANGING HUMAN BEHAVIORS

Overall, besides affecting the therapeutic relationship, social exchange theory is an important model to use in assessment and intervention. As social exchange occurs in the clinical situation, it also occurs in the daily interactions that clients have with the people in their environment. Clients constantly engage in social exchanges with different individuals, groups, organizations, and so forth. Social exchange theory can assist social workers in their efforts to assess clients and modify their ineffective and maladaptive behaviors. Clients can be taught social exchange theory and can be reinforced when they utilize effective social behaviors. This approach helps empower clients in their daily lives.

This approach can be easily integrated with system's theory, which suggests that clients engage in multiple, interacting systems in their daily lives. Social exchange theory simply helps clients conceptualize how to interact with these multiple systems in an effective manner. Social exchange theory adds a concrete, behavioral component to the vagueness of systems theory. For instance, system's theory asserts that systems are established and maintained on input and output functions. Social exchange theory would enhance this statement by specifying the type of interaction or exchange that reinforces the development or maintenance of the system. Both theories are helpful in understanding human behavior.

The social exchange model provides a framework that incorporates elements of many major learning paradigms—respondent, operant, and modeling. It provides a framework for viewing the social worker–client system as an interactional, reciprocal exchange process. Social work practice has often conceptualized treatment as a one-way process in which the clinician solely influences the client. The social exchange model emphasizes the interdependent influence of client and social worker behaviors. In addition, social exchange theory reminds social workers that power differentials must be mediated for the therapeutic relationship to be effective in inciting change. It is useful in assessing clients' behaviors and in helping empower them to be more effective in their daily lives.

## SOCIAL WORKER BURNOUT

For many social workers in the field, the word *burnout* is no stranger. For many social workers, job-related stress that is left unattended can lead to burnout. In terms of research, though burnout is known to exist, the definition of what it involves can vary. Therefore, the events that constitute burnout in one social worker may not have the same effect on another social worker. The diverse and varied circumstances that surround burnout make it difficult and subjective phenomena to address and it is no surprise that few have evaluated and looked closely at this issue. This lack of clarity, however, can prove to be fertile ground, and utilizing social exchange theory may assist in the explanation of this phenomenon. As mentioned previously, social workers consider relationship development as paramount, and, in trying to ensure that this process continues throughout the helping relationship, the social worker may face considerable pressure to either initiate or develop the relationships with all clients. In fact, the onus of the relationship development rests with social workers since they have been trained to complete this process and as professional helpers are being paid to do so. Consequently, in productive relationship fostering and building, the social worker must exert more effort and provide more reinforcers than the client. For some, the creation of this seemingly unbalanced relationship can be stressful and frustrating.

To continue relationship growth the social worker is expected to exert more effort in the maintenance of the relationship. After all, the social worker has been trained to tolerate negative client behaviors and is required to do so in all but the most dangerous circumstances. In contrast, clients who consider relationship important can simply terminate treatment if they find the relationship is not reinforcing. Consequently, social workers must supply many more rewards, especially in the beginning, to the relationship than they are receiving. Furthermore, when client termination occurs early it often happens in the first few sessions when the development of the relationship is emerging. Many times, social workers provide considerable energy, effort, and reinforcements to the client, only to have clients terminate treatment before the social worker is reinforced in turn. For the social work practitioner this dismissal may result in frustration, anger, and eventual burnout.

As the relationship develops and the client starts to benefit from treatment, the social worker begins to receive more rewards. However, those rewards are never equal to the rewards received by the client. For example, the client may have a reduction in depression, an increased pleasure in work and home life, and an increase in productive sleep. The social worker may receive satisfaction from the job, gratitude from the client, and praise from the client's family members. Although these rewards are pleasant, they are not an equal exchange for the amount of effort exerted into the relationship nor are they equal to the reinforcers the client received.

A study by Dressel, Waters, Sweat, and Clayton (1990) found that worker burnout occurred when social workers were unaware that their relationships with clients would, for the most part, require more energy (at least initially) for fewer rewards. In other words, those workers who acknowledged and predicted this unequal relationship were less likely to experience work stress, anxiety, frustration and anger as opposed to those workers who did not expect this unbalanced reciprocity (Dressel, Waters, Sweat, & Clayton).

Social exchange theory suggests that social work burnout can be reduced when social workers are trained to initially expect unequal relationships with their clients and a delay in rewards until later in the therapeutic process. To successfully prepare students for the field of social work, schools of social work have a responsibility to educate future social workers about the stress and inequality of therapeutic relationships.

## SUMMARY

Social exchange theory, though often underutilized, can provide an effective theoretical foundation for understanding growth and development for human interaction patterns. This theory can be used to explain and predict behavior in therapeutic relationships, mitigate social worker burnout, and guide intervention strategies at all levels of social work practice. The behavioral basis of this empirically based theory facilitates its integration with other frequently used theories, such as system's theory. Social exchange theory should not replace other practice modalities that social workers utilize. Rather, it can be used either as the theoretical basis of the therapeutic relationship or as one of many intervention strategies. Further research is needed to develop the conceptual framework of social exchange theory and expand its social work applications.

## REFERENCES

Altman, I., & Taylor, D. (1973). *Social penetration: The development of interpersonal relationships*. New York: Holt, Rhinehart, & Winston.

Azoulay, D. (1999). Encouragement and logical consequences versus rewards and punishment: A reexamination. *Journal of Individual Psychology, 55* (1), 91–99.

Bachrach, A. (1962). *Experimental foundations of clinical psychology*. New York: Basic Books.

Bandura, A. (1977). Cognitive processes mediating behavioral change. *Journal of Personality and Social Psychology, 35* (3), 125–139.

Bandura, A. (1986). *Social foundations of thought and action: A social cognitive theory*. Englewood Cliffs, NJ: Prentice-Hall.

Beutler, L., Machado, P., & Neufeldt, S. (1994). Therapist variables. In A. Bergin & S. Garfield (Eds.), *Handbook of psychotherapy and behavior change* (pp. 229–269). New York: John Wiley & Sons.

Blau, P. (1974). *On the nature of organizations*. New York: John Wiley & Sons.

Call, K., Finch, M., Huck, S., & Kane, R. (1999). Caregiver burden from a social exchange perspective: Caring for older people after hospital discharge. *Journal of Marriage and Family, 61* (3), 688–699.

Cate, R. (1981). An interpersonal resource exchange program for couples. *Social Casework: The Journal of Contemporary Social Work, 62* (4), 210–217.

Donovan, R., & Jackson, B. (1990). Deciding to divorce: A process guided by social exchange, attachment and cognitive dissonance theories. *Journal of Divorce, 13* (4), 23–35.

Dressel, P., Waters, M., Sweat, M., & Clayton, O. (1990). Exchange rules in the mediation of social welfare work. *Journal of Sociology & Social Welfare, 17* (4), 75–97.

Early, B. (1992). An ecological-exchange model of social work consultation within the work group of the school. *Social Work in Education, 14* (4), 207–214.

Elkind, D. (Ed.). (1971). *Learning: An introduction.* Genview, IL: Scott and Foresman.

Emerson, R. (1976). Social exchange theory. In M. Rosenberg & R. Turner (Eds.), *Social psychology: Sociological perspectives* (pp. 30–65). New York: Basic Books.

Glaser, R. (Ed.). (1971). *The nature of reinforcement.* New York: Academic.

Guttman, N. (1977). On Skinner and Hull: A reminiscence and projection. *American Psychologist, 32,* 321–328.

Kimble, G. (1961). *Hilgard and Marquis' "Conditioning and Learning."* New York: General Learning.

LaValle, D. (1999). Different types of social exchange: Homans, Becker and Parsons. Utilitarianism and rational choice in Sociology. *Studi di Sociologia, 37* (1), 3–23.

Lawler, E., & Thye, S. (1999). Bringing emotions into social exchange theory. *Annual Review of Sociology, 25,* 217–244.

Levine, S., & White, P. (1961). Exchange as a conceptual framework for the study of interorganizational relationships. *Administration Science Quarterly, 5,* 583–601.

Levinger, G., & Snoek, J. (1972). *Attraction in relationships: A new look at interpersonal attraction.* New York: General Learning.

Long, E., Hammack, J., May, F., & Campbell, B. (1958). Intermittent reinforcement of operant behavior in children. *Journal of Experimental Analysis of Behavior, 1* (4), 315–339.

Lysaught, E., Rapp, L., Wodarski, J., & Feit, M. (1999). An integrated human behavior theory: The exchange model. *Journal of Human Behavior in the Social Environment, 2* (3), 29–54.

MacNair, R. (1981). Citizen participation as a balanced exchange: An analysis and strategy. *Journal of the Community Development Society, 12* (1), 1–19.

Makoba, J. (1993). Toward a general theory of social exchange. *Social Behavior and Personality, 21* (3), 227–240.

Markovsky, B., Willer, D., & Patton, T. (1988). Power relations in exchange networks. *American Sociological Review, 53,* 220–236.

Martin, P. (1981). A critical analysis of power in professional-client relations. *Arete, 6* (3), 35–48.

Maypole, D., & Wright, W. (1979). The integration of services of a medical clinic and a community mental health center in a rural area. *Social Work in Health Care, 4* (3), 299–308.

Miller, W., & Rollnick, S. (1991). *Motivational interviewing: Preparing people to change addictive behavior.* New York: Guilford.

Molm, L., Quist, T., & Wisely, P. (1994). Imbalanced structures, unfair strategies: Power and justice in social exchange. *American Sociological Review, 59,* 98–121.

Orlando, R., & Bijou, S. (1960). Single and multiple schedules of reinforcement in developmentally retarded children. *Journal of Experimental Analysis of Behavior, 4,* 339–348.

Parke, R. (Ed.). (1972). *Recent trends in social language theory.* New York: Academic.

Ruben, D. (1998). Social exchange theory: Dynamics of a system governing the dysfunctional family and guide to assessment. *Journal of Contemporary Psychotherapy, 28* (3), 307–325.

Salzinger, K. (1969). The place of operant conditioning of verbal behaviors in psychotherapy. In C. Franks (Ed.), *Behavior therapy: Appraisal and status.* New York: McGraw-Hill.

Skinner, B. F. (1938). *The behavior of organisms.* Englewood Cliffs, NJ: Prentice-Hall.

Specht, H. (1986). Social support, social networks, social exchange, and social work practice. *Social Service Review, 60* (3), 218–240.

Tracy, L. (1995). Negotiation: An emergent process of living systems. *Behavioral Science, 40,* 41–55.

## CHAPTER 8

# Introduction to Human Behavior: Group-Level Variables

## Karen D. Smith, Claudia M. Leo, and Elaine M. Maccio

In the past the majority of clients that received services in social work practice were seen on an individual basis. Yet, a changing environment has challenged practitioners to develop effective strategies for prevention and treatment of most social and psychological problems (Corey, 1995). In many instances, groups represent a natural forum for treatment and prevention in social and professional arenas. Therefore, groups have become an avenue to influence human behavior and to provide a network for problem solving.

The provision of service in the group setting allows for an interactional situation that typifies many kinds of daily interactions. The behaviors learned in the group setting can empower people for better participation in larger society while helping them to learn social skills necessary to secure reinforcement (Feldman & Wodarski, 1975; Henry, 1992; Wodarski, 1981). Groups offer a forum for members to address issues and to participate in collective decision making, allowing for feedback from others (Brandler & Roman, 1991; Corey, 1995; Henry, 1992). According to social learning theory, when a behavior is learned as in a group context, it is likely to come under the control of a greater number of discriminative stimuli. This allows for greater generalization and maintenance of the behavior for a broader variety of interactional contexts.

In social work practice, utilizing groups as an intervention format can allow for service to a greater number of clients per session and help agencies to increase revenue and funding. Agencies are finding that utilizing a group format is practical, cost-effective, and allows for a broader distribution of resources (Adix, Kelly, & Rosenthal, 1984; Corey, 1995; Rohde & Stockton, 1993). In group settings, learning and benefits can be derived by merely being present and watching others interact. On the other hand, in individual therapy, interaction is limited to only the therapist and client (Sonstegard, 1998). Groups also allow for nonverbal expressions to be conveyed and interpreted by other group members, allowing for a greater flexibility of participation by group members. Although group therapy offers less privacy than does individual practice, mutual aid is found in the sharing and commonalties of difficulties and challenges. Since there is pressure to utilize group interventions whenever possible, social workers are expected to simultaneously advocate for the legitimate benefits of group therapy while monitoring outcomes (Hawkins, 1998; Henry, 1992).

## GROUPS AS A MEANS OF UNDERSTANDING HUMAN BEHAVIOR

Groups can provide an excellent forum for developing new or for modifying existing behaviors. Generally, the group setting provides a context in which new behaviors are tested in a realistic atmosphere. According to Bowman and Delucia (1993), groups are microcosms of the *real* world where clients have an opportunity to practice new skills and behaviors as they relate to others. Subsequently, clients can receive immediate peer feedback and support regarding their problem-solving behavior. They are provided with role models to facilitate the acquisition of requisite social behavior. Groups provide a more valid locus for accurate diagnosis and a more potent means for changing client behavior (Blank, 1996; Brandler & Roman, 1991; Henry, 1992; Holmes, 1978).

Moreover, the majority of clients that a social worker sees feels guilt, emptiness, social isolation, and a sense of failure, and could benefit from the support derived from the group (Brandler & Roman, 1991; Corey, 1995; Kruger, 1979; Seligman, 1993). The provision of services through groups greatly increases the number of clients served by an effective treatment program (Henry, 1992). Participating in and leading groups is requisite to professional life. This chapter reviews the components of groups that the social worker can employ to facilitate the execution of relevant tasks.

# DEVELOPING SUCCESSFUL GROUPS

To develop successful groups, a major determinant of group composition involves clearly identifying the purpose of the group. According to Henry (1992), Klein (1972), and Williams (1994), the group's purpose will bring members together, guide the composition of the group, and influence the selection of goal directed activities. It will further determine group composition by influencing the selection of members whose behavior will enable group cohesion and movement toward the group's goal.

As a result, groups can be either homogeneous (having like) members or heterogeneous (non-alike) members. The decision to conduct a homogeneous or heterogeneous group is determined by the group treatment environment and its effect on clients, and how it maximizes or minimizes inclusion and participation (Williams, 1994). Adler (1995) has suggested that a lack of awareness of the reciprocal action and reaction of homogeneity-heterogeneity variables in group construction can harness a counselor's therapeutic options. He recommends that homogeneity be sought in clients' tolerance of anxiety, motivation, mental and social abilities, and exclusion criteria, because it has been asserted that heterogeneity should be sought for nearly all dimensions.

## Issues of Diversity

Homogeneous groups can provide opportunities for group members to explore more effective and productive ways of dealing with fears and concerns as they build group alliances and cohesiveness (Gainor, 1992). These multidimensional groups are generally accepted as supportive and one-issue focused (Adler, 1995). For example, Williams (1994) facilitated a homogeneous group with African American men who abused their partners. It was discovered that homogeneity within this group (a) increased client involvement, (b) increased levels of trust, (c) allowed for greater identification with themes discussed in the group, and (d) encouraged members to collectively work on the social issues presented. On the other hand, Williams observed that in a heterogeneous group of men (8 Caucasians, 2 African Americans, and 1 Native American), who also had abused their partners, nonminority group members had a difficult time. These nonminority group members had a difficult time identifying with the minority members what stressors aggravated violence. As a result, the group divided and the minority group members formed a more cohesive group, identifying on issues foreign to the nonminority members. This phenomenon has been described as *in-groups* homogeneous effect and it is more common when the in-group is a minority group (Vanbeselaere, 1988, 1991).

To address this phenomenon, Vanbeselaere (1991) suggested that *out-group* homogeneity could mediate in-group favoritism and bias. Therefore, heterogeneity can set up barriers if a lack of clarity and understanding among fellow group members exists; also, benefits of the group approach are reduced with clients of color. Although Heckathorn (1993) suggests that heterogeneous groups can provide an opportunity for group members with diverse characteristics to facilitate collective actions, workers and members should take care not to set up barriers that will negatively influence treatment outcome.

Smith, Tindale, and Dugoni (1996) explored this concept further by studying undergraduate students ($n = 250$) for minority and majority influence within the context of freely interacting groups. The results supported the hypothesis that the contributions of minority group members could reduce the degree of polarization in majority members' attitudes. In addition, based on the principles of Tajfel and Turner's social identity theory and Brewer's optimal distinctiveness model, Lee and Ottati (1995) sought to demonstrate the perceptions of in-group homogeneity. These authors evaluated the salience of in-group membership of Chinese students and scholars ($n = 134$), with the nature of the stereotypic expressions directed toward them. Results indicated that perceived in-group membership lead to greater feelings of sameness.

In addition, utilizing a T-group model, McRae (1994) studied interracial group dynamics using graduate students ($n = 7$, ages 25–33) of a group counseling class facilitated by an African American female professor. The results demonstrated the formation of coalitions within and across racial groups and a shifting of racial identity attitude for in-group interactions. The researcher concludes that counselors should move away from stereotypical racial thinking and should focus more on understanding members in the context of the group environment. It is suggested that the facilitator's listening for comments reflecting racial identity attitudes is one way of understanding coalitions and levels of interaction.

Using Hofstede's four dimensions of culture (power distance, uncertainty avoidance, individualism, and masculinity), along with the factors of language, cultural norms, status, and politics, Bantz (1993) explored the relationship between cultural diversity and group dynamics. The author's analysis of 10 years of data derived from a cross-cultural team research project suggested that the diversity in work groups on these dimensions and issues influences the group dynamics of leadership, norms, roles, and conflict. Based on this analysis, the author suggests that the most effective tactics for managing the influence of differences on the work group involved are to (a) gather information, (b) adapt to differing situations, issues, and needs, (c) build social and task cohesion, and (d) identify clear, mutual long-term goals.

Watson, Kumar, and Michaelsen (1993) compared homogeneous and diverse task groups for cultural diversity's impact on interaction processes and performance. The study involved White American undergraduates ($n = 81$), working in 17 culturally homogeneous (CH) groups; and undergraduates ($n = 92$), working in 19 culturally diverse groups, all performing tasks at 5, 9, 13, and 17 weeks into the semester. Performance and group interaction process measurements were taken. The results indicate that, whereas initially, CH groups scored higher on process and performance effectiveness, over time, both groups improved on process and performance, and the between-group differences converged. At week 17, no differences were noted in process or overall performance; however, the culturally diverse groups scored higher on two task measures.

Chu and Sue (1984) and Davis and Proctor (1989) suggested that homogeneity of ethnic-specific groups are preferred by people of color, and often are more productive, especially when issues of racial identity, racism, and culture are the focus of discussion. For example, according to Davis and Proctor, in social work training White students favor *mixed* groups to learn from each other, whereas most students of color accept mixed groups but prefer their own groups when racism and oppression are likely to be high on the agenda. It was noted by Chu and Sue that members of a culturally homogeneous group can better understand one another's style of communication and can provide better support. In addition, Maharujeh (1984) described a study that compares a culturally heterogeneous group with a homogeneous group. The results of this study were such that the clients in the heterogeneous group had problems adjusting to the group process, were frequently absent, and were forced into the role of *spectator*. In contrast, the clients in the homogeneous group were more cohesive and expressive. Finally, Davis and Proctor suggest that heterogeneous groups, especially those that are mixed as to race and gender, are likely to *import* distrustful attitudes from women and people of color toward men and Caucasians.

In any event, successful behavioral treatments in groups most often are reported for adult clients who are similar in educational and social background (Lazarus, 1982). Rose (1974) reported that differences in educational and socioeconomic status were not barriers to successful treatment outcomes. The majority of the empirical studies reviewed, however, show greatest promise when adults have similar social attributes and exhibit similar presenting problems.

Oakes, Haslam, Morrison, and Grace (1995) conducted a field study that examined the impact of familiarity on perceptions of group homogeneity throughout a 26-day "Outward Bound" course. Of the 31 adult subjects in three interacting groups studied, results indicated that over time group members saw themselves as becoming more homogeneous. Moreover, subjects reported stronger characteristics of group qualities to group members over the duration of the course. The researchers maintain that stereotyping can be sensitive to reality when reality is defined appropriately at the group level.

To examine individual dissimilarity and group heterogeneity as correlates of recruitment, promotions, and turnover within the workplace, Jackson et al. (1991) conducted a study that used Schneider's attraction-selection-attrition model, and Pfeffer's organization demography model to generate individual-level and group-level hypotheses. Interpersonal context was operationalized as personal dissimilarity; group heterogeneity was operationalized as age, tenure, level of education, curriculum, alma mater, military service, and career experiences. Top management teams in bank holding companies ($n = 93$) were studied over a 4-year period. The results indicated that turnover rate was predicted by dissimilarity to other group members, whereas promotion was not. Furthermore, team heterogeneity was a comparatively strong predictor of team turnover rates, and reliance on internal recruitment predicted subsequent team homogeneity.

For mixing individuals of different genders, Home (1991) agreed that there is a need for women's groups to be conducted without men present since men often assume control and leadership roles, subordinating the needs of women. On the other hand, men often prefer and benefit from mixed groups because they use the presence of women to be in touch with their feelings, more so than if they were only with other men (Reed & Garvin, 1983).

In social work these studies support that homogeneity is an important variable for developing trust and building cohesion. Therefore, the challenge to group workers is to take the necessary steps to demonstrate their commitment to cultural diversity and to create an environment of trust (Bilides, 1990; Brown & Misty, 1994; Williams, 1994). Furthermore, group cohesion, fostered by homogeneity, has been shown to lead to greater client satisfaction (Perrone & Sedlacek, 2000), a correlate of successful outcomes.

In summary, more research is needed to more accurately determine whether a homogeneous or heterogeneous perspective, or a combination of both, might be the best way to serve group members. For example, Beeber (1991) recommends that schizophrenic patients (more specifically, those who are receiving in-patient hospitalization) be exposed to varying levels of group treatment. It was found that low-functioning persons with schizophrenia could benefit from participation in a (heterogeneous) group with high-functioning persons with the same diagnosis. Persons who are lower functioning have more appropriate social skills modeled for them by higher functioning persons, whereas those persons learn helping behaviors and positive reinforcement as models from their lower functioning peers. The balance comes from allowing each group, lower and higher functioning persons, to participate in homogeneous groups of their same-functioning peers.

Another example of the need for clarity in the homogeneity-heterogeneity beneficence dichotomy is Bowers, Pharmer, and Salas's (2000) meta-analysis that examined 57 effect sizes from 13 studies. The authors report that the success of heterogeneous versus homogeneous groups was affected by variables such as task type, task difficulty, and team size. These findings suggest that a complex interaction of mediating structural, contextual, and process variables affect group outcomes.

The inconsistent data on homogeneity and heterogeneity of group composition indicate the need for more research to isolate how such variables interact to produce behavioral change. Additional research in this area would determine under what conditions it is appropriate to match clients on relevant variables. The literature suggests that treating individuals who exhibit similar difficulties in the group setting may be beneficial if powerful behavioral change techniques such as progressive relaxation, systematic desensitization, and assertiveness training are employed. Data on matching client and social worker characteristics are similarly inconclusive (Gurman & Razin, 1977).

## GOALS AND PURPOSE, GROUP COHESION, AND LEADER ROLE

Effective group work, aside from an experienced leader and the proper setting with adequate environmental supports, is a delicate yet complex balance between the group's structure, composition, leader, and stage of development (Horne & Rosenthal, 1997). The following sections outline some of the factors that affect the progress and outcomes of therapeutic group work.

## Goals and Purpose

The functions of individual and group therapists, in many ways, are the same (Bergin & Garfield, 1994). Notwithstanding, the role taken by the social worker with any group of clients will depend upon the purpose for which the group is formed. According to Berman-Rossi (1993), the role of the social worker is to strengthen members as they pursue common tasks and gain a sense of collectiveness, and also to encourage them to gain a sense of *groupness*. The amount of direction offered by the social worker also will depend upon the needs of the group members for skills to be acquired and behaviors to be modified. Leadership roles will emerge through task needs and attributes of the group members.

The treatment techniques utilized by the social worker to achieve the desired behavioral changes will depend upon a variety of factors such as the ages of the clients, the clients' physical and intellectual limitations, and the agency setting in which treatment is to take place. For example, the treatment of institutionalized psychotic adults or autistic children who must acquire socially relevant behaviors and self-care skills to function outside of the institutional setting will require an extended period of monitoring and group work and a highly active and directive role on the part of the therapist. Group treatment contracts with such populations would have to be short, concise, and uncomplicated.

A greater reliance upon group contingencies and group sanctions over individual incentives may be required to build group cohesion and cooperation and maintain newly acquired behavioral patterns such as group cooperation, task mastery, and goal attainment. Such groups may require extended periods of practice, shaping, and repeated exposure to models before new behavioral skills are adopted. Group therapists may have to use primary reinforcers paired with social reinforcers initially before tokens can be introduced as a means of altering behavior.

These groups may have difficulty utilizing various behavioral techniques such as self-control methods and cognitive behavioral approaches that require symbolic modeling, patience, and vivid imagination of scenes, concentration, and a certain degree of abstract reasoning ability. On the other hand, different groups will have different needs. For example, a group of middle-class adults wanting to learn self-control at a neighborhood center or a church-affiliated agency will require a different strategy than a group of married couples who desire to learn more effective problem-solving skills and conflict-negotiating strategies. Furthermore, such groups may be expected to deposit an initial fee with the social worker. In turn the social worker may contract to refund a specific amount of money to each group member for such things as attendance; punctuality; completion of homework assignments (e.g., practicing newly acquired behaviors to increase the probability of transfer and generalization); reading specific books, pamphlets, and articles; charting and monitoring behavior; and correctly using contingencies and stimulus control procedures.

Aside from the specificity of purpose, designating the goals themselves may well affect group variables such as group identification, cohesion, and performance. Group participation in setting the goals reduces anxiety among members but does not necessarily improve cohesion or motivation (Wegge, 2000). However, setting short-term goals on the way toward achieving long-term goals results in choosing more difficult long-term goals, and challenging goals lead to enhanced group identification (Wegge, 2000) and improved group performance (Wegge, 2000; Weldon & Yun, 2000).

## Group Cohesion

The creation of a cohesive group bond may be less important in some groups, especially when the focus of treatment is on building each member's self-sufficiency or on strengthening a marital bond between spouses. Therefore, the role of the social worker in such groups would be that of a consultant or an advisor who functions more as an educator than as an active group director. Groups such as these may be able to employ filmed and videotaped models to achieve the desired skill level, and cognitive behavioral approaches may be used more effectively with such clientele. These individuals can also be expected to cognitively rehearse alternative behaviors while they are observing other group members practicing or role-playing behavioral assignments.

Nonetheless, a significant number of recent studies (Blumer & McNamara, 1985; Braaten, 1989; Budman, Demby, Feldstein, & Gold, 1984; Caple & Cox, 1989; Hurley, 1989; Jeffery, Snell, & Forster, 1985; Roark &

Sharah, 1989; Stokes, Fuehrer, & Childs, 1983; Wright & Duncan, 1986) suggest that group cohesion is seen not only as necessary and sufficient, but also as cause and effect as well as process and outcome. It is the universality of shared experiences that helps to develop group cohesion and member bonding (Sonstegard, 1998). In another study that examines cohesiveness as the role of faction size, Zdaniuk and Levine (1996) evaluate how anticipated membership in a majority or minority faction affects thought generation. In this study, undergraduates ($n = 313$) were led to believe one of five different circumstances regarding the topics of the anticipated 6-person discussion groups that they were about to enter. The results revealed that the smaller the subject's faction, the less biased the subjects were in their thoughts regarding their own position. The researchers concluded that the findings elucidate the influence of majority and minority, and suggest that more attention be paid to the cognitive consequences of anticipated interaction in the group setting.

Marziali and her colleagues (Marziali, Munroe-Blum, & McCleary, 1997) studied 79 men and women aged 18 to 65 years that were patients of a psychiatric hospital. Subjects were randomly assigned to two groups, one that received group therapy and the other that received individual therapy. The researchers hypothesized that the group cohesion and group alliance experienced by members in the group treatment setting would better the desired outcome for group participants. The results indicate that the two independent variables, cohesion and alliance, when combined did affect a positive impact on therapeutic outcome. This finding adds to the credibility of group versus individual therapy.

Annesi (1999) also found group cohesion can positively affect attrition and attendance rates. The researcher examined two exercise groups, one that participated in small-group warm-up/cool-down programs before and after the workout, and one that did not. Findings indicated that the small-group programs promoted group cohesion and thereby increased member attendance and decreased member dropout. This suggests that group cohesion may be effective not only for productivity but also for participation and retention.

Group cohesion, as a quantifiable variable, can be measured via standard paper-and-pencil assessment instruments. Recently, Bollen and Hoyle's Perceived Cohesion Scale (PCS) was adapted to small group settings and found to possess satisfactory reliability and validity ratings (Chin, Salisbury, Pearson, & Stollak, 1999). The PCS is a six-item instrument that captures sense of belonging (three items) and morale (three items) on a Likert-type agree-disagree scale.

## The Role of the Group Leader

Research has suggested that there is a mutual exchange between group leader and members (e.g., Curran & Loganbill, 1983; Fodor & Riordan, 1995; Morran & Hulse, 1984). However, the group is less about the leader and more about its members. Therefore, experienced leaders best lead groups, those who understand group processes and can anticipate the natural flow of progressive stages (Sonstegard, 1998). Furthermore, Stinchfield and Burlingame (1991) conducted a study, which evaluated *expert group leaders* ($n = 4$) involving a 15-week therapy group of 40 members. The resulting transcript analysis indicated that the leaders were more directive when they had more direct influence, and conversely, less directive when they had less influence. In another study (Albright & Forziati, 1995) examined cross-situational consistency and perpetual accuracy in leadership in which university student leaders ($n = 7$) interacted with nonleaders ($n = 24$) on four tasks requiring social organization and coordination. As hypothesized, the results reveal stability in leadership across the four tasks and some evidence for consistency across groups, as well as a high level of consensus and accuracy in perceptions of leadership.

Preliminary data on the type of leadership role and characteristics of social workers indicate that they should be attractive and possess good interpersonal communication skills; be similar to the client on relevant variables such as age, sex, educational level, and expectations for behavioral change; exhibit empathy, genuineness, and nonpossessive warmth; be able to provide initial structure necessary to motivate clients to change; and, possess behaviors that facilitate bargaining and negotiating between themselves and other clients (Lieberman, 1976). Moreover, the social worker chosen should be an exemplar of the behaviors the clients wish to acquire. Thus, variables affecting the process of modeling social worker behavior such as age, sex, and social attributes (Bandura, 1977) should be taken into account before a social worker is assigned to a group.

## Behavioral Group-Level Variables

Within the last decade, research results have indicated that group cohesion, commitment, performance, and effectiveness are related to the reward structure of the groups. Recently, there have begun to appear in the education and psychology literature a series of related small-group team techniques based on behavioral analysis that appear to have great promise in changing the basic structure of the group to achieve positive effects on many group dimensions at the same time such as performance, leadership effectiveness, cohesion, acceptance and liking of group members, norms, conformity proneness, power, acquisition of relevant skills, and commitment to group goals. These small-group techniques assist in increasing problem-solving behavior. Group members are provided with role models to facilitate the acquisition of behavior (Blank, 1996; Brandler & Roman, 1991; Henry, 1992; Holmes, 1978; Wodarski, 1983, 1992). In turn the relevant group behavior of each individual furthers group goals and increases individual support for group performance. Further, this increased group performance under a variety of circumstances and increased the frequency of relevant social behaviors, particularly interracial and gender liking (e.g., Fantuzzo, King, & Heller, 1992; Kouhara, 1990; Lloyd, Eberhardt, & Drake, 1996; Miller & Komorita, 1995).

## THEORETICAL BACKGROUND

A group may be composed of two essential elements that can be modified with ease: (a) a task structure, and (b) a reward structure (Kabanoff & O'Brien, 1979; Klaus & Glaser, 1970; Levine, 1991; Michaels, 1977). The task structure refers to the activities that make up the performance aspects of the group, that is, specifying what is to be done and how. The task may be performed individually by group members or by the group as a whole (Wodarski & Feit, 1994).

The reward structure of the group refers to the means (incentives) that leaders use to motivate individuals to perform tasks and with what frequency these means are used. Different types of rewards are employed to produce and maintain certain behaviors (i.e., norms of the group and the conformity pressures to maintain these norms). Thus, a reward structure is simply the rules under which rewards are dispensed. Every group has an explicit and implicit reward structure having a major impact on the group performance, peer norms, and relevant other social behaviors and attitudes of members. In most groups, the major rewards used are verbal and nonverbal praise and performance ratings. Leaders typically administer these rewards based on multiple criteria. For example, most ratings are given (consciously or unconsciously) on the basis of the comparison of members' performances with the leader's ideas of what members should have accomplished (that is, their *effort*) in addition to such factors as attitude, neatness, and the behavior of other group members. Informal praise is administered according to the same general criteria.

One important commonality in these criteria is that they are all examples of competitive or individual reward structures. That is, these criteria are determined either comparatively in situations where members are essentially in competition (competitive reward structure), or on a scale that is either absolute or relative to the member's own performance (individual reward structure). However, because few group leaders would be willing to give acceptable rewards to all their members regardless of how well each performed, the reward structure of the great majority of groups is primarily a competitive one in which members compete for a necessarily limited number of acceptable ratings (rewards).

## TYPICAL GROUP TASK-REWARD STRUCTURE

The traditional group may be characterized as consisting of an independent or individualistic task structure and a competitive reward structure (e.g., Friedman, Todd, & Kariuki, 1995; Rapoport & Bornstein, 1989). This particular task-reward structure has many virtues: it tends to be easily administered; it is *fair* in that an individual's reward depends almost entirely on self-performance, however defined; and it is easily understood by group members and personnel.

The traditional task-reward structure, however, has been questioned for many years based on several shortcomings. First, traditional reward structures do not motivate all members well, especially low-performing members. Since traditional reward structures are competitive by nature, many low-performing members have no chance of making acceptable ratings regardless of their performance or effort. On the other hand, many high-performing members could also have difficulty making acceptable ratings regardless of their effort.

Second, traditional reward structures "set members against one another," and in turn discourage group commitment and effective performance. Since the success of one member entails a decrease in the chances that another member will be able to make an acceptable performance (only a limited number of rewards are available for the top ratings), in actuality one member's success can require another's failure.

Third, a competitive reward structure disrupts interpersonal bonds between members leading members to discourage group performance on the part of their peers. This sets up a situation in which anti-group peer norms oppose institutional norms. For example, high school students who could achieve at a high level may reject this notion and look toward more peer-supported activities such as sports (Coleman, 1959). In many group situations where group performance requisites are high these anti-group norms can become so strong that members develop a reward structure in which peers more effectively punish group achievement than leaders reward it. Likewise, traditional group task structures provide few opportunities for active learning. For most members the large proportion of group task time is spent in either passive listening or individual work for which feedback may be far removed in time from performance (Ettin, Vaughan, & Fiedler, 1987; Wodarski & Feit, 1994).

In summary, research supports that running groups based on traditional task-reward structures can be nonproductive. These types of groups can lead to a decrease in the participant's social connectedness, self-esteem and self-image, social competence, norm commitment, interpersonal integration, and sense of belonging. Furthermore, decreases can occur in an individual's ability to relate to others, cross-racial and cross-gender liking and acceptance, interpersonal attraction, and sharing of requisite information for successful completion of group tasks (Buckholdt & Wodarski, 1978; Feldman & Wodarski, 1975; Niehoff & Mesch, 1991; Wheeler & Ryan, 1973; Wodarski & Feit, 1994).

## ALTERNATIVE GROUP TASK-REWARD STRUCTURES

There are numerous alternative group task-reward structures available to assist social work professionals in addressing group variables as part of human development and learning. For example, an alternative to assigning an individual task in the group setting is to utilize the assignment of a group team task. Further, alternatives to the direct use of competitive reward structures can involve individual reward structures as well as cooperative reward structures.

When working in a group environment a *group task* can be simply defined as one in which members are permitted or encouraged to aid each other in their learning activities. Peer tutoring, in which members help each other attain team goals, is one widely used example of a group task as are various group projects such as a jointly planned report, a discussion group, or joint problem solving. It is essential to remember that a group task does not always involve a group (or cooperative) reward structure. Oftentimes in developing a group task members are encouraged to work together but receive rewards (material reinforcers or praise) on an individual or competitive basis.

## GROUP REWARD STRUCTURE

There are three possible categories of group reward structures: (a) competitive, (b) independent, and (c) cooperative. If one member's receipt of rewards diminishes the probability that another will also be rewarded, the members are operating under a competitive group reward structure. Grading on a curve is an example of a competitive reward structure. For example, if one member works especially hard to receive an A and the number of A's is fixed, then that member's performance reduces the probability that other members will also receive A's. Likewise, in a team situation when a group is involved in competition for first place, the reward structure is competitive. If the probability of one member's receiving a reward is unrelated to the probability that any other member receives a reward, the members are in an individual group reward structure, as in individualized instruction or any setting in which there are fixed performance criteria for reinforcement (e.g., a piecework schedule in industry).

Finally, if an increase in the performance level of any member increases the probability that another will receive rewards, the members are in a cooperative group reward structure. According to Niehoff and Mesch (1991), cooperative reward structures should lead to the highest levels of member performance when the task presents opportunities for members to share resources. Most team sports include this sort of structure within the team. For example, on a football team, extra practice by a guard improves the chances that the quarterback or any other player will be reinforced (by winning), and vice versa. In addition, in group practice, participation of all members is required for all members to receive a reward. Cooperative reward structures may be further broken down into group competition (in which one group's performance is evaluated against a fixed standard) and group contingencies.

Group contingencies refer to reinforcements that are presented to all or most group members following the display of certain behaviors by the group or selected members. Such behaviors may be denoted by the group's accomplishment of certain tasks, such as increasing accuracy or productivity, or by the accomplishments of specific group members. In either case, a significant portion of the group membership receives reinforcement following manifestation of the desired behavior by the entire group or by certain of its members. Group contingencies modify behaviors most readily by producing the greatest group pressure (a) when all members have to exhibit a given behavior at a certain criterion rate or (b) when one or two group members are required to exhibit a certain rate of appropriate group task behaviors for each group member to receive reinforcement. The situation and the behaviors to be modified determine which of these contingencies the leader should employ. The effectiveness with which group contingencies modify behaviors decreases as the proportion of group members who receive reinforcement decreases (Hayes, 1976; Wodarski & Bagarozzi, 1979; Wodarski & Feit, 1994). Typically, groups have many different types of reward structures operating simultaneously (e.g., an individual reward structure for task A, a group reward structure for task B, and a combination of both at times for both tasks A and B). This separation is necessary for conceptualization purposes and as a means for providing the leader with a guide for structuring appropriate interventions.

Kohler et al. (1995) utilized a group-oriented contingency design in a study seeking to increase social interactions between children with autism and their peers. The researchers evaluated the effects of a group-oriented contingency on the social interactions of 4-year-old preschoolers ($n = 3$) diagnosed with autism, and 3- to 5-year-old socially competent peers ($n = 6$). All subjects experienced daily manipulative play activities in group settings of three (one target subject and two peer subjects). The results reveal that a group reward contingency increased the target subject's social interactions with peer subjects; however, it produced few if any corollary supportive exchanges.

## INDIVIDUAL REWARD STRUCTURES: PROS AND CONS

Individual reward structures have the advantage over traditional competitive structures in that all group members may, if they work hard enough, achieve a criterion level of performance that entitles them to rewards. However, if all members are given the same criterion to meet, meeting the standard will be much easier for some members than for others. In fact, some members may have less of a chance of earning an acceptable reward (by meeting a high criterion) in an individual reward structure than in a competitive one. Furthermore, although the effectiveness of a competitive reward structure does not depend on the difficulty of the material (members can be ranked regardless of their absolute level of performance), such difficulty is a major factor in an individual reward structure in which a criterion may well be too easy or too hard for many members to master or achieve. Reward structures that motivate all members would facilitate the acquisition of relevant task behavior.

Another advantage of individual reward structures is that they are completely *fair* because rewards are entirely dependent upon the individual's performance, whereas in competitive structures, rewards depend upon the skill or motivation of competitors. Individual reward structures, in which a set criterion must be reached, also have built-in quality control. If the criterion set of behaviors can be specified as essential, then it should not matter how much a member knows compared to other members as long as he or she can perform the requisite behaviors. However, supervisors and members easily understand comparative evaluation and praise, whereas individual, noncomparative evaluation may have little meaning, and thus little motivational value.

Individual reward structures frequently lead to dysfunctional or unanticipated outcomes in groups. For instance, structuring of competitive activities among group members may result in failure and rejection for certain members, lack of adequate learning of requisite skills, exclusion from power positions in the group, lower goal attainment for the group as a whole, and perhaps increased antisocial behavior by certain members. Likewise, by reinforcing only selected members in the presence of others, the leader, in effect, may withdraw available reinforcements from those who are not rewarded. The latter members may perceive such relative deprivation as a form of punishment, resulting in all the dysfunction thereof.

Hence, the utilization of individual reinforcement contingencies within groups may produce a number of undesired outcomes. It not only may entail adverse consequences for the reinforced members but also in addition may decrease the members' attraction to one another. It may also militate against group sharing and goal attainment and, in sum, may diminish the group's overall effectiveness as a prosocial influence vehicle. Moreover, the few members who receive individual reinforcements may acquire aversive stimulus or discriminate properties for the others. This may suggest to the others that further interpersonal exchanges with the *successful* members will be likely to result in their own continued failure to receive desired reinforcements. Consequently, as a number of nonreinforcing exchanges increase, the tendency for members to interact with their peers and to remain in the learning situation may decrease. Such a process may be one of the key variables in determining whether a member will remain active in the group.

On the other hand, by employing group reinforcement contingencies with group members, the leader can eliminate the likelihood that only a select number of members will receive reinforcement within the group. Hence, it becomes unnecessary to force competition for available reinforcers. Instead, members are encouraged to exhibit appropriate group tasks that contribute to the procurement of reinforcers for all. Moreover, they would be likely to exert strong conformity pressures upon their peers to exhibit such behaviors. These behaviors can lead to additional reinforcers after a number of pairings with the original reward and, therefore, to the acquisition of secondary reinforcing properties. As the task group develops valuable reinforcing properties, its effectiveness for being a viable learning vehicle is likely to be enhanced.

## COOPERATIVE REWARD STRUCTURES: PROS AND CONS

Cooperative reward structures, regardless of whether they are group contingencies or group competitions, have several advantages over individual competition. First, they motivate all members equally well. An extra point contributed to a group score is just as useful when it comes from a low performer as it is when it comes from a high achiever. Second, cooperative reward structures completely reverse the process inherent in competitive reward structures in which members are *set against* each other and come to oppose group performance efforts on the part of their peers. In a cooperative reward structure, the effective performance of a group member always improves the chances that others will be rewarded. As a result, performance-effective members gain in sociometric status in a cooperative reward structure, but lose status in either a competitive reward structure (Stevens, Slavin, & Farnish, 1991; Wodarski & Feit, 1994) or an individual reward structure (Slavin, 1977; Wodarski & Feit). Furthermore, cooperative reward structures motivate members to help (tutor) each other with the group task (Buckholdt & Wodarski, 1978; DeVries & Edwards, 1974; Slavin, 1977;

Stevens et al., 1991; Williamson, Williamson, Watkins, & Hughes, 1992; Wodarski & Feit, 1994; Wodarski, Hamblin, Buckholdt, & Ferritor, 1972, 1973).

According to Pigott and Heggie (1986), group reinforcement contingencies are generally superior to individual contingencies when academic behavior is targeted for modification. Group reinforcement can function to promote a cooperative environment whereby students learn to work together toward mutual goal attainment and thereby improve group performance (Pigott & Heggie; Slavin, 1990; Stevens et al., 1991; Williamson et al., 1992).

In addition to efforts on achievement-related dimensions, cooperative reward structures have had strong and consistent positive impacts on the social connectedness of members such as mutual concern (for reviews see Buckholdt & Wodarski, 1978; Feldman & Wodarski, 1975; Johnson & Johnson, 1974; Slavin & Karweit, 1984; Stevens et al., 1991; Wodarski & Bagarozzi, 1979; Wodarski & Feit, 1994). These effects of cooperative teams on social and attitudinal variables appear to consistently increase members' mutual attraction and respect for one another. Unfortunately, this outcome of group reward structures has been exploited by the use of teams in desegregated settings to facilitate interracial and gender friendship, helping, and respect (Blaney, Stephen, Rosenfield, Aronson, & Sikes, 1977; Stephan & Rosenfield, 1978; Wodarski & Feit, 1994).

On the other hand, cooperative reward structures must be carefully structured if they are to have positive effects on group performance. First, they must be designed so that no individual is allowed to sit back and let the rest of the group do the work. That is, each team member must be individually accountable to the group regarding individual behavior. Second, the group task must be one in which the participation of all team members is necessary. A frequently used group reward and task structure that may not meet this criterion is the *group report* in which several members are expected to write one paper. Unless the work is carefully divided, this nearly always becomes essentially an individual task. Third, cooperative reward structures can cause group members to have a negative self-perception. Harris and Covington (1993) completed a study on the role of cooperative rewards. Their findings suggest that often, low performers and high performers rate themselves as less smart in cooperative conditions.

A major difficulty with cooperative reward structures is that they may not be *fair*. Each member's reward usually depends on the luck at being put on a skilled or motivated team. However, weighing procedures that equalize different academic abilities or skill levels in groups can alleviate this dysfunction and provide the requisite incentives for achievement by all members. Remember: The larger the group, the less the behavior of any individual determines the outcome.

# APPLICATIONS OF GROUP CONTINGENCIES TO GROUP PERFORMANCE

## Measuring the Effectiveness of Groups

Substantial research is accumulating to indicate that structuring individual reinforcement contingencies may not be the most productive means for achieving desired group effectiveness and social outcomes. Group contingencies, in particular, have far-reaching effects to the larger whole based on the acts of all members regardless of how few. Romeo (1998) exemplified this in her work on group contingencies within classroom settings. In the context of contingencies as discipline, an entire classroom of children can be denied a reward because of the disruption of a single classmate. A series of studies support the idea that children from various socioeconomic classes (ranging in age from 3 to 18 in classrooms comprising 4 to 17 members) can work together effectively in group reinforcement instructional situations. These situations can involve curricula such as mathematics, social studies, vocabulary development, reading, and nutrition, and group members can serve to teach one another. Moreover, the studies indicate that when appropriate reinforcement is provided for cooperative behavior, helping behaviors as well as academic performance can be increased and disruptive behavior decreased. Thus, group contingencies are particularly applicable in helping low-achieving team members acquire requisite skills. Group contingencies create a learning situation in which necessary tutoring is provided with ample incentives for the low-achieving individuals and others to learn.

## Interpersonal Relationships

An interesting by-product of using group contingencies in academic environments, as opposed to individual reinforcement contingencies, is the finding that liking or caring about other group members increases. Research evidence suggests that structuring classroom situations such that reinforcement of a group's performance is dependent upon the whole group's performance increases the liking of each individual member by the group. Thus, one strategy for increasing liking among individuals of different races, academic abilities, genders, physical attributes, and so forth is to place them in contexts where the reinforcers that each individual secures are dependent upon other group members' performance. Likewise, sharing and enjoying positive reinforcers increases the frequency of positive behavior exchanges among individuals (Aronson, Blaney, Sikes, Stephen, & Snapp, 1975; Feldman & Wodarski, 1975; Lucker, Rosenfield, Sikes, & Aronson, 1976; Wodarski & Feit, 1994).

## The Components of Effective Group Reward Structures

The reward structure of the group is at least one of the most important manipulatable features of group process that can facilitate effective problem solving. How should an ideal system be constructed? Literature in educational and organizational psychology indicates that certain reward structures can facilitate group cohesion, leader effectiveness, productivity, and group effectiveness. In applying the given principles tasks have to be chosen that are appropriate to the ability level of the group members, are attractive, and are feasible.

The social worker should analyze the following points in developing a relevant reward system:

1.  Appropriate behavior must be reinforced. The failure of pass-fail experiments in universities (Johnson, 1975; Wodarski & Feit, 1994) question whether students study for the sake of learning alone. Students often study because they are rewarded for studying, and when not rewarded the incidence of this behavior will be quite low (Bandura, 1969). Thus, appropriate social behavior in groups is dependent on reinforcement (rewards) from peers as well as from the leader. Disruptive behavior, a major problem in groups, will decrease when it is not reinforced, and leaders must therefore structure rewards that are contingent upon appropriate behavior. Token economies are one example of ways in which appropriate behaviors can be reinforced (Wodarski & Bagarozzi, 1979; Wodarski & Feit).

2. Reinforcers must be available to all members, but not too easily available. As obvious as this sounds, this is the major failing of traditional reward systems. When frequently or easily rewarded, it is not surprising that a substantial number of members turn themselves off as learners and do only what is required to be a member, which at most is not much (Schultz & Sherman, 1976). Thus, reinforcement systems must be structured in such a manner as to require effort according to each member's ability to attain the criterion.

3. To be maximally effective, reinforcers (feedback) should be delivered close in time to the occurrence of the behavior. For younger members, less able members, and members who have not yet learned to delay gratification, a reward delivered every 6 to 9 weeks is not feasible. When rewards are delayed too long, members may decide that primarily fate or leader preference determines rewards. In addition, the reward system may not be sensitive enough to recognize and reinforce an increase in performance level in a member who has been a low performer. Accumulated research indicates that feedback is one of the most significant variables that increase individual performance in a group (Glassman & Kates, 1990; Wodarski & Feit, 1994). Feedback on group tasks initially should occur daily and should be faded (phased out) as members acquire necessary social and academic skills. Feedback can occur through credits on posters and charts, in daily newsletters, and so forth.

4. Consistent application is needed. Members should know what behaviors are going to be reinforced and how often (i.e., the structure facilitates the attainment of group goals). Additionally, leaders must be consistent in their application of reward systems. Inconsistent application leads to ineffective acquisition of relevant academic and social behaviors. Therefore, contingencies must be specified in such a manner that members understand what is involved in securing rewards (DeRisi & Butz, 1975; Wodarski & Feit, 1994). Members should possess a record (preferably in written form) of the reward system, and this communication can occur in contract form.

5. Effectiveness of reinforcement is needed. Reinforcers should be selected individually and it is important to make sure that the reinforcer is not weak when compared with other reinforcers that are currently maintaining the behavior. Three critical questions

center on how appropriate are the incentives. (a) How much of the reinforcer has the member had in the past? (b) How much of the reinforcer does the member currently possess? and (c) How much of the reinforcer do other members in the group possess? The power of the reinforcer is inversely related to the answer to all three of these questions. For example, the reinforcer may be appropriate, but the amount is not proportional to the effort involved in changing the behavior. Likewise, the amount or the size of the reinforcer may be appropriate, but the reinforcer is not provided at a high enough frequency or the schedule of reinforcement is too erratic to override the cost involved in the member's changing the behavior. Leaders can isolate relevant reinforcement by asking the members what they would like, observing them in free time periods, and giving the Reinforcement Survey (Cautela, 1972; Cautela & Kastenbaum, 1967). Such research ensures that the leader possesses the requisite information for structuring an effective reinforcement system.

6. Patterns of reinforcement by significant others must be established. When appropriate reinforcers and delivery conditions are sufficient, significant others in the client's environment are not forgotten. These members can provide the reinforcement that maintains the behaviors or can punish behaviors that are being reinforced. Also, the significant others or members of the peer group chosen to participate in the modification plan may be inconsistently applying the agreed-upon plan of behavioral change or may not be attractive enough to facilitate the behavioral changes. These reinforcement systems encourage peer support for appropriate group behavior (Wodarski & Feit, 1994).

## Generalization and Maintenance

The primary objective of the social work practitioner is that the group members terminate successfully and achieve their endpoint goal. In other words, the members must transfer the appropriate behavior learned within the group context to their natural environment and have that treatment effect extend past the termination of the group. According to Nelson and Politano (1993), generalization and maintenance are two fundamental concepts that address issues related to after-treatment progress that can influence the treatment outcome. Though group members acquired knowledge of their problems and possible solutions, they have not always had the opportunity to practice in their natural environment the appropriate problem-solving skills. Therefore, termination from the group environment provides an opportunity for the members to transfer and maintain appropriate observable behavior into their natural environment without the external support of the group leader.

A major area addressing generalization is the social competence of children. Chandler, Lubeck, and Fowler (1992) completed a descriptive analysis in which they reviewed 51 studies that assessed generalization of preschool children's peer-directed social skills. Their findings showed that studies able to produce generalization appeared to use a combination of antecedent and consequence strategies (prompting and positive reinforcement), and the studies that failed to produce generalization primarily employed combinations of antecedent strategies (modeling and rehearsal). The authors further said that a combination of antecedent and consequent strategies may be more likely to produce generalization because they address both ends of the three-term contingency (antecedents, behaviors, and consequences).

Though the literature is limited in the area of generalization and maintenance, behavioral group therapists have successfully used maintenance groups with obsessive-compulsive disordered (OCD) patients. In a study conducted by Fals-Stewart and Lucente (1994), 10 OCD patients were assigned to groups for a 9-week course. After completion of the intensive therapy phase, the patients met in a behavior therapy group (booster sessions) once weekly for 2 months. The booster sessions provided support and encouraged the patients to develop exposure assignments so that they could do without extensive therapist supervision. The booster sessions strongly influenced the maintenance of treatment gains and relapse prevention.

According to Rhode, Morgan, and Young (1983), research in psychology and special education focuses on the use of self-management training for facilitating generalization and maintenance of treatment gains. Rhode and colleagues also state that self-management training is a viable means of promoting generalization in students with learning and behavioral problems.

Pierce and Schreibman (1994) investigated the efficacy of pictorial self-management to teach daily living skills to low-functioning children with autism. The children received books with picture prompts for various target behaviors (i.e., removal of pajama top, retrieve shirt, put on shirt). The results of their study showed that children with autism can successfully use pictures to manage their behavior independently, can generalize their behavior across settings and tasks, and can maintain the newly acquired behaviors at follow-up sessions.

Glynn (1990) strongly supports the use of a token economy but stressed that generalization and maintenance are critical aspects of this strategy. Some programs attempt to address generalization issues with a level or tier system by which patients are slowly weaned away from immediate reinforcement (the payment of tokens). The author further suggests that social reinforcement replace the payment of tokens because it is more natural and more likely to be available in the community. Providing social reinforcement lavishly to clients during and immediately after the task is complete will better ensure generalization and maintenance of desired behavioral changes.

There is a need for additional empirical research in the area of behavioral views of generalization and maintenance of the treatment effect. Although the literature discusses the use of self-efficacy, booster groups, self-reporting, feedback, peer interventions, and social reinforcement, there is a great need to explore the effects of generalization and maintenance over a longer period.

## SUMMARY

As stated at the beginning of this chapter, understanding group level variables are essential to human growth and development because much of what an individual does is either learned or reinforced in the group setting. In practice, addressing health and mental health issues in a group format remains a practice necessity (Sonstegard, 1998). Today, groups once considered adjunctive treatment are often the primary intervention of choice. This may well impact the nature and structure of group therapy, and understanding the most effective methods of administering group treatment has become tantamount.

How important is the reward structure of the group? One can argue that it is the most important manipulatable feature of the group setting. Studies on tasks, leader style, methods of delivery, and the like have been notoriously ineffective in demonstrating important changes in member behavior because of variations on these dimensions (Hamblin, Buckholdt, Ferritor, Kozloff, & Blackwell, 1971). On the other hand, major changes in reward structures have been associated with changes in behavior. By implementing simple, highly contingent leader's praise in groups, researchers in the behavior modification tradition have been consistently successful in increasing members' on-task behavior (Kazdin & Klock, 1973), group performance (Johnson, 1975), adherence to group rules (Ayllon & Roberts, 1974), and with teaching individuals who have failed in school because of verbal, reading, and arithmetic deficiencies.

Whereas accumulated research on cooperative reward structures indicates consistent positive effects on academic performance, time on task, proacademic peer norms, and other variables produce a set of behaviors that are clearly undesirable such as cheating, lack of tutoring, and concern only for one's self-learning (DeVries & Slavin, 1976). Furthermore, they produce a set of peer norms that oppose exhibition of the academic behaviors that the institution seeks to increase (e.g., studying, participating in class, etc.). In elementary and secondary schools, these antiacademic norms may be quite strong, creating for certain students a reward structure in which peers more effectively punish academic achievement than teachers and parents reward it. Group reward structures provide social workers with effective procedures for altering such destructive learning processes.

Finally, maximal generalization and maintenance will occur when therapeutic efforts are geared toward teaching new skills, then transferring those skills to the client's environment (Nelson & Politano, 1993). Although the client may experience setbacks, the success of a particular treatment intervention is determined by clients' abilities to cope with the challenges and experiences confronting them within the natural environment after the treatment intervention, and by their abilities to use the newly acquired skills.

## REFERENCES

Adix, R. S., Kelly, T., & Rosenthal, D. (1984). Substance abuse prevention: A developmental skills approach. *Journal for Specialists in Group Work, 9* (1), 32–37.

Adler, M. (1995). Homogeneity or heterogeneity of groups: When, and along what dimensions? *Canadian Journal of Counseling, 29* (1), 14–21.

Albright, L., & Forziati, C. (1995). Cross-sectional consistency and perceptual accuracy in leadership. *Personality and Social Psychology Bulletin, 21* (12), 1269–1276.

Annesi, J. J. (1999). Effects of minimal group promotion on cohesion and exercise adherence. *Small Group Research, 30* (5), 542–557.

Aronson, E., Blaney, N., Sikes, J., Stephen, C., & Snapp, M. (1975, February). Busing and racial tension: The jigsaw route to learning and liking. *Psychology Today, 8,* 43–50.

Ayllon, T., & Roberts, M. D. (1974). Eliminating discipline problems by strengthening academic performance. *Journal of Applied Behavior Analysis, 7* (1), 71–76.

Bandura, A. (1969). *Principles of behavior modification.* New York: Holt, Rinehart & Winston.

Bandura, A. (1977). *Social learning theory.* Englewood Cliffs, NJ: Prentice-Hall.

Bantz, C. R. (1993). Cultural diversity and group cross-cultural team research. *Journal of Applied Communication Research, 21* (1), 1–20.

Beeber, A. R. (1991). Psychotherapy with schizophrenics in Team Groups: A systems model. *American Journal of Psychotherapy, 45* (1), 78–86.

Bergin, A. E., & Garfield, S. L. (Eds.). (1994). *Handbook of psychotherapy and behavior change* (4th ed.). New York: John Wiley & Sons.

Berman-Rossi, T. (1993). The tasks and skills of the social worker across stages of group development. *Social Work with Groups, 16* (1–2), 69–81.

Bilides, D. G. (1990). Race, color, ethnicity, and class: Issues of biculturalism in school-based adolescent counseling groups. *Social Work with Groups, 13* (4), 43–58.

Blaney, N. T., Stephen, C., Rosenfield, D., Aronson, E., & Sikes, J. (1977). Interdependence in the classroom: A field study. *Journal of Educational Psychology, 69* (2), 121–128.

Blank, L. (1996). *Changing behavior in individuals, couples, and groups: Identifying, analyzing, and manipulating the elements involved in change in order to promote or inhibit alteration of behavior.* Springfield, IL: Charles C Thomas.

Blumer, C. H., & McNamara, R. J. (1985). Preparatory procedures for videotaped feedback to improve social skills. *Psychological Reports, 57* (2), 549–550.

Bowers, C. A., Pharmer, J. A., & Salas, E. (2000). When member homogeneity is needed in work teams: A meta-analysis. *Small Group Research, 31* (3), 305–327.

Bowman, V. E., & Delucia, J. L. (1993). Preparation for group therapy: The effects of preparer and modality on group process and individual functioning. *Journal for Specialists in Group Work, 18* (2), 67–79.

Braaten, L. J. (1989). Predicting positive goal attainment and symptom reduction from early group climate dimensions. *International Journal of Group Psychotherapy, 39* (3 Spec. Issue), 377–387.

Brandler, S., & Roman, C. P. (1991). *Group work: Skills and strategies for effective interventions.* New York: Haworth.

Brown, A., & Misty, T. (1994). Group work with 'mixed membership' groups: Issues of race and gender. *Social Work with Groups, 17* (3), 5–21.

Buckholdt, D. R., & Wodarski, J. S. (1978). The effects of different reinforcement systems on cooperative behaviors exhibited by children in the classroom contexts. *Journal of Research and Development in Education, 12* (1), 50–68.

Budman, S. H., Demby, A., Feldstein, M., & Gold, M. (1984). The effects of time-limited group psychotherapy: A controlled study. *International Journal of Psychotherapy, 34* (4), 587–603.

Caple, R. B., & Cox, P. L. (1989). Relationships among group structure, member expectations, attraction to group, and satisfaction with the group experience. *Journal for Specialists in Group Work, 14* (1), 16–24.

Cautela, J. R. (1972). Reinforcement survey schedule: Evaluation and current applications. *Psychological Reports, 30* (3), 683–690.

Cautela, J. R., & Kastenbaum, R. (1967). A reinforcement survey schedule for use in therapy, training, and research. *Psychological Reports, 20* (3, Pt. 2), 1115–1130.

Chandler, L. K., Lubeck, R. C., & Fowler, S. A. (1992). Generalization and maintenance of preschool children's social skills: A critical review and analysis. *Journal of Applied Behavior Analysis, 25* (2), 415–428.

Chin, W. W., Salisbury, W. D., Pearson, A. W., & Stollak, M. J. (1999). Perceived cohesion in small groups: Adapting and testing the Perceived Cohesion Scale in a small-group setting. *Small Group Research, 30* (6), 751–766.

Chu, J., & Sue, S. (1984). Asian/Pacific-Americans and group practice. *Social Work with Groups, 7* (3), 23–36.

Coleman, J. S. (1959). Academic achievement and the structure of competition. *Harvard Educational Review, 29* (4), 330–351.

Corey, G. (1995). *Theory and practice of group counseling* (4th ed.). Pacific Grove, CA: Brooks/Cole.

Curran, J., & Loganbill, C. R. (1983). Factors affecting the attractiveness of a group leader. *Journal of College Student Personnel, 24* (4), 350–355.

Davis, L., & Proctor, E. (1989). *Race, gender, and class: Guidelines for practice with individuals, families, and groups.* Englewood Cliffs, NJ: Prentice-Hall.

DeRisi, W., & Butz, G. (1975). *Writing behavioral contracts: A case simulation practice manual.* Champaign, IL: Research.

DeVries, D. L., & Edwards, K. J. (1974). Student teams and learning games: Their effects on cross-race and cross-sex interaction. *Journal of Educational Psychology, 66* (5), 741–749.

DeVries, D. L., & Slavin, R. E. (1976). *Teams-Games-Tournament: A final report on the research* (Center for Social Organization of Schools Report No. 217). Baltimore: John Hopkins University Press.

Ettin, M. F., Vaughan, E., & Fiedler, N. (1987). Managing group process in nonprocess groups: Working with the theme-centered psychoeducational group. *Group, 11* (3), 177–192.

Fals-Stewart, W., & Lucent, S. (1994). Behavioral group therapy with obsessive-compulsives: An overview. *International Journal of Group Psychotherapy, 44* (1), 35–51.

Fantuzzo, J. W., King, J. A., & Heller, L. R. (1992). Effects of reciprocal peer tutoring on mathematics and school adjustment: A component analysis. *Journal of Educational Psychology, 84* (3), 331–339.

Feldman, R. A., & Wodarski, J. S. (1975). *Contemporary approaches to group treatment.* San Francisco: Jossey-Bass.

Fodor, E. M., & Riordan, J. M. (1995). Leader power motive and group conflict as influences on leader behavior and group member self-affect. *Journal of Research in Personality, 29* (4), 418–431.

Friedman, A., Todd, J., & Kariuki, P. W. (1995). Cooperative and competitive behavior of urban and rural children in Kenya. *Journal of Cross Cultural Psychology, 26* (4), 374–383.

Gainor, K. A. (1992). Internalized oppression as a barrier to effective group work with Black women. *Journal for Specialists in Group Work, 17* (4), 235–242.

Glassman, U., & Kates, L. (1990). *Group work: A humanistic approach.* San Francisco: Sage.

Glynn, S. M. (1990). Token economy approaches for psychiatric patients: Progress and pitfalls over 25 years. *Behavior Modification, 14* (4), 383–407.

Gurman, A. S., & Razin, A. M. (Eds.). (1977). *Effective psychotherapy.* New York: Plenum.

Hamblin, R. L., Buckholdt, D., Ferritor, D. E., Kozloff, M., & Blackwell, L. (1971). *Humanization process: A social behavioral analysis of children's problems.* New York: John Wiley.

Harris, A. M., & Covington, M. V. (1993). The role of cooperative reward interdependency in success and failure. *Journal of Experimental Education, 6* (12), 151–168.

Hawkins, D. M. (1998). An invitation to join in difficulty: Realizing the deeper promise of group psychotherapy. *International Journal of Group Psychotherapy, 48* (4), 423–438.

Hayes, L. A. (1976). The use of group contingencies for behavioral control: A review. *Psychological Bulletin, 83* (4), 628–648.

Heckathorn, D. D. (1993). Collective action and group heterogeneity: Voluntary provision versus selective incentives. *American Sociological Review, 58* (3), 329–350.

Henry, S. (1992). *Group skills in social work: A four dimensional approach* (2nd ed.). Pacific Grove, CA: Brooks/Cole.

Holmes, S. (1978). Parents Anonymous: A treatment method for child abuse. *Social Work, 23* (3), 245–247.

Home, A. M. (1991). Mobilizing women's strengths for social change group connection. *Social Work with Groups, 14* (3/4), 153–173.

Horne, A. M., & Rosenthal, R. (1997). Research in group work: How did we get where we are? *Journal for Specialists in Group Work, 22* (4), 228–240.

Hurley, J. R. (1989). Affiliativeness and outcome in interpersonal groups: Member and leader perspectives. *Psychotherapy, 26* (4), 520–523.

Jackson, S. E., Brett, J. F., Sessa, V. I., Cooper, D. M., Julin, J. A., & Peyronnin, K. (1991). Some differences make a difference: Individual dissimilarity and group heterogeneity as correlates of recruitment, promotions, and turnover. *Journal of Applied Psychology, 76* (5), 675–689.

Jeffery, R. W., Snell, M. K., & Forster, J. L. (1985). Group composition in the treatment of obesity: Does increasing group homogeneity improve treatment results? *Behavioral Research & Therapy, 23* (3), 371–373.

Johnson, D. W., & Johnson, R. T. (1974). Instructional structure: Cooperative, competitive, or individualistic. *Review of Educational Research, 44* (2), 213–240.

Johnson, J. M. (Ed.). (1975). *Behavior modification and technology in higher education.* Springfield, IL: Charles C Thomas.

Kabanoff, B., & O'Brien, G. E. (1979). The effects of task type and cooperation upon group products and performance. *Organizational Behavior & Human Decision Processes, 23* (2), 163–181.

Kazdin, A. E., & Klock, J. (1973). The effect of nonverbal teacher approval on student attentive behavior. *Journal of Applied Behavior Analysis, 6* (4), 643–654.

Klaus, D. J., & Glaser, R. (1970). Reinforcement determinants of team proficiency. *Organizational Behavior & Human Decision Processes, 5* (1), 33–67.

Klein, A. (1972). *Effective group work.* New York: Association Press.

Kohler, F. W., Strain, P. S., Hoyson, M., Davis, L., Donina, W. M., & Rapp, N. (1995). Using a group-oriented contingency to increase social interactions between children with autism and their peers: A preliminary analysis of corollary supportive behaviors. *Behavior Modification, 19* (1), 10–32.

Kouhara, S. (1990). An experimental study on deviation behavior which promotes group outcome. *Japanese Journal of Experimental Social Psychology, 30* (1), 53–61.

Kruger, L. (1979). Group work with abusive parents. *Social Work, 24* (4), 337–338.

Lazarus, A. A. (1982). Multimodal group therapy. In G. M. Gazda (Ed.), *Basic approaches to group psychotherapy and group counseling* (3rd ed., pp. 213–234). Springfield, IL: Charles C Thomas.

Lee, Y. T., & Ottati, V. (1995). Perceived in-group homogeneity as a function of group membership salience and stereotype threat. *Personality and Social Psychology Bulletin, 21* (6), 610–619.

Levine, B. (1991). *Group psychotherapy: Practice and development.* Prospect, IL: Waveland.

Lieberman, M. A. (1976). Change induction in small groups. In M. R. Rosenzweig & L. W. Porter (Eds.), *Annual review of psychology: Vol. 27* (pp. 217–250). Palo Alto, CA: Annual Reviews.

Lloyd, J. W., Eberhardt, M. J., & Drake, G. P., Jr. (1996). Group versus individual reinforcement contingencies within the context of group study conditions. *Journal of Applied Behavior Analysis, 29* (2), 189–200.

Lucker, G. W., Rosenfield, D., Sikes, J., & Aronson, E. (1976). Performance in the interdependent classroom: A field study. *American Educational Research Journal, 13* (2), 115–123.

Maharujeh, H. (1984). Alice in Wonderland: The multi-racial small group in clinical practice. *International Journal of Social Psychiatry, 30* (1–2), 85–88.

Marziali, E., Munroe-Blum, H., & McCleary, L. (1997). The contribution of group cohesion and group alliance to the outcome of group psychotherapy. *International Journal of Group Psychotherapy, 47* (4), 475–497.

McRae, M. B. (1994). Interracial group dynamics: A new perspective. *Journal for Specialists in Group Work, 19* (3), 168–174.

Michaels, J. W. (1977). Classroom reward structures and academic performance. *Review of Educational Research, 47* (1), 87–98.

Miller, C. E., & Komorita, S. S. (1995). Reward allocation in task-performing groups. *Journal of Personality and Social Psychology, 69* (1), 80–90.

Morran, D. K., & Hulse, D. (1984). Group leader and member reactions to selected intervention statements: A comparison. *Small Group Behavior, 15* (2), 278–288.

Nelson, W. M., III, & Politano, P. M. (1993). The goal is to say "goodbye" and have the treatment effects generalize and maintain: A cognitive-behavioral view of termination. *Journal of Cognitive Psychotherapy: An International Quarterly, 7* (4), 251–263.

Niehoff, B. P., & Mesch, D. J. (1991). Effects of reward structures on academic performance and group processes in a classroom setting. *Journal of Psychology, 125* (4), 457–467.

Oakes, P. J., Haslam, S. A., Morrison, B., & Grace, D. (1995). Becoming an in-group: Re-examining the impact of familiarity on perceptions of group homogeneity. *Social Psychology Quarterly, 58* (1), 52–60.

Perrone, K. M., & Sedlacek, W. E. (2000). A comparison of group cohesiveness and client satisfaction in homogeneous and heterogeneous groups. *Journal for Specialists in Group Work, 25* (3), 243–251.

Pierce, K. L., & Schreibman, L. (1994). Teaching daily living skills to children with autism in unsupervised settings through pictorial self-management. *Journal of Applied Behavior Analysis, 27* (3), 471–481.

Pigott, H. E., & Heggie, D. L. (1986). Interpreting the conflicting results of individual versus group contingencies in classrooms: The targeted behavior as a mediating variable. *Child and Family Behavior Therapy, 7* (4), 1–15.

Rapoport, A., & Bornstein, G. (1989). Solving public good problems in competition between equal and unequal size groups. *Journal of Conflict Resolution, 33* (3), 460–479.

Reed, B. G., & Garvin, C. D. (Eds.). (1983). Group work with women/Group work with men: An overview of gender issues in social groupwork practice [Special issue]. *Social Work with Groups, 6* (3/4).

Rhode, G., Morgan, D. P., & Young, R. K. (1983). Generalization and maintenance of treatment gains of behaviorally handicapped students from resource rooms to regular classrooms using self-evaluation procedures. *Journal of Applied Behavior Analysis, 16* (2), 171–188.

Roark, A. E., & Sharah, H. S. (1989). Factors related to group cohesiveness. *Small Group Behavior, 20* (1), 62–69.

Rohde, R. I., & Stockton, R. (1993). Working with groups: The group as an effective medium for working with children of chemically dependent families. *Journal for Specialists in Group Work, 18* (4), 182–188.

Romeo, F. E. (1998). The negative effects of using a group contingency system of classroom management. *Journal of Instructional Psychology, 25* (2), 130–133.

Rose, S. D. (1974). Group training of parents as behavior modifiers. *Social Work, 19* (2), 156–162.

Schultz, C. B., & Sherman, R. H. (1976). Social class, development, and differences in reinforcer effectiveness. *Review of Educational Research, 46* (1), 25–59.

Seligman, M. (1993). Group work with parents of children with disabilities. *Journal for Specialists in Group Work, 18* (3), 115–126.

Slavin, R. E. (1977). Classroom reward structure: An analytic and practical review. *Review of Educational Research, 47* (4), 633–650.

Slavin, R. E. (1990). General education under the regular education initiative: How must it change? *Remedial and Special Education, 11* (3), 40–50.

Slavin, R. E., & Karweit, N. L. (1984). Mastery learning and student teams: A factorial experiment in urban general mathematics classes. *American Educational Research Journal, 21* (4), 725–736.

Smith, C. M., Tindale, R. S., & Dugoni, B. L. (1996). Minority and majority influence in freely interacting groups: Qualitative versus quantitative differences. *British Journal of Social Psychology, 35* (1), 137–149.

Sonstegard, M. A. (1998). A rationale for group counseling. *The Journal of Individual Psychology, 54* (2), 164–175.

Stephan, W. G., & Rosenfield, D. (1978). Effects of desegregation on racial attitudes. *Journal of Personality & Social Psychology, 36* (8), 795–804.

Stevens, R., Slavin, R., & Farnish, A. (1991). The effects of cooperative learning and direct instruction in reading comprehension strategies on main idea identification. *Journal of Educational Psychology, 83* (1), 8–16.

Stinchfield, R. D., & Burlingame, G. M. (1991). Development and use of the directives rating system in group therapy. *Journal of Counseling Psychology, 38* (3), 251–257.

Stokes, J., Fuehrer, A., & Childs, L. (1983). Group members' self-disclosures: Relation to perceived cohesion. *Small Group Behavior, 14* (1), 63–76.

Vanbeselaere, N. (1988). Reducing intergroup discrimination by manipulating ingroup/outgroup homogeneity and by individuating ingroup and outgroup members. *Communication and Cognition, 21* (2), 191–198.

Vanbeselaere, N. (1991). The impact of in-group and out-group homogeneity/heterogeneity upon intergroup relations. *Basic & Applied Social Psychology, 12* (3), 291–301.

Watson, W. E., Kumar, K., & Michaelsen, L. K. (1993). Cultural diversity's impact on intersection process and performance: Comparing homogeneous and diverse task groups. *Academy of Management Journal, 36* (3), 590–602.

Wegge, J. (2000). Participation in group goal setting: Some novel findings and a comprehensive model as a new ending to an old story. *Applied Psychology: An International Review, 49* (3), 498–516.

Weldon, E., & Yun, S. (2000). The effects of proximal and distal goals on goal level, strategy development, and group performance. *Journal of Applied Behavioral Science, 36* (3), 336–344.

Wheeler, R., & Ryan, F. L. (1973). Effects of cooperative and competitive classroom environments on the attitudes and achievement of elementary school students engaged in social studies inquiry activities. *Journal of Educational Psychology, 65* (3), 402–407.

Williams, O. J. (1994). Group work with African American men who batter: Toward more ethnically sensitive practice. *Journal of Comparative Family Studies, 25* (1), 91–104.

Williamson, D. A., Williamson, S. H., Watkins, P. C., & Hughes, H. H. (1992). Increasing cooperation among children using dependent group-oriented reinforcement contingencies. *Behavioral Modification, 16* (3), 414–425.

Wodarski, J. S. (1981). *The role of research in clinical practice.* Austin: PRO-ED.

Wodarski, J. S. (1983). *Rural community mental health practice.* Austin: PRO-ED.

Wodarski, J. S. (1992). Social work perspectives on human behavior. *Journal of Health and Social Policy, 4* (2), 93–112.

Wodarski, J. S., & Bagarozzi, D. (1979). *Behavioral social work.* New York: Human Sciences.

Wodarski, J. S., & Feit, M. D. (1994). Applications of reward structures in social group work. *Social Work with Groups, 17* (1/2), 123–142.

Wodarski, J. S., Hamblin, R. L., Buckholdt, D. R., & Ferritor, D. E. (1972). The effects of low performance group and individual contingencies on cooperative behaviors exhibited by fifth graders. *Psychological Record, 22* (3), 359–368.

Wodarski, J. S., Hamblin, R. L., Buckholdt, D. R., & Ferritor, D. E. (1973). Individual consequences versus different shared consequences contingent on the performance of low-achieving group members. *Journal of Applied Social Psychology, 3* (3), 276–290.

Wright, T. L., & Duncan, D. (1986). Attraction to group, group cohesiveness, and individual outcome: A study of training groups. *Small Group Behavior, 17* (4), 487–492.

Zdaniuk, B., & Levine, J. M. (1996). Anticipated interaction and thought generation: The role of faction size. *British Journal of Social Psychology, 35* (1), 201–218.

## CHAPTER 9

# Macro-Level Variables as Factors in Human Growth and Development

## Sophia F. Dziegielewski and John S. Wodarski

Macro-level variables cover the range of influences on client behavior that cannot be addressed by individual (micro) and group (mezzo) interventions. Macro-level variables are crucial to the understanding how humans develop within an environmental context as well as the social work helping process. These interventions include broad-based organizational and societal efforts that include the alleviation of problems that continue to occur despite our best efforts with individuals, groups, families, and communities (Popple & Leighninger, 2001). Macro issues generally represent systemic problems that can create insurmountable hurdles for individual clients (Colby & Dziegielewski, 2001).

This chapter examines macro-level variables that can help individual clients get what they need, while exploring the need for intervention at the broader societal and political arenas. The historical and contextual foundations of macro-level practice along with the problems associated with it will be outlined. Recommendations for the further development in the area are presented.

## UNDERSTANDING MACRO-LEVEL VARIABLES

Numerous strategies have developed in the field of social work, targeting individuals, institutions, and society as the focus of change (Connaway & Gentry, 1988; Egan, 1994; Haynes & Mickelson, 1991). Macro-level social

The authors would like to thank James M. Haitz and Linda Schlichting-Ray for earlier contributions to this chapter.

work practice is interested in examining variables related to organizations and communities within social, political, historical, economic, and environmental contexts (Barker, 1999; Meenaghan, 1987). Meenaghan, in the *Encyclopedia of Social Work*, states that macro-level practice concerns itself primarily with four basic applications: "planning, administration, evaluation, and community organizing" (p. 83). Barker defines macro-level practice as practice that focuses on improvements and changes in general society.

Kirst-Ashman and Hull (1997) define macro-level practice using four dimensions. The first includes the following tasks to meet client needs: (a) changing or improving policies and procedures that regulate the distribution of resources, and (b) creation of new resources. The second dimension focuses on *the system* to determine where and how changes can be made. Systems include, for example, political, legal, and service delivery systems. The third dimension of macro-level practice includes advocacy on behalf of clients assisting them to get needed resources and services. The final dimension of macro-level practice includes an organizational perspective, since most services provided to clients are carried out within agencies or organizations.

According to Zastrow (1999), social workers practice at three levels: (a) micro—working on a one-to-one basis with an individual, (b) mezzo—working with families and other small groups, and (c) macro—working with organizations, communities, or seeking changes in legislation and social policies. Netting, Kettner, and McMurtry (1993) discuss the emergence of macro-level practice in response to societal prejudice aimed at vulnerable and oppressed populations. The impact of macro-level variables on minority groups and vulnerable populations continues to be profound (Brenner, 1977; Cohen & Wagner, 1992; DuBois & Miley, 1999; Gordon, 1975; Herrick, 1978; Hopkins, 1980; Korchin, 1980; Mulroy & Lane, 1992; Netting et al., 1993; Rothman, 1994; Weil, 1989).

Although macro-level variables may be seen by many as separate and distinct from micro and mezzo practice, the importance in solving problems of individuals cannot be overstated. In fact, micro and mezzo approaches are extremely limited when there are interfering practices and policies at the macro level. For example, services provided for clients may not adequately address their needs if clients have no transportation to receive it. The advocacy inherent in this activity has broader based implications than simply arranging for a ride. How will the client get there in the future and is the lack of adequate transportation prohibitive from others utilizing the service? If so, the social worker (often referred to as the change agent) must then decide whether to engage in organizational or institutional change. This may include advocating for changing social policy and regulations, organization policies and procedures, and other strategies such as mass media appeals, activism, confrontation, grass-roots approaches, and social programs (Schneider & Lester, 2001).

Certain practices related to macro-level variables that are adverse to client social functioning include: (a) the failure of agencies to readily change to meet clients' needs (Cohen & Austin, 1994; Cole & Pilisuk, 1976; Fugii, 1976; Kettner, Moroney, & Martin, 1990); (b) the tendency of agencies to retain certain clientele and their failure to increase clients' social functioning because of vested interests (Daly, 1972; McRoy, 1989; Resnick & Menefee, 1993); (c) the reluctance of agencies to implement new programs that would provide essential services for clients (Carlton & Jung, 1972; Fabricant, 1986; Feldman, 1978; Gummer, 1975); (d) the administration's choice of bureaucratic rather than humanistic modes of operation (Lewis, Lewis, & Souflee, 1991; Rothman, 1994); and (e) the manipulation of the institutions of education, law, health, economics, housing, politics, and employment to prevent the social advancement of various groups, thus adding impetus to the belief in the superiority of one group (Beauregard, 1977; Deegan, 1981; Hauser, 1975; Miller, 1993). Such practices result in the denial of social services or their substandard delivery to vulnerable populations and minority groups (Lide, 1973; Netting et al., 1993; Rothman, 1994).

Many theories utilized in the profession of social work do not lend themselves to the alleviation of the effects of macro-level variables. Macro social work has received far less attention than micro and mezzo levels, and consequently, an integrated macro-level social work theory is lacking (Schwartz, 1977). Historically, macro-level social work education was seen as a specialization, and student enrollment and interest in macro-level practice was declining (Schwartz & Dattalo, 1990). However, today, an integrated practice approach needs to include intervention at all three levels.

The need for macro-level approaches is evident when considering the extent to which macro variables help to create and perpetuate disenfranchised and powerless groups. Hasenfeld (1992) discusses the levels of power exerted over individuals, from the simple A has power over B, with B being dependent on A because B has no power because of inability to negotiate or change the system. This is evident where various disenfranchised groups have been denied the right to vote, or they were excluded from voting because of procedures that totally ignored segments of society. In essence, the group's power was diminished by total exclusion from the powerful majority. Therefore, to fully address and support social work's values of empowerment and self-determination, macro variables must be addressed.

A number of theories place blame on clients for their own problems (Brown, 1974; Cowger, 1994; Glenn & Kunner, 1973; Saleebey, 1992; Weick, Rapp, Sullivan, & Kisthardt, 1989). Literature in the field reveals limited attempts at conceptualizing how social systems might be responsible for individual afflictions (Rothman, 1979; Saleebey, 1992; Shaffer, 1972; Tidwell, 1971; Yeich & Levine, 1992). Theories that place blame on the individual preclude the development of knowledge pertaining to how institutions of the social system encourage discrimination and what strategies could be utilized to modify these institutions (Balgopal, Munson, & Vassil, 1979; Hendricks, Howard, & Gary, 1981; Hogan & Siu, 1988; Longres, 1972; Nichols-Casebolt, 1988; Ryan, 1976; Yeich & Levine). The impact on social work education and practice is twofold: (a) The client suffers because we do not provide intervention that addresses the underlying cause of the client's problem, and (b) the profession suffers because macro practice is not developed to its fullest extent.

Hence, agencies and schools of social work must explore in depth how various institutions of the social system contribute to discriminatory practices. Schools of social work should maintain a curriculum which will ensure that students are provided with adequate education and training in macro-level social work to acquire the knowledge and skills needed to address this task and alleviate the discriminatory practices (Abel & Kazmerski, 1994; Gamble, Shaffer, & Weil, 1994). To explore this issue in depth it will necessitate a study of the legal, political, educational, and economic institutions (Allen-Meares, 1990; Gutierrez, 1990; Proctor & Davis, 1994; Robinson, 1989).

Macro variables have a special importance in providing interventions to minority, culturally diverse, and disenfranchised populations. Most of the institutions that provide human services have been organized using the values, mores, and intuitive and intellectual processes familiar to the dominant culture. Frequently, discriminatory practices and ways of thinking and approaching work are built into the system. For example, predominant culture theories may posit that nonwhites have "no delayed gratification," "low educational expectations," and "low verbal ability." These ways of thinking, and processes to support them, may be deeply ingrained into the organization. Replacing approaches based on such bias must be supplanted by theories that emphasize strengths of various minorities, emphasizing their ability to adapt and survive under severe social stress (Carter, 1978a, 1978b; Cooper, 1973; Longres, 1972; Smith, 1973; Tuck, 1971).

To summarize, macro-level variables include those characteristics of organizations, society, the environment, and the community, which can be supportive to individual client and group interventions, but frequently pose significant barriers to providing optimum service. In fact, repeated attempts to resolve insurmountable obstacles in the macro environment sometimes thwart client problems at the individual (micro) and group (mezzo) levels. Macro variables involve the political, economic, educational, and social arenas. Macro variables have significant influence on interventions with minority, culturally diverse, and disenfranchised populations, because the aforementioned arenas are often built upon the knowledge and beliefs of the predominant culture. To facilitate real and lasting change macro variables cannot be ignored (Colby & Dziegielewski, 2001; Popple & Leighninger, 2001).

## MACRO INTERVENTIONS

Interventions in macro arenas vary to the extent of the problems introduced. A number of substantive models for macro intervention provide knowledge, skills, and frameworks for initiating change in macro variables. Kettner, Daley, and Nichols (1985) proposed a nine-step process of change: (a) identifying and analyzing the change opportunity, (b) setting goals and objectives, (c) structuring the change effort, (d) planning for resources, (e) implementing, (f) monitoring, (g) evaluating, (h) reassessing the change effort, and (i) stabilizing the situation.

Other models include planning, administrative, and community organization models (Meenaghan, Washington, & Ryan, 1982), and *environmental practice* models, including community resource coordination, social support, and organizational environments (Neugeboren, 1996). William Brueggemann (1996) discusses "An Action Model" (p. 39) in dealing with social problems. Although traditional social science attempts to remain value-neutral, and avoids making recommendations about society's responsibility for social betterment, the action model in macro social work takes a highly critical stance. Accordingly, from the macro perspective, every social worker must be a discerning social critic (Brueggemann, 1996).

A generalist social worker may explore intervention alternatives at the micro, mezzo, and macro levels. For example, a practitioner may have a number of elderly clients who are experiencing problems living alone in their own homes. A macro level intervention might include initiating a new program to assist these clients, or initiating a change in policy, which would provide access to existing services for these clients. Kirst-Ashman and Hull (1997) provide a wide range of intervention approaches that include use of micro-mezzo skills in the macro environment, and step-by-step processes for changing organizations and agency policy, implementing and developing programs, and intervening in neighborhoods and communities. It is important to note there is interdependency between macro and micro approaches. For example, a caseworker who is coordinating resources for a specific client must be aware of the array of services available to the client and must convey to administrators needs that are not being met. At the macro level, administrators must be aware of the service needs of clients to use macro approaches to the best benefit of clients (Neugeboren, 1996). The skills used for micro interventions can be used in macro practice as well. In macro practice the micro skills of building relationships, listening, and empathy are extremely important (Kirst-Ashman & Hull, 1997).

An intervention in the organizational and educational arenas might include the hiring of teachers and supervisors who provide positive role models for novice social workers. People tend to model behaviors of others whom they wish to emulate. Modeling is even greater when: (a) Competent behaviors are exhibited by high-status models; (b) models are similar to observers in essential characteristics such as race, age, sex, social history, and attitudes; (c) models control resources for the observer or are important to the observer in another manner; and (d) models are reinforced for their behaviors (Bandura, 1971a, 1971b; Goldstein & Sorcher, 1974). If the assumption can be made that novice social workers desire to emulate certain prestigious professionals such as social welfare administrators, supervisors, faculty members, and practitioners, then it would seem that attention to the type of role model provided is warranted. For a variety of reasons, professionals at times do not exhibit behaviors reflecting the accepted values of the profession such as conviction in the inherent worth, integrity and dignity of the individual, and the belief in the right of self-determination (Connaway &

Gentry, 1988; Proctor & Davis, 1994; Reeser, 1992). Poor role models may fail to provide the incentives for new social workers to exhibit behaviors that are aimed at alleviating such macro-level problems as discrimination. Professionals must exhibit noncontradictory behaviors. In addition, for an agency to deal with practices that are discriminatory the agency's administration must have a clear, firm policy and maintain the ability to monitor and impose sanctions when the policy is violated (Compton & Galaway, 1989).

Many social workers will find employment in agencies in which the environment is not necessarily conducive to assisting clients, and may in fact employ discriminatory practices (Frey, 1990; Hurst, 1971; Jansen & Von Glinow, 1985). For example, economic aspects of administering many agencies often induce administrators to respond to the demands of the agency system rather than to the needs of clients. Agencies wield considerable power in providing incentives for the social worker's exhibition of behaviors favorable to the system when economic conditions create a tight job market. Research data suggest that individuals more readily engage in social change strategies when economic conditions are favorable, thus minimizing one agency gaining control due over all the employment possibilities (Miceli, 1984).

Professional organizations have opportunities to intervene and encourage macro intervention in agencies. Three major professional organizations—the National Conference of Social Welfare (NCSW), the Council on social Work education (CSWE), and the National Association of Social Workers (NASW)—have set forth policies aimed at the alleviation of practices that are often discriminatory and counter to client assistance. Accurate accountability procedures should be developed and implemented. It has been proposed that these agencies monitor the practices of the profession through on-site agency evaluations and impose sanctions when these policies are not being met. Likewise, to provide an incentive for agencies to involve themselves in the alleviation of institutional practices that prevent client assistance, bonuses or special recognition through citations could be given by the agencies.

The enormity of the task of developing accountability procedures is evidenced by the difficulties schools of social work have encountered with one aspect of institutional procedure—the lack of minority context in curriculum for reading entries, lecture content, and assignments. The development of criteria to assess the adequacy of programs and to monitor behaviors is a substantial task and will require diligent effort (Harrison, Thyer, & Wodarski, 1996).

A discussion of macro interventions would be incomplete without noting the primary importance of research. Brueggemann (1996) discusses research that is involved in the actual practice of macro interventions. Research may be used in the actual practice of macro intervention, such as doing an extensive investigation to understand a community, including a wide range of variables that may impact the target problem in the community. This approach is applied research. Ethnographic research, interviews, and participant observation might be used in preparing for social reform and program development. Research questions may be descriptive, for example, What is the setting like? What people are involved and what roles do they play? Where are the power influences? What are the politics, financial base, and the social milieu? Predictive questions might include: Why are things done in a certain way? Why are there no services to meet a specific need? Why are services not available to a specific clientele? Prescriptive questions are the "how to" questions: How can change best be facilitated? What are the alternative strategies? (Brueggemann, 1996).

Neugeboren (1996) calls for research related to a number of environmental practices. Included are research to study the effectiveness of various skills used in macro practice, including multi-dimensional practice skills, and the effects of macro interventions in achieving consumer benefit. Other areas suggested for research include the impact of collaboration among micro and macro practitioners in the coordination of community resources, the relationships between lay citizens and professionals in the delivery of services, how organizational environments impact the needs of service users, and research into specific strategies for macro practice with vulnerable populations (Brueggemann, 1996).

Much research pertaining to minority groups has provided evidence to support theories that focus more on individual responsibility and blame, with little on strengths of minority populations and societal responsibility (Moynihan, 1968). There is a need for research on the strength of minority groups and vulnerable populations to survive and even excel under stressful conditions. Willie (1974), for example, suggests that minority groups hold values quite similar to the majority of White Americans. Literature on resilience does suggest that attention is focusing on variables that account for strengths in various populations who have faced adverse life situations (Blocker & Copeland, 1994; Garmezy, Masten, & Tellegen, 1984; Kobasa, 1979).

In addition, research into the causes of discriminatory practices in agencies deserves further study (Herzog, 1971; Smith, 1973). Such research might investigate variables involved in changing discriminatory attitudes of various groups and the study of organizational policies of institutions that promote discriminatory practices. It is hoped that research into a wide range of macro variables will lead us further in the direction of developing theories and intervention models in the area of micro practice.

In many instances it may be necessary to acquaint practitioners with the means of changing the present state of practice in agencies. At times, activist change strategies may be required. Four strategies are suggested for generating change: (a) pressure from within the organization, (b) pressure from clients, (c) pressure from outside through imposition of sanctions or incentives by various groups, and (d) employment of practitioners as change agents (Kotler, 1971; Kutner, 1976).This will necessitate that practitioners be trained to make organizational diagnoses that will yield data from which they can choose the appropriate course of action. The social worker must be able to ascertain what type of change agent would be successful in a particular agency. Several questions are presented that need to be answered. What are the appropriate change techniques for this particular context? Who makes the important decisions in the agency? Who gets the reinforcers? What are the networks of reinforcement and communication? Who controls the incentives in the organization? How much support is there for change among practitioners, clients and professional organizations? What reinforcers and sanctions do they possess (Frey, 1990; Netting et al., 1993; Stevens, 1981)?

If the social worker clearly perceives these processes then he or she can begin to assess how much pressure for organizational change can be brought from within the organizations or from other sources. If a strategy of pressure from within the organization is chosen to change institutional discriminatory practices, it must be kept in mind that the more people involved in pressuring the agency to change its practices, the higher the probability of success (Hugman & Hadley, 1993). It has been suggested that support for change usually come from young, active, professionally educated social workers.

If it is decided that pressure from clients is necessary, the possibility that conflict can be kept within the agency is eliminated and instead the greater public becomes involved. Additional support for the proposed change may be gained through the organizer's skillful use of the various media to inform the public of the proposal for change. Bringing in professional organizations to assess the agency's current practices may provide additional pressure; however, specific criteria as to when this and other avenues used by the change agent need further development.

The prudent and effective use of media such as television, radio, newspapers, and professional periodicals may be used to bring about change in social work agencies and institutions of education, law, health, economics, housing, politics, and employment. The decision to put to use any of the various media should be calculated according to the desired results. Data indicate that television is the easiest to comprehend and better reaches the general public, whereas newspapers reach a smaller segment of the population. Professionals tend to put more merit into professional periodicals. Furthermore, the message must be geared to the characteristics of the people who will receive it (Chong, 1993; Haynes & Mickelson, 1991; Kahn, 1991). The following are three rules practitioners might adhere to when engaging the media: (a) There must be consistency in the message, and it must be addressed in the most attractive manner to the constituency it is to influence; (b) the message should be expounded by a person having prestige within the target group; and (c) the message must indicate how individuals exhibiting requisite behaviors will be reinforced (McGuire, 1969; Zimbardo & Ebbesen, 1969).

The literature reflects a variety of studies focusing on social change (Burghardt, 1977; Cnaan & Rothman, 1986). As the area of social change develops an empirical base, it will be necessary to isolate what techniques should be combined with what characteristics of the change agent and in what contexts they should be used, what level of commitment is necessary, and how one develops and maintains the necessary level of commitment to carry out the change process.

For social workers there are two realistic avenues open for effecting change in an agency. First, a practitioner can work with the agency, building up what Hollander (1958) referred to as *idiosyncrasy credits*. Building these credits allows social workers to increase progress up the bureaucratic ladder, achieving a level in which they are high enough to change the agency's policies (Dozier & Miceli, 1985; Fiedler, 1960; Hollander, 1958; Homans, 1961; Parmerlee, Near, & Jensen, 1982). There are various pros and cons to this type of approach. For example, these types of change agents are within the agency and have helped the agency attain its current status. Therefore, people will more likely listen to them, and there is less risk because of their seniority in the agency.

A major drawback to this type of situation is that the practitioners may have become so involved with the agency and socialized to its goals that they can no longer objectively assess the current state of practice. They therefore reinforce the system and, consequently, bring about little change. The longer it takes practitioners to achieve a leadership position, the less likely it is that they will act as change agents. Likewise, social workers who are recently introduced into an agency and wish to become change agents are hampered unless they can organize large portions of that agency for change, or gain influence with the decision makers. If the social worker gains a position of leadership, the techniques of influence and persuasion derived from attitude, attraction, reaction theory, contingency theory, and cognitive dissonance can be used to reduce practices that support bias in the organization (Argyris, 1975; Jansen & Von Glinow, 1985; Kiesler, 1971; Netting et al., 1993).

The action of whistle-blowing has been briefly studied to determine under what conditions workers will speak out in opposition to organizational wrongdoing and discriminatory practices (Dozier & Miceli, 1985; Miceli, 1984; Parmerlee et al., 1982). Change agents within an organization who are viewed as credible based upon years of experience, knowledge of intra-agency practices, and altruistic motives to prevent further harm of coworkers or clients may be in a position to reframe the act of whistle-blowing into a prosocial behavior of seeking assistance to improve and strengthen the functioning of the organization (see Dozier & Miceli). Additional research in this are may be warranted to further legitimize the action of whistle-blowing.

The organizational constraints placed on an internal change agent may often be too great for that agent to achieve significant change. In this instance the second avenue for change could be used. That is, for various social work organizations, such as the NCSW, the CSWE, and the NASW, to set aside funds to employ professionals as external change agents. These change agents would make periodic site visits to assess the current status of practice in agencies wishing to become members of these organizations or to maintain memberships. Because the external change agent's economic base would be outside the agency being evaluated, economic and social constraints in making assessments or decisions would be eliminated. Such agents would have to employ various mechanisms to secure reliable data, such as interviews with clients, employees, and data on services being provided.

Social entities such as groups, complex organizations, and social institutions can be characterized as being composed of a series of interconnected reinforcers and punishers. Acknowledgment and manipulation of these factors in combination with individuals who have the power to make organizational changes can control reinforcers, both positive and negative, regardless of the size of the unit. The social entities communicate the conditions of reinforcement and punishment (consequences) through the provision of discriminative stimuli to individuals. Formal discriminative stimuli of social entities are: signed contracts, policy manuals of rules and regulations, and informal norms and folkways of the entities. For example, through taxation governments secure a generalized reinforcer from citizens' money and then welfare departments and other agencies redistribute these reinforcers through guidelines (contingencies) set forth by Congress. There is no desire to deemphasize the complexity of this process, but for the purposes of this text this definition suffices. In the future a more sophisticate model will include other essential variables.

An increasing call for social workers to engage in social action with their clients has been noted. Behavior analysis presents us with a beginning methodology for social action. We can ask and determine what reinforcers social workers and their clients possess that can be utilized to manipulate other individuals who distribute reinforcers such as housing, jobs, medical care, and other social services. Social workers' collective reinforcers, such as knowledge and money, and their availability to effective organize, may be used to exert considerable force on politicians. Once organized, social action strategies may begin by asking an official to secure more adequate social conditions for certain disadvantaged groups, for example. If this strategy did not work, the next strategy might be to utilize a punishment contingency such as a demonstration or use of the media to secure public outcry. Finally, the ultimate strategy might be a type of economic boycott.

Social action can also contribute to the empowerment of vulnerable and oppressed groups through education and consciousness raising. Action movements and citizen advocacy efforts can refocus the target for change from individual deficiency to environmental and system deficiency (Ezell, 2001). As macro-level change occurs through improved responsiveness of social, economic, educational, employment, legal, and other institutions, individual growth and resource development can simultaneously occur (Cox, 1991; Henderson, 1993; Pearlman & Edwards, 1982).

It is important to note that while available literature discusses the social worker's role in organizing and implementing social change movements, empirical guidelines are still being developed that will indicate appropriate choices within the change strategy. The selected approach is applicable only to the extent that targets of social action consist of recurrent and habituating behaviors on the part of accessible agency officials. However, some of the most intolerable situations involve relatively inaccessible decision makers engage in ad hoc behaviors. Methods of influencing such targets need additional theoretical and empirical development.

## THE VALUE OF MACRO-LEVEL INTERVENTION

There have been many attempts to discredit the value of social work interventions, and assaults on the profession have occurred at the organizational and political level. Encouraging the investment in human social services that will help prepare citizens to develop to their fullest potential can reduce these attempts. It is hoped that society will realize from the results of empirical studies that reductions in social services are extremely costly to individuals and to society. Data indicate that as the economy falters, the incidence of admissions to mental hospitals and prisons, child abuse, spouse abuse, suicide, and so forth are dramatically increased (Hamburg, 1994; Weinert, 1982).

The more we, in the social work profession, can demonstrate the effectiveness of macro and micro interventions, the more we build the credibility of the profession as we effectuate changes that are people enhancing and cost effective. Likewise, as a profession we need to learn more about political processes and activities. We have witnessed dramatically how political processes can affect clients and the ability to serve them. Social workers must become more sophisticated in influencing the political structure if we are to create environments conducive to client change. When we do, we open new avenues for clients that heretofore have been impossible, we enhance the profession, and we benefit society and its organizations and institutions. We also create environments that will be less likely to discriminate with other client populations and with employees because we help to raise the consciousness or the macro target to a higher level.

## PROBLEMS IN MACRO-LEVEL INTERVENTION

Many of the problems have been addressed in the discussion of interventive techniques. To summarize, intervention at the macro level can produce the greatest good for the most people, but not without risk. Action within organizations can be a threat to one's job and livelihood, as well as to promotion opportunities, job assignment preferences, and a myriad of other impacts on one's life within the organization. Interventions must be weighed carefully against potential risks, choosing those that can effect the required change at the lowest risk.

Efforts to initiate macro change can be very time consuming. As noted earlier, one must thoroughly assess the macro target and garner support for change. Underlying forces may require a few steps backward, and regrouping, to target unforeseen challenges. Political forces are strong and frequently have no basis in reality; therefore, they are difficult to account for in planning strategy. Especially in bureaucratic environments, even if change is ultimately agreed upon, there will frequently be a multitude of horizontal and vertical approvals required before implementation. Therefore, involving from the start all known entities that will be impacted by the change will help to cut down on the amount of time for approvals and concurrence.

Another problematic area is the strong resistance to change on the part of organizational entities and individuals. Without anticipation and knowledge of strategies to overcome resistance, a macro intervention can be doomed from the start. On the positive side, many of the skills used in micro practice to deal with resistance to change on the part of individuals, families, and groups can be effectively used to overcome resistance in macro targets of intervention. Too frequently, social workers see macro and micro practice as very separate, with theories that diverge significantly. In reality, the micro level skills can be extremely effective in macro change efforts.

Finally, one of the greatest barriers to change can be monetary cost. Politicians and society at large are very attuned to costs and sources of revenue (most often taxes). A well-designed intervention plan, with well-documented positive results anticipated, may fail due to high cost or lack of funding. Social workers must be aware of the cost of interventions to society. A good plan will demonstrate planned effectiveness, cost benefit, and sources of revenue. When possible, social workers should apply for grants and they should have the skills necessary for grant writing. Social workers must have a basic understanding of how their organizations fund initiatives and, when new funding is not available, how funds might be shifted to accomplish the intended goal.

# SUMMARY

Attention to macro variables, and interventions to improve outcome probability for clients, is the first step in using macro approaches to intervene on behalf of clients. Social workers should develop good micro skills and see their usefulness in working directly with clients, other employees in the organization, and with entities that can facilitate larger macro change. Practitioners must use culturally relevant clinical skills to assist clients, to better understand client needs, and to communicate to others the relevance of culture and disadvantage in effecting client change. The message conveyed must be one of professional respect and courtesy, and the elimination of discriminatory barriers hampering delivery of services (Proctor & Davis, 1994).

Agencies must become more receptive environments for the display of social work values. This might be accomplished if public and private agencies would incorporate clients into their governing bodies, thereby ensuring that professionals do not isolate themselves from client needs (Colby & Dziegielewski, 2001; McDaniel & Balgopal, 1978; Young, 1968). Likewise, client involvement ensures feedback on client concerns and provides for communication channels, whereby clients may discuss agency practices and policies that interfere with client service.

Educational institutions must include macro-practice variables and interventions in the social work curriculum. Recognizing the integration of macro and micro interventions will help prevent the division in the two approaches that has been a detriment to the profession historically.

Finally, more research is needed on macro variables and interventions and how they are coordinated with micro-level variables and interventions to effect positive and lasting client outcomes. Additional research on organizations, environments, and politics as well as their impact on client services and outcomes are necessary. In the whole process, empowerment of clients should be an ultimate goal. Further use of participatory research methods to involve vulnerable and oppressed population in social problem-solving methods should be examined. Direct client involvement in the creation and implementation of the intervention plan offers opportunities that further empower people, rather than blame victims, is another step in the direction of sound macro practices and client strength perspective (Yeich & Levine, 1992).

This chapter has discussed how behavior can be controlled through intervention at various levels, that is, individual, group, organizational, institutional, and societal interventions. Adequate control will be achieved, however, only through coordination of these components. The social work professional needs to become equipped to provide such coordination. The intent of this chapter has been to define macro-level variables, review the scope of possible interventions at the macro level, identify problems in implementing macro-level interventions, and demonstrate the importance of macro-level change in maximizing social work outcomes with clients and with the larger society. With these in mind, social workers will be better equipped to help clients toward behavioral change and positive outcomes by addressing the full spectrum of factors influencing that change.

## REFERENCES

Abel, E. M., & Kazmerski, K. J. (1994). Protecting the inclusion of macro content in generalist practice. *Journal of Community Practice, 1* (3), 59–72.

Allen-Meares, P. (1990). Educating black youths. The unfulfilled promise of equality. *Social Work, 35* (3), 283–286.

Argyris, C. (1975). Danger in applying results from experimental social psychology. *American Psychologist, 30* (4), 469–485.

Balgopal, P. P., Munson, C. E., & Vassil, T. V. (1979). Developmental theory: A yardstick for ethnic minority content. *Journal of Education for Social Work, 15* (3), 28–35.

Bandura, A. (Ed.). (1971a). *Psychological modeling: Conflicting theories.* Chicago: Aldine-Atherton.

Bandura, A. (1971b). Psychotherapy based upon modeling principles. In E. Bergin & L. Garfield (Eds.), *Handbook of psychotherapy and behavior change.* New York: Wiley.

Barker, R. L. (1999). *The social work dictionary* (4th ed.). Silver Spring, MD: The National Association of Social Workers.

Beauregard, R. A. (1977). From isolation to organization: Structural barriers to client-induced accountability in the human services. *Journal of Sociology and Social Welfare, 4* (7), 1109–1121.

Blocker, L. S., & Copeland, E. P. (1994). Determinants of resilience in high stressed youth. *High School Journal,* April/May, 86–293.

Brenner, M. H. (1977). Personal stability and economic security. *Social Policy,* May/June.

Brown, P. (1974). *Toward a Marxist psychology.* New York: Harper Colophon.

Brueggemann, W. G. (1996). *The practice of macro social work.* Chicago: Nelson Hall.

Burgest, D. R. (1973). Racism in everyday speech and social work jargon. *Social Work, 18,* 20–25.

Burghardt, S. (1977). A community organization typology of group development. *Journal of Sociology and Social Welfare, 4* (7), 1086–1108.

Carlton, T. O., & Jung, M. (1972). Adjustment or change: Attitudes among social workers. *Social Work, 17* (6), 64–71.

Carter, L. H. (1978a). The black instructor: An essential dimension to the content and structure of social work curriculum. *Journal of Education for Social Work, 14* (1), 16–22.

Carter, L. H. (1978b). How do black graduate social work students benefit from a course on institutional racism? *Journal of Education for Social Work, 14* (3), 27–33.

Chong, D. (1993). Coordinating demands for social change. *Annals,* July, 126–141.

Cnaan, R. A., & Rothman, J. (1986). Conceptualizing community intervention: An empirical test of "Three Models" of community organization. *Administration in Social Work, 10* (3), 44–55.

Cohen, B. J., & Austin, M. J. (1994). Organizational learning and change in a public child welfare agency. *Administration in Social Work, 18* (1), 1–19.

Cohen, M. B., & Wagner, D. (1992). Acting on their own behalf: Affiliation and political mobilization among homeless people. *Journal of Sociology and Social Welfare, 19* (4), 21–39.

Colby, I., & Dziegielewski, S. F. (2001). *Introduction to social work: The people's profession.* Chicago: Lyceum.

Cole, O. J., & Pilisuk, J. M. (1976). Differences in the provision of mental health service by race. *American Journal of Orthopsychiatry, 46* (3), 510–525.

Compton, B., & Galaway, B. (1989). *Social work processes* (4th ed.). Belmont, CA: Wadsworth.

Connaway, R. S., & Gentry, M. E. (1988). *Social work practice.* Englewood Cliffs, NJ: Prentice-Hall.

Cooper, S. A. (1973). A look at the effect of racism on clinical work. *Social Casework, 54* (2), 76–84.

Cowger, C. D. (1994). Assessing client strengths: Clinical assessment for client empowerment. *Social Work, 39* (3), 262–268.

Cox, E. O. (1991). The critical role of social action in empowerment oriented groups. *Social Action in Group Work, 4* (3–4), 77–90.

Daly, D. B. (1972). National planning for public social services. *The social welfare forum, 1972.* New York: Columbia University Press.

Deegan, J. J. (1981). Multiple minority groups: A case study of physically disabled. *Journal of Sociology and Social Welfare, 8* (2), 274–292.

Dozier, J. B., & Miceli, J. P. (1985). Potential predictors of whistle blowing: A prosocial behavior perspective. *Academy of Management Review, 10* (4), 823–836.

DuBois, B., & Miley, K. K. (1999). *Social work: An empowering profession.* Needham Heights, MA: Allyn and Bacon.

Egan, G. (1994). *The skilled helper: A problem-management approach to helping* (5th ed.). Pacific Grove, CA: Brooks/Cole.

Ezell, M. (2001). *Advocacy in the human services.* Belmont, CA: Brooks/Cole.

Fabricant, M. (1986). Creating survival services. *Administration in Social Work, 10* (3), 71–84.

Feldman, S. (1978). Promises, promises or community mental health services and training: Ships that pass sin the night. *Community Mental Health Journal, 14,* 83–91.

Fiedler, F. E. (1960). The leader's psychological distance and group effectiveness. In D. Cartwright & A. Zander (Eds.), *Group Dynamics: Research and theory* (2nd ed.). Evanston, IL: Row, Peterson.

Frey, G. A. (1990). A framework for promoting organizational change. *Families in Society: The Journal of Contemporary Human Services, 72* (2), 142–147.

Fugii, S. (1976). Elderly Asian Americans and use of public services. *Social Casework, 57* (3), 202–207.

Gamble, D. N., Shaffer, G. L., & Weil, M. O. (1994). *Assessing the integrity of community organization and administration content in field practice.* School of Social Work, CB#3550, University of North Carolina.

Garmezy, N., Masten, A. S., & Tellegen, A. (1984). The study of stress and competence in children: A building bloc for developmental psychopathology. *Child Development, 55*, 97–111.

Glenn, M., & Kunner, R. (1973). *Repression or revolution.* New York: Harper Colophon.

Goldstein, A. P., & Sorcher, M. (1974). *Changing supervision behavior.* New York: Pergamon.

Gordon, D. M. (1975). Digging up the roots. *The social welfare forum, 1974.* New York: Columbia University Press.

Gummer, B. (1975). The interorganizatinal relationships of a public welfare agency. *Journal of Sociology and Social Welfare, 3* (1), 34–47.

Gutierrez, K. L. M. (1990). Working with women of color: An empowerment perspective. *Social Work, 35* (2), 149–153.

Hamburg, D. A. (1994). *Today's children: Creating a future for a generation in crisis.* New York: Times Books.

Harrison, D. F., Thyer, B. A., & Wodarski, J. S. (1996). *Cultural diversity and social work practice.* Springfield, IL: Thomas Books.

Hasenfeld, Y. (Ed.). (1992). *Human services as complex organizations.* Newbury Park, CA: Sage.

Hauser, P. M. (1975). Mobilizing for a just society. *The social welfare forum, 1974.* New York: Columbia University Press.

Haynes, K. S., & Mickelson, J. S. (1991). *Affecting change: Social workers in the political arena* (2nd ed.). New York: Longman.

Henderson, H. (1993). Social innovation and citizen movements. *Futures.* April, 322–338.

Hendricks, L. E., Howard, C. S., & Gary, L. R. (1981). Help-seeking behavior among urban black adults. *Social Work, 26* (2), 161–163.

Herrick, J. E. (1978). The perpetuation of institutional racism through ethnic and racial minority content in the curriculum of schools of social work. *Journal of Sociology and Social Welfare, 5* (4), 527–537.

Herzog, E. (1971). Who should be studied? *American Journal of Orthopsychiatry, 16* (1), 4–12.

Hogan, P. T., & Siu, S. F. (1988). Minority children and the child welfare system: An historical perspective. *Social Work, 33* (6), 493–498.

Hollander, E. P. (1958). Conformity, status, and idiosyncrasy credit. *Psychological Review, 65*, 117–127.

Homans, G. C. (1961). *Social behavior: Its elementary forms.* New York: Harcourt, Brace, & World.

Hopkins, T. J. (1980). A conceptual framework for understanding the three "isms." Racism. Ageism. Sexism. *Journal of Education for Social Work, 16* (2), 63–72.

Hugman, R., & Hadley, R. (1993). Involvement, motivation, and reorganization in a social services department. *Human Relation, 46* (11), 1319–1348.

Hurst, C. H. (1971). The time of crisis—A challenge for social work education everywhere. *Journal of Education for Social Work, 7* (2), 19–24.

Jansen, E., & Von Glinow, M. A. (1985). Ethical ambivalence and organizational reward systems. *Academy of Management Review, 10* (4), 814–822.

Kahn, S. (1991). *Organizing: A guide for grassroots leaders* (Rev. ed.). Silver Spring, MD: National Association of Social Workers.

Kettner, P. M., Daley, J. M., & Nichols, A. W. (1985). *Initiating change in organizations and communities. A macro practice model.* Monterey, CA: Brooks/Cole.

Kettner, P. M., Moroney, R. M., & Martin, L. L. (1990). *Designing and managing programs: An effectiveness-based approach.* Newbury Park: Sage.

Kiesler, C. A. (1971). *The psychology of commitment.* New York: Academic.

Kirst-Ashman, K. K., & Hull, G. H., Jr., (1997). *Understanding generalist practice.* Chicago: Nelson-Hall.

Kobasa, S. C. (1979). Stressful life events, personality, and health: an inquiry into hardiness. *Journal of Personality and Social Psychology, 37* (1), 1–11.

Korchin, S. J. (1980). Clinical psychology and minority problems. *American Psychologist, 35* (3), 262–269.

Kotler, P. (1971). The elements of social action. *American Behavioral Scientist, 14* (5), 691–717.

Kutner, N. G. (1976). Low income, ethnicity, and voluntary association involvement. *Journal of Sociology and Social Welfare, 3* (3), 311–321.

Lewis, J. A., Lewis, M. D., & Souflee, F., Jr. (1991). *Management of human service programs* (2nd ed.). Pacific Grove, CA: Brooks/Cole.

Lide, P. (1973). The national conference on social welfare and the black historical perspective. *The Social Service Review, 47* (2), 197–207.

Longres, J. (1972). The impact of racism on social work education. *Journal of Education for Social Work, 8* (1), 31–41.

McDaniel, C. O., & Balgopal, P. R. (1978). Patterns of black leadership: Implications for social work education. *Journal of Education for Social Work, 14* (1), 87–93.

McGuire, W. J. (1969). The nature of attitudes and attitude change. In G. Lindzey & E. Aronson (Eds.), *The handbook of social psychology* (2nd ed., Vol. 3). Reading, MA: Addison-Wesley.

McRoy, R. G. (1989). An organizational dilemma: The case of transracial adoptions. *Journal of Applied Behavioral Science, 25* (2), 145–160.

Meenaghan, T. M. (1987). Macro practice: Current trends and issues. *Encyclopedia of Social Work* (18th ed., Vol. 2). Silver Spring, MD: National Association of Social Workers.

Meenaghan, T. M., Washington, R. O., & Ryan, R. M. (1982). *Macro practice in the human services. An introduction to planning, administration, evaluation, and community organizing components of practice.* New York: The Free Press.

Miceli, M. P. (1984). The relationships among beliefs, organizational position, and whistle blowing status: A discriminant analysis. *Academy of Management Journal,* 27 (4), 687–705.

Miller, S. M. (1993). The politics of respect. *Social Policy,* Spring, 44–51.

Moynihan, D. P. (1968). *The Negro family: The case for national action.* New York: Bantam.

Mulroy, E. A., & Lane, T. S. (1992). Housing affordability, stress and single mothers: Pathway to homelessness. *Journal of Sociology and Social Welfare, 19* (3), 51–63.

Netting, F. E., Kettner, R. M., & McMurtry, S. L. (1993). *Social work macro practice.* New York: Longman.

Neugeboren, B. (1996). *Environmental practice in the human services. Integration of micro and macro roles, skills, and contexts.* New York: Haworth Press.

Nichols-Casebolt, A. M. (1988). Black families headed by single mothers: growing numbers and increasing poverty. *Social Work, 33* (4), 306–313.

Parmerlee, M. A., Near, J. P., & Jensen, T. C. (1982). Correlates of whistle-blowers' perceptions of organizational retaliation. *Administrative Science Quarterly,* 27, 17–34.

Pearlman, M. H., & Edwards, M. G. (1982). Enabling in the eighties: The client advocacy group. Social Casework: *The Journal of Contemporary Social Work,* November, 532–539.

Popple, P. R., & Leighninger, L. (2001). *The policy-based profession: An introduction to social welfare policy analysis for social workers.* Boston: Allyn and Bacon.

Proctor, E. K., & Davis, L. E. (1994). The challenge of racial difference: Skills for clinical practice. *Social Work, 39* (3), 314–323.

Reeser, L. C. (1992). Professional role orientation and social activism. *Journal of Sociology and Social Welfare, 19* (3), 190–194.

Resnick, H., & Menefee, D. (1993). A comparative analysis of organization development and social work, with suggestions for what organization development can do for social work. *Journal of Applied Behavioral Science, 29* (4), 432–445.

Robinson, J. B. (1989). Clinical treatment of black families: Issues and strategies. *Social Work, 34* (4), 323–329.

Rothman, J. (1979). Macro social work in a tightening economy. *Social Work,* 24, 274–281.

Rothman, J. (1994). *Practice with highly vulnerable clients: Case management and community-based service.* Englewood Cliffs, NJ: Prentice-Hall.

Ryan, W. (1976). *Blaming the victim* (Rev. ed.). New York: Vintage.

Saleebey, D. (1992). *The strengths perspective in social work practice.* New York: Longman.

Schneider, R. L., & Lester, L. (2001). *A new framework for action: Social work advocacy.* Stamford, CT: Brooks/Cole.

Schwartz, E. E. (1977). Macro social work: A practice in search of some theory. *Social Service Review, 5* (2), 207–227.

Schwartz, S., & Dattalo, P. (1990). Factors affecting student selection of macro specializations. *Administration in Social Work, 14* (3), 83–96.

Shaffer, A. (1972). Community organization and the oppressed. *Journal of Education for Social Work, 8* (3), 65–75.

Smith, J. F. (1973). Who should do minority research? *Social Casework, 54* (7), 393–397.

Stevens, C. (1981). Poor urban blacks and community participation. *Journal of Sociology and Social Welfare, 8* (1), 132–149.

Tidwell, B. J. (1971). The black community's challenge to social work. *Journal of Education for Social Work, 7* (3), 59–65.

Tuck, S., Jr. (1971). Working with black fathers. *American Journal of Orthopsychiatry, 41* (3), 465–472.

Weick, A., Rapp, C., Sullivan, W. P., & Kisthardt, W. (1989). A strengths perspective for social work practice. *Social Work, 34* (4), 350–354.

Weil, M. (1989) Research on vulnerable populations. *Journal of Applied Behavioral Science, 25* (4), 419–437.

Weinert, B. A. (1982). A dialogue for change: Policy, politics and advocacy. *Administration in Social Work, 6* (2/3), 125–137.

Willie, C. V. (1974). The black family and social class. *American Journal of Orthopsychiatry, 44* (1), 50–60.

Yeich, S., & Levine, R. (1992). Participatory research's contribution to a conceptualization of empowerment. *Journal of Applied Social Psychology, 22,* 1894–1908.

Young, W. M. (1968). Tell it like it is. *Social Casework, 49* (4), 207–212.

Zastrow, C. (1999). *The practice of social work* (6th ed.). CA: Brooks-Cole.

Zimbardo, P., & Ebbesen, E. B. (1969). *Influencing attitudes and changing behavior.* Reading, MA: Addison-Wesley.

# Conclusions

---

## CHAPTER 10

---

# Human Behavior Theory: Emerging Trends and Issues

## Peter Lyons and Marvin Feit

T he advent of the new millennium is a powerful catalyst to reflections on the past, and projections for the future. However, predicting the future is fraught with peril, particularly in this age of continuously accelerating change. In recognition of the potential pitfalls and to minimize sheer speculation this text extrapolates current trends in human behavior theory with special reference to those trends relevant to the practice of social work. This chapter summarizes many of the ideas presented in this book and specific topics include: (a) the importance of diversity and empirical evaluation when applying all theoretical frameworks (addressed in chapter 1), (b) biological variables (chapter 2), (c) cognitive variables (chapter 3), (d) life span development (chapter 4), and (e) labeling theory (chapter 5). In Part II of the text an introduction to the mezzo and macro principles is highlighted with an emphasis on (a) learning theory (chapter 6), (b) exchange theory (chapter 7), (c) group-level variables (chapter 8), and (d) macro-level variables (chapter 9). The nature of the social work endeavor is such that all theories of human behavior have some relevance for the profession, whether they owe their ontogenesis to psychiatry, psychology, economics, sociology, anthropology, medicine, political science, or to the newer biological and neurological sciences. The complexities of the human condition and commensurate social problems, however, with which social work is concerned, mean that to date, no single theory can offer an overall integrative framework for the profession. The current prevailing ideologies in social work in North America have been greatly influenced by the micro-level analyses discussed in Part I of this book. These frameworks are often credited to psychiatry, psychology, and medicine but used extensively in the field of social work (Specht & Courtney, 1994). It is clear, however, that a large proportion of the evils, which inflict themselves upon individuals and families, are a function of the mezzo and macro system as discussed in Part II. Therefore, as described in chapter 5 on labeling theory, the emphasis upon individual remediation of these problems often leads to interventions that support victim blaming (Brown, 1974; Glenn & Kunnes, 1973).

The purpose of this text is to examine emerging trends and issues in human behavior theory; however, the authors believe it is not possible to isolate these trends from their political, economic, demographic, philosophical, and scientific context. In political terms for example, despite projected budget surpluses, there is still a trend in federal fiscal policies toward a reduction in the availability of services, particularly since the advent of the George W. Bush administration (Atherton 1990a, 1990b; Hopps, 1989). This concern, and the commensurate erosion of resources, has led to greater scrutiny of the outcome effectiveness of social work intervention. Social welfare reform, managed care, and health care reform have all contributed to demands for short-term therapies of proven effectiveness. These pressures are likely to lead to a reverse construction, which places greater emphasis upon the necessity to elaborate theories of human behavior, which are supportive of brief, effective interventions.

This trend of demonstrated effectiveness is reflected in the drive toward a research-oriented profession (Reid, 1993; Task Force on Social Research, 1991). This direction is to be applauded, provided the profession recognizes that the *bottom line* should be demonstrated in a difference to clients and that there is often a great difference between statistical and clinical significance (Jayaratne, 1990).

It has been argued that the level of psychotherapeutic sophistication, therefore by implication the level of human behavior theory sophistication, is not yet sufficient to allow for total integration (Lazarus, 1989; Silverman, 1994; Wodarski, 1992). However, the theme of integration, or at least convergence, arises frequently in this analysis of trends. Even so, it is likely that the gap between the sophistication of our theorizing and the complexity of the human condition will lead to almost equal and opposite fragmentation, and divergence.

## DIVERSITY ISSUES

The necessity for social work and human behavior theorists to take firm action to resist, and repel racist, sexist, and homophobic attitudes has been articulated previously (Wodarski, 1992; Zuckerman, 1990). However, the need to supplant theories that promulgate the negative attributes of non-Whites [e.g., "The Bell Curve" (Hernstein & Murray, 1994), is still evident. Research that is insensitive to diversity issues must be counterbalanced by culturally sensitive and accurate research. In order to achieve this goal research strategy must be improved. Sampling methods on culturally diverse groups have frequently depended upon non-random samples, or samples of convenience; comparative norms have too often been those of the White middle class (see Eichler, 1988; Stewart & Napoles-Springer, 2000; Tidwell, 1990; Zuckerman, 1990). In addition, Jones and Jacklin (1988) have called for the specification of those variables that would facilitate changes in the racist and sexist attitudes of different groups. This is a direction that research is increasingly likely to take. Calls to develop culturally sensitive research and practice, to develop strategies to combat institutional racism (Wodarski, 1992), and to establish course content that is reflective of the historical and cultural context of urban Black settings (Daniels, Wodarski, & Davies, 1987) must be heeded. In addition, the increasing recognition of the difference between the surface and core features of ethnicity (Green, 1995; Nash, 1989; Pinderhughes, 1994) is worthy of further exploration. Green has suggested that the study of ethnicity should focus on boundaries, control, and the construction of meaning. Consequently, one of the crucial tasks for social work is the need to understand how the dominant group uses ethnic differences to exclude minorities, and to incorporate this knowledge into strategies for individual and social change.

Ethnicity and race are not the only areas of cultural diversity to which human behavior theory must address itself. The theme of integration is evident in the feminist literature, in several different manifestations. The congruence of feminism and the mission of social work have led to suggestions of an integration of feminist theory and social work (DiNitto & McNeece, 1990; Hammer & Statham, 1989). Writers who identify the problems that occur when race and gender are separated also have expanded the role of feminist thought in a different direction. Feminist theory sees gender as a socially constructed phenomenon, which is a function of societal systems, rather than individuals. This theory has contributed to our historical differentiation between men and women (Hooyman & Gutierrez, 1994), and is therefore likely to have an increased impact upon macro human behavior theory and macro social work practice. Feminism itself is likely to continue the trend away from essentialism and make more room for women of color (Collins, 1989) and older women (Browne, 1994). As a stance that views the disproportionate number of social injustices inflicted upon women as structurally imposed rather than individually, feminism is increasingly likely to return to its roots in social activism. As a cautionary note, however, social work itself has not been exempt from gender differentiation. Petchers (1996) reviewed employment trends in social work education from 1972 to 1993 and found that despite increasing numbers of females in social work education they were still clustered in nontenure and nontenure track positions.

A recent text bridges individual, interactional, and institutional levels of analysis, while examining issues of gender, work, family, sexuality, culture, race, and class (Myers, Anderson, & Risman, 1998). This broadening of the net provides increased recognition of the complexity of gender roles that are reflected in several themes identified in the literature. These cryptically named, chronological themes include, in the order in which they appeared: (a) Women and men are different aren't they? (b) People think men and women are different don't they? and (c) Maybe this is all more complicated then we think (Deaux, 1999). Again for social work practice this reinforces the need for recognition of the complexity of the human condition and to respond appropriately, that is without oversimplification, or assumption. Indeed Padgett (1997) has suggested that the tremendous in-group diversity among women must always be considered when assessing and treating mental health. Thus, age, life stage, birth cohort, socioeconomic status, ethnicity, strengths, and protective factors should all be factored into individual and institutional level decision making.

## BIOLOGICAL VARIABLES

As outlined in chapter 2, the unfolding fields of genetics, molecular biology, biochemistry, and neuroscience are also likely to pose new opportunities, new explanations, and new challenges to social work as advances in human behavior derive from these vibrant fields of research. The gradual unraveling of the chromosomal structure and greater understanding of brain function have brought new insights into the development of devastating afflictions such as schizophrenia, Parkinson's disease, manic depressive illnesses, and Alzheimer's disease. These advances are providing new strategies to caregivers and social workers for the management and care of the sufferers (Carlsson & Carlsson, 1990; Gershon, Martinez, Goldin, & Gejman, 1990; Gill, Taylor, & Murray, 1989; Nemeroff, 1997, 1998).

The new drive toward cost effectiveness and the concomitant trend toward briefer therapies are likely to lead to an increased use of psychotherapeutic approaches to medical issues for prevention, treatment, and maintenance (of both health and behavior change). Cummings (1987) has indicated the potential reducing effect on health care costs of the application of brief psychotherapies. The learning theory literature is replete with demonstrations of the efficacy of cognitive behavior therapy and behavior therapy on health care issues. These demonstrations have been shown to be effective in the area of oncology (Boynton & Thyer, 1994); depression (Sher, Baucom, & Lazarus, 1990); asthma (Dahl, Gustafsson, & Malin, 1990); skill acquisition in schizophrenia (Wirshing, Marder, & Eckman, 1992); and accommodations to address the limitations of chronic illness (Rybarczyk, Gallagher, & Rodman, 1992).

Biobehavioral research has increasingly identified the role of stress in society and its devastating contribution to conditions including infectious diseases; coronary heart disease (Cebelin & Hirsch, 1980); the hypertensive diseases; peptic ulcers (Tennant, 1988); depression; general ill health; and poor birth outcomes (Lobel, 1994; Moss, 1986; Schwartz, Gramling, & Mancini, 1994). This is likely to ensure both a continued place for social work in the prevention of these "diseases of culture" and the amelioration of stress and pain (Gramling, 1992; Leukenfield, 1989a, 1989b), as well as maintain the impetus toward further elaboration of the psychosomatic correlates of many conditions.

Increasingly, there emerges a consensus that major advances in human behavior and mental disorder will come about through research in the new neurosciences, and in genetics and molecular biology (Gershon & Reider, 1992; Lenfant & Schweitzer, 1985; Peele, 1981; Straus, 1988). Biology is also providing a partial integrative framework for theories of learning. For example, the cellular basis of classical conditioning is being unraveled. Research into a simple organism, the *Aplysia*, a 20,000-neuron marine snail, has provided the opportunity to observe the connections between the sensory neurons and their target cells. It has been possible to pair an unconditioned stimulus in this creature and then monitor the secretions of serotonin within the neural network (Hawkins, Abrams, Carew, & Kandel, 1983).

Neurobiological advances are also forming a link to cognitive psychology as aspects of learning and cognition are gradually being linked to specific neural functions. For example, the study of subjects with specific brain lesions has led to the elaboration of two different types of learning. One type involves largely automatic tasks and the other is dependent upon conscious awareness and cognitive processes (Kandel & Hawkins, 1992). This information can help to provide a valuable link between radical behaviorism and cognitive psychology as the cognitive aspects of learning become more and more tangible.

## COGNITIVE VARIABLES

One of the significant trends in cognitive therapy has been in the specification and testing of cognitive models for particular conditions such as panic disorders (Beck & Greenberg, 1988); eating disorders (Goldfein, Devlin, & Spitzer, 2000; Wilson & Fairbairn, 1993); depression (Beck, Rush, Shaw, & Emery, 1979; Lenz & Demal, 2000); and childhood problems (Corcoran, 2000; Kendall, 1993). As outlined in chapter 3, the increasing body of research into the efficacy of cognitive approaches is somewhat akin to the self-efficacy deemed crucial to success for individuals. The emergence of condition-specific models and therapeutic approaches has much to offer to the practice of social work if practitioners can be persuaded to consult the literature.

The themes of convergence and divergence are also evident in the area of cognitive psychology in the postmodernist manifestation of *constructivism.* The evolution of cognitive psychotherapies since the *cognitive revolution* of the mid 1970s (Neimeyer, 1993, p. 159) has made for difficulty in conceptualizing the field as a consolidated, or monolithic entity. Mahoney (1991) has described an "evolution within the revolution," which contains the potential for two bipolar expressions of cognitive therapy. At one end, it is representative of the constructivist position and based upon the assertion that "humans actively create and construe their personal realities" (Mahoney & Lyddon, 1988, p. 200). While at the other end, it becomes the province of the objectives or rationalist, proclaiming that there is a true, stable, and external reality that will gradually yield to inquiry.

To validate this two-factor classification DiGiuseppe and Linscott (1993) elicited some qualified support for the dichotomy; however, they were unable to support the bipolar nature, and posited a continuum with therapists able to hold beliefs from each *pole* simultaneously. This has some features in common with the false dichotomy often posited in research, between qualitative and quantitative methods, postmodernism and empiricism. Most researchers recognize that each methodology has something to offer, depending upon the research question and the context. Social workers should also be able to adopt intervention strategies based upon "where the client is at" and guided by evidence of effectiveness.

The constructivist model differs from the traditional model for its conceptualization of: the nature of reality, knowledge, problem definition, treatment goals, assessment, and intervention (Granvold, 1996). Neimeyer (1993) has characterized the constructivist approach as comprising several traditions of psychotherapy: (a) personal construct theory, (b) narrative psychology, (c) structural developmental approaches, and (d) constructivist family therapy. He sees constructivism as providing the potential for synthesis with other clinical traditions (psychoanalysis, family therapy, cognitive behavioral therapy, and existential humanistic therapies), as post modernist thought permeates each. He suggests that cross-fertilization with other constructivist fields such as cognitive science, developmental psychology, and cultural studies may also result. However, unless constructivist concepts can lend themselves to empirical verification, their value to social work is likely to be inhibited.

Another area of integration is represented by the combination of neurobiology and cognitive psychology (den Boer, 2000; Post et al., 2000). Windmann (1998) suggested the juxtaposition of these might provide a useful framework for understanding panic disorders, because this framework can provide a heuristic for the conceptualization of many types of mental health problems, while demonstrating how to integrate previously conflicting theories.

The theme of integration is also present in the unraveling of the genetics of cognitive abilities and disabilities (e.g., Reiss & Neiderhiser, 2000). During the earlier part of the twentieth century, psychology was dominated by environmental explanations of cognitive abilities. In recent times a more balanced view has prevailed in which nature and nurture interact in cognitive development. The notions that the environment is influential are not in doubt. However, genetics may determine how easily we learn through the contribution of genetics to understanding of reading ability and intelligence, for example. Molecular genetics, however, while offering the opportunity to identify the genes for specific disorders and thus the opportunity for early intervention, brings with it a host of ethical issues. What new choices, challenges, and opportunities for use and misuse arise from our new understandings? How social work acts to influence policy and individual decisions in response to new developments must all be guided by the core values of the profession. The year 1998 alone saw the unraveling of genes associated with speech, stamina, smell, baldness, some psychiatric problems, one type of muscular dystrophy, and several types of mental retardation (Glausiusz, 1999).

## LIFE SPAN DEVELOPMENT

Life span development as outlined in chapter 4, allows theorists to propose various stage models of development. The utility of these models lies in their support for intervention at various points in the life span, as opposed to models that saw early development as both paramount and insurmountable (Davison & Neale, 1982). They also are helpful for their elaboration of stage appropriate interventions for social work. However, the stage model developmental theories also have their detractors who see them as outdated and not truly reflective of the complexities of modern interactionally determined causality (Dannefer, 1984; Germaine, 1987) or the complexities of modern culture (Breslow, 1988; Germaine).

Life span development theory must expand its horizons and accommodate the new demographic realities such as the increasing number of elderly persons, and the old demographic realities, women and minorities, which had previously been largely ignored. Criticisms of the male bias of life span development as it relates to the concept of identity formation, for example, have been raised by Archer (1992) and Patterson, Sochting, and Marcia (1992). Furthermore, the gender progression of identity formation may be different for males and females (Josselson, 1973). Research is also now beginning to unravel the specific dimensions of the life span as it relates to the experiences of women (Snyder, 2000). Esterberg and associates demonstrated the social exchange aspects of the transitional phases of marriage and divorce for women (Esterberg, Moen, & Dempster-McCain, 1994). They point to the circumstances that facilitate the transition to divorce for women, such as return to school, availability of options, and other structural factors as being more significant than attitudinal factors. Research such as this on women's life transitions must also contribute to the life span perspective.

Inclusion must also be extended to minorities, such as African Americans. Their experience has some features typical of many of the other minority groups in North American society. For example, they continue to remain one of the most disadvantaged sectors (Jaynes & Williams, 1989). The explanations for this disadvantage include (a) the legacy of past discrimination, (b) differences in human capital, and (c) experience and the cumulative impact of past discrimination (Thomas, Herring, & Horton, 1994). Although they found no explanation totally consistent with their results, Thomas et al. report that the cumulative effects of discrimination over the life course was the formulation that conformed most closely to the results of a synthetic cohort study which reviewed data from 1940–1990. The implications of this type of research for life stage theories centers upon the need to accommodate that which is not, stereotypically, White, male, and middle class.

In addition to the need to develop theories on a broader base, there is a need to extend the concept of stage development further through the life course. Olshansky, Carnes, and Grahn (1998) have suggested that new technologies and improved living conditions are creating what might be considered "manufactured time" toward the end of people's lives. For this and other reasons the elderly are the fastest growing population in the United States, and included in this population are increasing numbers of the oldest old (Longino, 1988; Rosenwaike, 1985). There is likely to be increased emphasis upon life span development as it relates to this group. Johnson (1994) has warned against assuming that the oldest old (not simply the old) are a homogeneous group. She reviews the demographic data on the elderly and advises that they too must be understood relative to their social and cultural diversity. In addition, she stresses that there are misconceptions about the old that must be dispelled to more fully understand the life span. Misconceptions tend to be associated first with conceptions about loneliness and family abandonment, which have led to a view that engendered substitute care is the primary option for care of the elderly. Second, further examination must take place regarding the view that disengagement and lack of social involvement is damaging (Palmore, 1979). Although this may be the case for the youngest old, it may not be for the oldest old.

Corman and Kingson (1996) emphasized the need to broaden the discussion on aging with respect to several issues including: (a) the complexity of old age, (b) the diversity of the Baby Boom cohort, and (c) commensurate health care issues. With the increase in the elderly population they suggest the need for a national dialogue on age that addresses the aforementioned issues, as well as issues associated with stereotypes and diversity, early and late Baby Boomers, and race. Social work is uniquely placed to play a major role in this national dialogue, and all of these have profound consequences for social work practice that is intimately involved with decisions about placement and support of the elderly as well as policy development on our aging population. Jackson and Sellers (1996) have also suggested an ecological framework for examining poor mental and physical health outcomes for African Americans, which encompasses major health issues across the life span.

## LABELING AND THE PERCEPTUAL PROCESS

Beckett has demonstrated how the labeling process operates at the macro level (1994). She demonstrated support for the contention that it is the "definitional activities of the state and the media, rather than the reported incidence of crime or drug use and abuse that has shaped public concern about those issues" (Beckett, p. 425). These findings are supported by other writers in respect to drug use and drug related crime (Jensen, Gerber, & Babcock, 1991; Lyons & Rittner, 1998; Reinarman & Levine, 1989). This *constructionist* account on the wider level is akin to the process of labeling at the individual level. As explained in depth in chapter 5, the powerless are labeled as deviant in some way by the powerful in society. Their retention of this label is a function of their incapacity to shed it. This process has important ramifications for social work at both macro and micro levels. At the societal level, social work must determine the relative weight to attribute to actual incidence of social problems, and the public concern about those problems, which may not always be in accord with each other. At the micro level social workers must be aware of their own power to label individual clients, with both internal and external effects. Externally the social worker has the capacity to attach labels to a client that may then be transferred to other aspects of the client's life (Klassen, 2000). The problem of what has been termed "designer diagnosis" is a very cogent manifestation of this process (Bentley, Harrison, & Hudson, 1993). Bentley and colleagues posit, along with many others (Gambrill, 1990; Walters, 1990; Wetzel, 1991), that the use of "popular labels and clinical concepts" has detrimental effects in stigmatizing and presenting clients as pathological. This has a particularly devastating effect upon women and minorities.

These authors tend not to deny the utility of using concepts, but rather their concern is with the uncritical application of labels without reference to the errors in reasoning that is often contraindicated with their use. These errors include: "the failure of clinicians to consider the behavioral referents of concepts they use, the tendency to use concepts as labels to explain causality, and the tendency to make erroneous assumptions about the origin of concepts" (Bentley, Harrison, & Hudson, 1993, p. 463). As the spectrum and level of external criticism of social work services grows (Ofshe & Watters, 1994; Wakefield & Underwager, 1994; Yapko, 1994), there is likely to be continued emphasis upon the need for critical thought about all aspects of the profession, particularly uncritical application of damaging labels. Further, social work attention must focus on the empirical unraveling of the intricacies of human memory because the profound impact of suggestibility is becoming more apparent. Social workers are in a tremendously powerful position with respect to vulnerable, victimized, and suggestible populations and should be aware of the intricacies and foibles of human perception, particularly as it relates to memory and suggestibility.

Despite some evidence to the contrary (Neimeyer, Neimeyer, & Landfield, 1983), there seems to be a relationship between cognitive complexity and integration, and information processing in social judgment situations, which is precisely what a social worker client interview is (Ferguson & Fletcher, 1989; Raphael, Moss, & Rosser, 1979). However, further work is needed to elaborate the relationship between cognitive complexity and integration because this has implications for the way social workers view their clients and subsequently make decisions about them. Social workers must be aware of the impact of the labeling process and their perceptual screen on their own perceptions of the client.

## LEARNING THEORIES

One of the trends evident in the field of learning theory that chapter 6 highlights is the perennial interest in the maintenance and generalization of learned behavior (see Bernard, 1990; Wodarski, 1987). This interest is being pursued in several different ways. Nelson and Politano (1993) have identified a paucity of research into the issue of treatment termination within the behavioral therapy literature, finding only one article in a review of more than 14,000 that dealt with the process of termination. They suggest that this is in part because the minimization of the role of the client-therapist relationship by early behaviorists. They suggest that generalization and maintenance are so significant that the issues of termination and relationship are important areas to study, insofar as they impact upon the two former concepts. Further, both traditional behavioral therapies and cognitive behavioral therapies have been criticized in the past for the lack of long-term follow-up studies (Keeley, Shemberg, & Carbonell, 1976). This is reflected in the lack of research on the process issues, which contribute to transfer and durability of learning. There is likely to be an increase in the interest and consequent research efforts to examine process issues in treatment and posttreatment. These process areas will include the client-therapist relationship as it relates to termination and interaction generally, and will benefit from the explicatory power of social exchange theory. Inevitably this will require long-term follow-up, or built-in relapse prevention. In practice implications social workers are ideally placed as professionals to provide longer term environmental or circumstantial changes in reinforcement contingencies based upon the profession's role in such services as home visiting (Wodarski, 1992).

The convergence and divergence themes also will be seen in learning theories as evidenced by moves toward the integration of the respondent, operant, and modeling frameworks that have been previously suggested (Wodarski 1992), with the further suggestion that a new integrated paradigm may arise from this. In addition, the relationship between behavior theory and behavior therapy has also been promulgated with specific emphasis on areas of commonality (Cahill, Carrigan, & Evans, 1998). Indeed there has been some research support for the suggestion that the difference between the learning theory paradigms is not so great as was previously believed (Wolpe, 1990).

Further debate is likely to take place with respect to the encroachment of "rationally deduced but unverified theories" on the field of behaviorism (Acierno, Hersen, Van Hasselt, & Ammerman, 1994, p. 179). This may be characterized by criticism of behaviorism for its limitations. From the opposite perspective, however, it is suggested that these limitations are in fact strengths. Therefore, the demand to replace or enhance the empirical stance of behaviorism arises from poor implementation of behavioral techniques and a failure to follow recommendations made by behavioral theorists (Goldfried & Castonguay, 1993; Plaud & Vogeltanz, 1993; Wolpe, 1977). An important question raised by Paul (1967, p. III) still must be addressed: "What treatment by whom is most effective for this individual with that specific problem, under which set of circumstances?" This question must be answered for all treatment or intervention models; however, an emphasis on the learning theories may hold the key to helping address this earliest in this field.

This brings us to another trend—which is associated with many treatment perspectives—the prescriptive matching of treatment intervention and client problem. Several writers have pointed out the necessity for appropriate matching of clients with treatment (Aceirno et al., 1994; Wodarski, 1992; Wolpe, 1993). Wolpe (1993) has summed up the prerequisite steps as the assessments of the symptom presentation, maintaining factors, etiological factors, and subject characteristics and history. Attempts to mitigate what Wolpe has described as this "Achilles heel" (1977) of behaviorism are also likely to lead to greater emphasis on research as attempts are made to answer Paul's critical question. Ducharme and Van Houten (1994) have also demonstrated the importance of the identification of the discriminative stimuli in the person's natural environment that contributes to the production of problem behaviors. As long ago as 1975, Kallman, Hersen, and O'Toole demonstrated the necessity of analysis of both the symptomatology and the environmental maintaining variables in the client's system. Kallman and colleagues also reported that the zeitgeist of interest in outcome is likely to lead to a much greater emphasis on this in the future.

## EXCHANGE THEORY

Exchange theory, as discussed in chapter 7, has great potential to provide a unifying schema for human behavior theory in its capacity to accommodate both the large-scale economic political structures and the small-scale behavioral transactions, which take place between individuals. The mathematical elaboration of the exchange theory paradigm is an immense task; however, the possibility that chaos theory will contribute to its explication and its predictive power is likely to be explored in the near future. One of the major features of current exchange theory is the extrapolation of Emerson's (1972) original analysis of recurring dyadic interactions to the broader scope of exchange networks. Exchange theory had originally been focused on contingencies and was a highly testable set of concepts. However, a shift away from testability had occurred in recent years. It appears that we are now seeing a return to the high level of testability (e.g., Tallman, Burke, & Gecas, 1998).

As an example of this trend Molm (1991) has distinguished two types of behavioral strategies that are identified as involving contingent action. These are classified as reciprocal and nonreciprocal strategies. The former referring to contingencies between what is described as functionally equivalent behavior, and which would take place in power-balanced relations. The latter referring to contingencies used in nonreciprocal power, imbalance relations. This latter is consistent with the clinical setting in many instances in which the social worker has the power. Molm hypothesizes that nonreciprocal contingency strategies will be more effective because they are not expected. Molm also stated that an experimental test of this theory and the relationship of the contingencies used to satisfaction provide some support for this analysis. This type of analysis should be integrated into our conceptualization of the clinical setting and the elements that exist therein.

These basic elements have previously been identified and include client and worker interactions and behaviors, the context in which this interaction takes place including the structure of the interaction, and finally, the attempts made by the social worker to achieve behavioral change in the client (Wodarski, 1992). Exchange theory carries with it the potential to shed greater light on the clinical setting, particularly as this setting fits the archetype of the power imbalanced relationship identified by Emerson (1972). Indeed social exchange theory has been applied to family dynamics and alcoholism within the family and, again following the theme of integration, has been combined with operant principles to predict family dysfunction and breakdown (Ruben, 1998; Tallman et al., 1998).

## GROUP-LEVEL VARIABLES

The demand for cost effectiveness is also leaning toward greater accountability and increased demand for programs and interventions of proven outcome effectiveness in group work. Chapter 8 serves to reflect the current trends of group-level variables including the utilization of effective outcome measures, which in turn is leading to increased sophistication of research design utilizing multiple measures (e.g., Wodarski, 1989). In an examination of trends in methodology, theory, and program development Tolman and Molidor (1994) report several indicators of the trend toward increasing methodological sophistication. The indicators included greater use of multiple measures and balancing of group leadership across comparison group conditions. Approximately 36 of the 54 studies reviewed used multiple outcome measures. However, the authors note that only one third included some kind of follow-up. There is likely to be an increase in the number of follow-up studies to examine the efficacy of the group in the maintenance of behavior. They also note there has so far been little effort aimed at determining the process elements of success in group treatment (for an exception see Whitney and Rose, 1990).

Wodarski and Feit (1994) have also stressed the signal importance of reward structures in groups, and since cognitive behavioral groups tend to be the most prevalent (Tolman & Molidor, 1994), it seems not only likely but also important that there be further examination of the relationship and efficacy of competitive and cooperative reward structures and individual and group task rewards. In addition, the role of the peer group in the maintenance of behavior is likely to receive more attention as the emphasis on treatment maintenance evaluation grows. A two-year follow-up study on the use of the Teams, Gaines, Tournaments approach to alcohol education demonstrated the effectiveness of this behaviorally based method (Wodarski & Bordnick, 1994). The reinforcement structure manifested in the peer group appears to be one of the likely ingredients that contributed to successful maintenance.

Another trend in the use of groups may be in the client population for whom groups are used. Though many forms of groups aimed at many different types of clients exist, the typical group in the United States is most likely to be offered to children for social skill development or behavioral problems (Tolman & Molidor, 1994). The use of groups may broaden to include diverse populations from Britain, Australia, Canada, and Israel. In these areas the literature shows that groups are more likely to be offered focusing on domestic violence, problems of aging, and human and civil rights as they affect new immigrants, women, and minorities (Forte, 1994).

The increased use of matching the appropriate clientele with the appropriate treatment methodology will be expressed for research to determine what is effective with whom, as well as in practice in which attempts are made to utilize existing and accumulating knowledge to match appropriately. Feldman's (1986) comment that "the research base for social group work is growing, but much remains to be done before group workers can safely claim that their practice is grounded in scientific research" remains cogent today (p. 13).

## MACRO-LEVEL VARIABLES

"We must have a vision of social work that enables us to direct our energies to the creation of healthy communities. That is how we make healthy people" (Specht, 1990, p. 356). This vision of the impact of community-level (macro) variables upon the individual has implications for both social work and human behavior theory. As outlined in chapter 9, no comprehensive, integrative theory of human behavior can ignore the macro level of analysis. Clearly, a large proportion of the social inequities in our society are a function of the operation of large-scale community (and larger) forces, and yet the general stance of social work has been to work at an individual level (Specht & Courtney, 1994). The prevailing ideology of demand for outcome effectiveness will lead to a greater role for social workers. This will continue to manifest itself both in attempts to ameliorate the conditions leading to unhealthy communities and in efforts to create environments, which make behavioral change more durable and transferable (e.g., Kanazawa, 2000).

Several writers (Morris, 1980; Taylor & Roberts, 1985) have commented that there is a lack of adequate theory for community level practice. However, behavior analysis and learning theories generally have made contributions in numerous areas; for example, increased participation in community activities (Rothman & Thyer, 1984), attendance at self-help meetings (Miller & Miller, 1970), and increased immunization (Yokley & Glenwick, 1984).

It is ironic that behavior theory, with its roots in the analysis of individual micro-level interactions, also has utility, as yet largely untapped, at the broader level. Mattaini eloquently summarized the contribution that behavior analysis can make to community-level practice (Mattaini, 1993); in this he echoed the view expressed by Fellin, Rothman, and Meyer (1967) that the sociobehavioral approach could make a major contribution to community-level practice in its demand for behavioral specificity. Mattaini outlines three decades of literature that elaborate the roles of behavior analysis in the provision of services to increase community participation, build positive community practices, and reduce negative community practices as well as to build new communities. In these endeavors he suggests that social workers must utilize and develop appropriate assessment, reinforcement, group work, and evaluation skills. If behavior analysis continues to demonstrate effectiveness in relation to outcome, then the outcome-effectiveness paradigm is likely to contribute to further demand for research on the application of these principles to macro-level variables.

## CONCLUSIONS

Despite many references in the literature to integration, there is often an uncomfortable fit between theories and application to the helping process. Sometimes the demand for inclusion and integration may lead to an inevitable fragmentation or overdilution of a theoretical position. In the areas of biology, however, learning theories and social exchange appear to offer promising potential for a more comprehensive partial solution.

Human behavior theory is developing in the fields of medical, biological, psychological, and sociological research and theory. There are numerous elements with some explanatory power that are not necessarily consistent with one another. Often their utility lies not in how closely they approximate reality but as heuristic devices lending the capacity to better interpret or understand reality. Even so, the theories and interventions that they spawn must be amenable to empirical testing if they are to be of practical value to social work, because their utility is closely related to their predictive and transformational power. Perhaps, from a social work perspective, the unifying or integrating feature of human behavior theory should be related to the basic premise of effectiveness. "Does it work?" may be a more important question for social workers at the current level of human behavior theory sophistication than "How or why does it work?"

## REFERENCES

Acierno, R., Hersen M., Van Hasselt, V. B., & Ammerman, R. T. (1994). Remedying the Achilles Heel of behavioral research and therapy: Prescriptive matching of intervention and psychopathology. *Journal of Behavior Therapy and Experimental Psychiatry*, 25 (3), 179–188.

Archer, S. L. (1992). A feminist's approach to identity research. In G. R. Adams, T. P. Gullota, & R. Montemayor (Eds.), *Adolescent identity formation* (pp. 25–49). Newbury Park, CA: Sage.

Atherton, C. R. (1990a). A pragmatic defense of the welfare state against the ideological challenge from the right. *Social Work, 35* (1), 41–45.

Atherton, C. R. (1990b). Liberalism's decline and the threat to the welfare state. *Social Work, 35* (2), 163–167.

Beck, A. T., & Greenberg, R. L. (1988). Cognitive therapy of panic disorder. In A. J. Frances & R. E. Hales (Eds.), *Review of psychiatry* (Vol. 7, pp. 571–583). Washington, DC: American Psychiatric Press.

Beck, A. T., Rush, J., Shaw, B., & Emery, G. (1979). *Cognitive therapy of depression.* New York: Guilford.

Beckett, K. (1994). Setting the public agenda: "Street crime" and drug use in American politics. *Social Problems, 41* (3), 425–447.

Bentley, K. J., Harrison, D. J., & Hudson, W. W. (1993). The impending demise of "designer diagnosis": Implications of the use of concepts in practice. *Research on Social Work Practice, 3* (4), 462–470.

Bernard, T. J. (1990). Twenty years of testing theories: What have we learned and why? *Journal of Research on Crime and Delinquency, 27* (4), 325–347.

Boynton, K. E., & Thyer, B. A. (1994). Behavioral social work in the field of oncology. *The Journal of Applied Social Sciences, 18* (2), 189–197.

Breslow, L. (1988). Possibilities and pitfalls in clinical application and cognitive-developmental theory. *New Directions for Child Development, 39,* 147–164.

Brown, P. (1974). *Towards a Marxist psychology.* New York: Harper Colophon.

Browne, C. (1994). Feminist theory and social work: A vision for practice with older women. *The Journal of Applied Social Sciences, 18* (1), 272–276.

Cahill, S. P., Carrigan, M. H., & Evans, I. M. (1998). The relation between behavior theory and behavior therapy: Challenges and promises. In J. K. Plaud & G. H. Eifert (Eds.), *From behavior theory to behavior therapy* (pp. 249–329). Boston: Allyn and Bacon.

Carlsson, M., & Carlsson, A. (1990). Interactions between glutamatergic and mono-aminergic systems within the basal ganglia—implications for schizophrenia and Parkinson's disease. *Trends in Neurosciences, 13* (7), 272–276.

Cebelin, M. S., & Hirsch, C. S. (1980). Human stress cardio-myopathy-myocardial lesions in victims of homicidal assaults without internal injuries. *Human Pathology, 11,* 123–132.

Collins, P. H. (1989). The social construction of black feminist thought. *Signs, 14* (4), 745–773.

Corcoran, J. (2000). Family treatment of preschool behavior problems. *Research on Social Work Practice, 10* (5), 547–588.

Corman, J. M., & Kingson, E. R. (1996). Trends, issues, perspectives, and values for the aging of the baby boom cohort. *Gerontologist, 36* (1), 15–26.

Cummings, N. A. (1987). The future of psychotherapy: One psychologist's perspective. *American Journal of Psychotherapy, 41,* 349–360.

Dahl, J., Gustafson, D., & Malin L. (1990). Effects of behavioral treatment programs on children with asthma. *Journal of Asthma, 27,* 41–46.

Daniels, M., Wodarski, J. S., & Davies, K. (1987). Education for community mental health practice with minorities. *Journal of Social Work Education, 23* (1), 40–47.

Dannefer, D. (1984). Adult development and social therapy: A paradigmatic reappraisal. *American Sociological Review, 49* (1), 100–116.

Davison, G. C., & Neale, J. M. (1982). *Abnormal psychology.* New York: Wiley.

Deaux, K. (1999). An overview of research on gender: Four themes from three decades. In W. B. Swann & J. H. Langlois (Eds.), *Sexism and stereotypes in modern society: The gender science of Janet Taylor Spence* (pp. 11–33). Washington, DC: American Psychological Association.

den Boer, J. A. (2000). Social anxiety disorder/social phobia: Epidemiology, diagnosis, neurobiology, and treatment. *Comprehensive Psychiatry, 41* (6), 405–415.

DiGiuseppe, R., & Linscott, J. (1993). Philosophical differences among cognitive behavioral therapists: Rationalism, constructivism, or both? *Journal of Cognitive Psychotherapy, 7* (2), 117–130.

DiNitto, D. M., & McNeece, C. A. (1990). *Social work: Issues and opportunities in a challenging profession.* Englewood Cliffs, NJ: Prentice-Hall.

Ducharme, J. M., & Van Houten, R. (1994). Operant extinction in the treatment of severe maladaptive behavior: Adapting research to practice. *Behavior Modification, 18* (2), 139–170.

Eichler, M. (1988). *Non-sexist research methods: A practical guide.* Boston: Allen & Unwin.

Emerson, R. M. (1972). Exchange theory part II: Exchange relations and networks. In J. Berger, M. Zelditch, & B. Anderson (Eds.), *Sociological theories in progress* (Vol. 2, pp. 58–87). Boston: Houghton Mifflin.

Esterberg, K. G., Moen, P., & Dempster-McCain, D. (1994). Transition to divorce: A life course approach to women's marital duration and dissolution. *The Sociological Quarterly, 5* (2), 289–307.

Feldman, R. (1986). Groupwork knowledge and research: A two-decade comparison. *Social Work with Groups, 9* (3), 7–13.

Fellin, P., Rothman, J., & Meyer, H. J. (1967). Implications of the sociobehavioral approach for community organization practice. In E. J. Thomas (Ed.), *The sociobehavioral approach and applications to social work* (pp. 73–86). New York: Council on Social Work Education.

Ferguson, J., & Fletcher, C. (1989). An investigation of some cognitive involved in person-perception during selection interviews. *Psychological Reports, 64,* 735–745.

Forte, J. A. (1994). Around the world with social group work: Knowledge and research contributions. *Social Work with Groups, 17* (12), 143–162.

Gambrill, E. (1990). *Critical thinking in clinical practice.* San Francisco: Jossey-Bass.

Germaine, C. B. (1987). Human development in contemporary environments. *Social Service Review, 51,* 565–580.

Gershon, E. S., Martinez, M., Goldin, L. R., & Gejman, P. J. (1990). Genetic mapping of common diseases: The challenge of manic-depressive illness and schizophrenia. *Trends in Genetics, 6* (9), 282–287.

Gershon, E. S., & Reider, R. O. (1992, September). Major disorders of mind and brain. *Scientific American, 267,* 127–133.

Gill, M., Taylor, C., & Murray, R. M. (1989). Schizophrenia research: Attempting to integrate genetics, neurodevelopment and nosology. *International Review of Psychiatry, 1* (4), 277–286.

Glausiusz, J. (1999). The genes of 1998. *Discover, 20* (1), 33.

Glenn, M., & Kunnes, R. (1973). *Repression or revolution.* New York: Harper Colophon.

Goldfein, J. A., Devlin, M. J., & Spitzer, R. L. (2000). Cognitive behavioral therapy for the treatment of binge eating disorder: What constitutes success? *American Journal of Psychiatry, 157* (7), 1051–1056.

Goldfried, M. R., & Castonguay, L. G. (1993). Behavior therapy: Redefining strengths and weaknesses. *Behavior Therapy, 24,* 505–526.

Gramling, S. E. (1992). Efficient pain assessment in clinical settings. *Behavior Research and Therapy, 30,* 71–75.

Granvold, D. K. (1996). Constructivist psychotherapy. *Families in Society, 77* (6), 345–359.

Green, J. W. (1995). *Cultural awareness in the human services: A multi-ethnic approach.* Boston: Allyn and Bacon.

Hammer, J., & Statham, D. (1989). *Women and social work.* Chicago: Lyceum.

Hawkins, R. D., Abrams, T. W., Carew, T. J., & Kandel, E. R. (1983). A cellular mechanism of classical conditioning in aplysia: Activity dependent amplification of presynaptic facilitation. *Science, 219,* 400–405.

Hernstein, R. J., & Murray, C. (1994). *The Bell Curve: Intelligence and class structure in American life.* New York: Free Press.

Hooyman, N. R., & Gutierrez, L. M. (1994). Introduction to feminist thought, social policy and social work practice. *The Journal of Applied Social Sciences, 18* (1), 2–4.

Hopps, J. G. (1989). Securing the future—What will we risk? (Editorial). *Social Work, 34* (4), 291–292.

Jackson, J. S., & Sellers, S. L. (1996). African-American health over the life course: A multi-dimensional framework. In P. M. Kato & T. Mann (Eds.), *Handbook of diversity issues in health psychology* (pp. 301–317). New York: Plenum.

Jayaratne, S. (1990). Clinical significance: Problems and new developments. In L. Videka-Sherman & W. J. Reid (Eds.), *Advances in clinical social work research.* Silver Spring, MD: National Association of Social Workers.

Jaynes, G., & Williams, R. (1989). *A common destiny: Blacks in American society.* Washington, DC: National Academy Press.

Jensen, E. L., Gerber, J., & Babcock, G. M. (1991). The new war on drugs: Grass roots movement or political construction? *The Journal of Drug Issues, 3,* 651–667.

Johnson, C. L. (1994). Social and cultural diversity of the oldest old. *International Aging and Human Development, 38* (1), 1–12.

Jones, G. P., & Jacklin, C. N. (1988). Changes in sexist attitudes towards women during introductory women's and men's studies courses. *Sex Roles, 18* (9–10), 611–622.

Josselson, R. (1973). Psychodynamic aspects of identity formation in college women. *Journal of Youth and Adolescence, 2,* 3–52.

Kallman, W. M., Hersen, M., & O'Toole, D. H. (1975). The use of social reinforcement in a case of conversion reaction. *Behavior Therapy, 6,* 411–413.

Kanazawa, S. (2000). A new solution to the collective action problem: The paradox of voter turnout. *American Sociological Review, 65* (3), 433–442.

Kandel, E. R., & Hawkins, R. D. (1992, September). The biological basis of learning and individuality. *Scientific American, 267* (3), 78–88.

Keeley, S. M., Shemberg, K. M., & Carbonell, J. (1976). Operant clinical interventions: Behavior management of beyond? Where are the data? *Behavior Therapy, 7*, 292–305.

Kendall, P. C. (1993). Cognitive approaches to children's problems. *Journal of Consulting and Clinical Psychology, 61*, 235–247.

Klassen, H. (2000). A name, what's in a name? The medicalization of hyperactivity, revisited. *Harvard Review of Psychiatry, 7* (6), 334–344.

Lazarus, A. A. (1989). Why I am an eclectic (not an integrationist). *British Journal of Guidance and Counseling, 17*, 258.

Lenfant, C., & Schweitzer, M. (1985). Contribution of health-related biobehavioral research to the prevention of cardiovascular diseases. *American Psychologist, 40* (2), 217–220.

Lenz, G., & Demal, U. (2000). Quality of life in depression and anxiety disorders: An exploratory follow-up study after intensive inpatient cognitive behaviour therapy. *Psychopathology, 33* (6), 297–302.

Leukenfield, C. G. (1989a). The future of social work in public health. *Health and Social Work, 14* (1), 9–11.

Leukenfield, C. G. (1989b). Prevention message for social workers. *Health and Social Work, 14* (2), 87–89.

Lobel, M. (1994). Conceptualizations, measurement and effects of prenatal maternal stress on birth outcomes. *Journal of Behavioral Medicine, 17* (3), 225–272.

Longino, C. (1988). Who are the oldest Americans? *The Gerontologist, 28*, 515–523.

Lyons, P., & Rittner, B. (1998). The construction of the crack baby's phenomenon as a social problem. *American Journal of Orthopsychiatry, 68* (2), 313–320.

Mahoney, M. J. (1991). *Human change processes.* New York: Basic Books.

Mahoney, M. J., & Lyddon, W. J. (1988). Recent developments in cognitive approaches to counseling and psychotherapy. *The Counseling Psychologist, 16*, 190–234.

Mattaini, M. A. (1993). Behavior analysis and community practice: A review. *Research on Social Work Practice, 3* (4), 420–447.

Miller, L. K., & Miller, O. L. (1970). Reinforcing self-help group activities of welfare recipients. *Journal of Applied Behavior Analysis, 3*, 57–64.

Molm, L. D. (1991). Affect and social exchange: Satisfaction in power dependence relations. *American Sociological Review, 56*, 475–493.

Morris, E. K. (1980). Applied behavior analysis for criminal justice practice: Some current dimensions. *Criminal Justice and Behavior, 7*, 131–145.

Moss, R. (1986). The role of learning history in current sick role behavior and assertion. *Behavior Research and Therapy, 24*, 681–683.

Myers, K. A., Anderson, C. D., & Risman, B. J. (1998). *Feminist foundations: Towards transforming sociology.* Thousand Oaks, CA: Sage.

Nash, M. (1989). *The cauldron of ethnicity in the modern world.* Chicago: University of Chicago Press.

Neimeyer, R. A. (1993). Constructivism and the cognitive psychotherapies: Some conceptual and strategic contrasts. *Journal of Cognitive Psychotherapy: An International Quarterly, 7* (3), 159–171.

Neimeyer, R. A., Neimeyer, G. J., & Landfield, A. W. (1983). Conceptual differentiation, integration, and empathic prediction. *Journal of Personality, 51,* 185–191.

Nelson, W. M., & Politano, P. M. (1993). The goal is to say "Good-bye" and have the treatment effects generalize and maintain: A cognitive-behavioral view of termination. *Journal of Cognitive Psychotherapy: An International Quarterly, 7* (4), 251–263.

Nemeroff, C. B. (1997). The corticotropin-releasing factor (CRF) hypothesis of depression: New findings and new directions. *Molecular Psychiatry, 1* (4), 336–342.

Nemeroff, C. B. (1998). The neurobiology of depression. *Scientific American, 278* (6), 42–58.

Ofshe, R., & Watters, E. (1994). *Making monsters: False memories, psychotherapy, and sexual hysteria.* New York: Scribners.

Olshansky, S. J., Carnes, B. A., & Grahn, D. (1998). Confronting the boundaries of human longevity. *American Scientist, 86* (1), 52–61.

Padgett, D. K. (1997). Women's mental health: Some directions for research. *American Journal of Orthopsychiatry, 67* (4), 522–534.

Palmore, E. (1979). Predictors of successful aging. *The Gerontologist, 19,* 427–431.

Patterson, S. J., Sochting, I., & Marcia, J. E. (1992). The inner space and beyond: Women and identity. In G. R. Adams, T. P. Gullotta, & R. Montemayor (Eds.), *Adolescent identity formation* (pp. 9–24). Newbury Park, CA: Sage.

Paul, G. L. (1967). Outcome research in psychotherapy. *Journal of Consulting Psychology, 31,* 109–118.

Peele, S. (1981). Reductionism in the psychology of the 80's. *American Psychologist, 36,* 807–818.

Petchers, M. K. (1996). Debunking the myth of progress for women social work educators. *Affillia: Journal of Women & Social Work, 11* (1), 1–38.

Pinderhughes, E. (1994). Diversity and populations at risk: Ethnic minorities and people of color. In F. G. Reamer (Ed.), *The foundations of social work knowledge.* New York: Columbia University Press.

Plaud, J., & Vogeltanz, N. D. (1993). Behavior therapy and the experimental analysis of human behavior: Contributions of the science of human behavior and radical behavioral philosophy. *Journal of Behavior Therapy and Experimental Psychiatry, 24,* 119–127.

Post, R. M., Denicoff, K. D., Leverich, G. S., Huggins, T., Post, S. W., & Luckenbaugh, D. (2000). Neuropsychological deficits of primary affective illness: Implications for therapy. *Psychiatric Annals, 30* (7), 485–494.

Raphael, D., Moss, S. W., & Rosser, M. E. (1979). Evidence concerning the construct validity of conceptual self as a personality variable. *Canadian Journal of Behavioral Science, 11,* 427–439.

Reid, W. J. (1993). Towards a research oriented profession. *Research on Social Work Practice, 3* (1), 103–113.

Reinarman, C., & Levine, H. (1989). Crack in context: Politics and media in the making of a drugs scare. *Contemporary Drug Problems, 16,* 535–577.

Reiss, D., & Neiderhiser, J. M. (2000). The interplay of genetic influences and social processes in developmental theory: Specific mechanisms are coming into view. *Development & Psychopathology Special Issue: Reflecting on the past and planning for the future of developmental psychopathology, 12* (3), 357–374.

Rosenwaike, I. (1985). A demographic portrait of the oldest old. *The Millbank Memorial Fund Quarterly, 63*, 187–205.

Rothman, J., & Thyer, B. A. (1984). Behavioral social work in community and organizational settings. *Journal of Sociology and Social Welfare, 11*, 294–326.

Ruben, D. J. (1998). Social exchange theory: Dynamics of a system governing the dysfunctional family and guide to assessment. *Journal of Contemporary Psychotherapy, 28* (3), 307–325.

Rybarczyk, B., Gallagher, C. D., & Roman, J. (1992). Applying cognitive-behavioral psychotherapy to the chronically ill elderly: Treatment issues and case illustration. *International Psychogeriatrics, 4*, 127–140.

Schwartz, S. M., Gramling, S. E., & Mancini, A. (1994). The influence of life stress, personality and learning on illness behavior. *Journal of Behavior Therapy and Experimental Psychiatry, 25* (2), 135–142.

Sher, T. G., Baucom, D. H., & Lazarus, J. M. (1990). Communication patterns and response to treatment among depressed and nondepressed maritally distressed couples. *Journal of Family Psychology, 4*, 63–79.

Silverman, W. H. (1994). Major trends in psychotherapy: Implication for priorities for psychotherapy. *Psychotherapy, 31* (2), 227–233.

Snyder, C. S. (2000). Generating a mutually informing dialogue: Collaboratively constructed grounded theory and testing a priori psychosocial theory. *Smith College Studies in Social Work, 70* (2), 329–353.

Specht, H. (1990). Social work practice and the popular psychotherapies. *Social Services Review, 64*, 345–357.

Specht, H., & Courtney, M. E. (1994). *Unfaithful angels: How social work has abandoned its mission.* New York: Free Press.

Stewart, A. L., & Napoles-Springer, A. (2000). Health-related quality-of-life assessments in diverse population groups in the United States. *Medical Care, 38 (Suppl 9),* September 2000, 102–124.

Straus, R. (1988). Interdisciplinary biobehavioral research on alcohol problems: A concept whose time has come. *Drugs & Society, 2* (3–4), 33–48.

Tallman, I., Burke, P. J., & Gecas, V. (1998). Socialization into marital roles: Testing a contextual developmental model of marital functioning. In N. Thomas (Ed.), *The developmental course of marital dysfunction* (pp. 312–342). New York: Cambridge University Press.

Task Force on Social Work Research. (1991). *Building social work knowledge for effective services and policies: A plan for research development.* Austin: University of Texas School of Social Work.

Taylor, S. H., & Roberts, R. W. (1985). The fluidity of practice theory: An overview. In S. H. Taylor & R. W. Roberts (Eds.), *Theory and practice of community social work* (pp. 30–29). New York: Columbia University Press.

Tennant, C. (1988). Psychosocial causes of duodenal ulcer. *Australia and New Zealand Journal of Psychiatry, 22*, 195–201.

Thomas, M. E., Herring, C., & Horton, H. D. (1994). Discrimination over the life course: A synthetic cohort analysis of earnings differences between black and white males, 1940–1990. *Social Problems, 41* (4), 608–628.

Tidwell, B. (1990). Research on black families. In S. Logan, E. Freeman, & R. McRoy (Eds.), *Social Work Practice With Black Families* (pp. 259–272). New York: Longman.

Tolman, R. M., & Molidor, C. E. (1994). A decade of social group work research: Trends in methodology, theory and program development. *Research on Social Work Practice, 4* (2), 142–159.

Wakefield, H., & Underwager, R. (1994). *Return of the furies: An investigation into recovered memory therapy*. Peru, IL: Open Court.

Walters, M. (1990, July/August). The co-dependent Cinderella who loves too much . . . fights back. *Family Therapy Networker, 18* (3), 53–57.

Wetzel, J. W. (1991). Universal mental health classification systems: Reclaiming women's experience. *Affilia, 6* (3), 8–31.

Whitney, D., & Rose, S. (1990). The effects of process and structured content on outcome in stress management groups. *Journal of Social Service Research, 13* (2), 89–104.

Wilson, G. T., & Fairbairn, C. (1993). Cognitive treatments of eating disorders. *Journal of Consulting and Clinical Psychology, 61,* 261–269.

Windmann, S. (1998). Panic disorder from a monistic perspective: Integrating neurobiological and psychological approaches. *Journal of Anxiety Disorders, 12* (5), 485–507.

Wirshing, W. D., Marder, S. R., & Eckman, T. A. (1992). Acquisition and retention of skills training methods in chronic schizophrenic outpatients. *Psychopharmacology Bulletin, 28,* 241–245.

Wodarski, J. S. (1987). *Social work practice with children and adolescents*. Springfield, IL: Charles C Thomas.

Wodarski, J. S. (1989). Evaluating a social learning approach to teaching adolescents about alcohol and driving: A multiple variable evaluation. *Journal of Social Service Research, 10* (2), 121–144.

Wodarski, J. S. (1992). Social work perspectives on human behavior. *Journal of Health & Social Policy, 4* (2), 93–112.

Wodarski, J. S., & Bordnick, P. S. (1994). Teaching adolescents about alcohol and driving: A two-year follow-up study. *Research on Social Work Practice, 4* (1), 28–39.

Wodarski, J. S., & Feit, M. D. (1994). Application of reward structures in social group work. *Social Work with Groups, 17* (1/2), 123–142.

Wolpe, J. (1977). Inadequate behavior analysis: The Achilles heel of outcome research in behavior therapy. *Journal of Behavior Therapy and Experimental Psychiatry, 8,* 1–3.

Wolpe, J. (1990). *The practice of behavior therapy* (4th ed.). Elmsford, NY: Pergamon.

Wolpe, J. (1993). Commentary: The cognitivist oversell and comments on the symposium contributions. *Journal of Behavior Therapy and Experimental Psychiatry, 24,* 141–147.

Yapko, M. D. (1994). *Suggestions of abuse: True and false memories of childhood sexual trauma*. New York: Simon and Schuster.

Yokley, J. M., & Glenwick, D. S. (1984). Increasing the immunization of preschool children: An evaluation of applied community interventions. *Journal of Applied Behavior Analysis, 17,* 313–325.

Zuckerman, M. (1990). Some dubious premises in research and theory on racial differences: Scientific, social and ethical issues. *American Psychologist, 45* (12), 1297–1303.

# Curriculum Suggestions for Human Behavior

## Lori A. Reyes

The philosophical underpinnings of social work practice and theory are founded on a commitment to enhancing, protecting, and preserving the integrity of the total person (Whitaker & Tracy, 1989). Summarized by Heffernan, Shuttlesworth, and Ambrosino (1996), "social work practice is based on values, ethics, knowledge of human behavior, practice skills, and planned change. Each of these attributes is important to professional social workers." Sound theoretical foundations are needed simultaneously with solid empirical infrastructures that can be implemented into social work curriculums. However, before implementation can be achieved, the content of human behavior courses must be scrupulously assessed and evaluated. Theories considered for selection should adhere to strict scientific criteria and the principles of research methodology. The means to achieve this end can only be accomplished through empirical research, testing, retesting of theories, and person-in-situation observation. In this appendix we shall offer a rudimentary framework for the implementation of content in human behavior courses at the graduate and undergraduate levels.

### PART I: MICRO AND MEZZO PERSPECTIVES

#### Learning Objectives

It is imperative that the student of social work practice has ample knowledge of the ideas that underlie various human behavior theories.

The editors would like to thank Karolin E. Davis Meggett for earlier contributions to this Appendix.

A working knowledge and understanding of the basic tools of science regarding theories and their elements are essential to acquiring knowledge and proficiency in social work practice. What are the three general purposes of a theory? What are the elements of a theory? What are the relationships between science, theory, and social work practice? Once students have a basic understanding of the principles that guide these concepts, students should develop tools for evaluating the philosophies of social work practice founded on scientific criteria. They should develop the ability to apply the concepts to clinical situations, develop and apply skills in the use of behavioral concepts that will empower them to delineate targets for intervention systematically whether it be with an individual, family, community, or agency.

Additionally, the capacity to understand the burgeoning research base of social work practice, the ability to assess treatment effects rigorously, and the knowledge to understand concepts—through participation in simulation exercises that illustrate these concepts—will allow the student and practitioner to develop their own level of expertise in the study of human behavior. Acquiring such knowledge should serve as a stimulus, which in turn will generate subsequent research in the profession (Wodarski, 1981).

## Course Objectives

*Students will:*

1.  Evaluate human behavior theories and concepts on scientific and practice criteria.
2.  See the sequential steps in building human behavior theory for social work practice.
3.  Translate theory and concepts into practice interventions.
4.  Know how theory relates to assessment, intervention, and choice of outcomes, that is, how it provides the rationale for practice.

## Outlines of Topics Covered

1.  Introduction—critical thinking regarding current issues in human behavior theory and research
2.  Analyzing the phenomena social workers deal with.

3. Models of behavior
4. Labeling and assessment of behavior
5. Relation of theories to therapy
6. Critical evaluation of the relationships between theories of human behavior, behavioral assessment, and techniques of therapy, that is, behavioral change
7. The effectiveness of psychotherapy or social work practice in bringing about change in human behavior
8. New models of human behavior
9. Development of personality: birth, early childhood, later childhood
10. Adolescence
11. Young adulthood
12. Early adulthood
13. Middle adulthood
14. The older years and death

## Simulation Exercises

*Students may:*

1. Read a case history and determine how different theoretical frameworks can account for causation of behavior, treatment interventions, context of interventions, duration of treatment, outcomes chosen, and so forth.
2. Complete various scales designed to measure an attribute and then assess the merits of such means of studying the phenomena. Use of assessment tools such as genograms and ecomaps (Longres, 1995).
3. Secure data on a concept through various means such as questionnaires, interview schedules, and behavioral observations. (This exercise helps students assess how various measurement techniques can affect theory building.)
4. Observe a behavior and participate in class discussions on causation of behavior and appropriate intervention, by whom, where, and for how long.
5. Observe a behavior with another individual or small group and reach a consensus on what happened. (This helps students see how difficult it is to communicate correspondingly about an observation of behavior.)

## Performance Criteria

A final examination on class lectures and on the required texts is appropriate. Two papers are required, one involving assessment of a child's behavior and the other assessment of an adult's behavior, along with a group presentation focusing on group dynamics, theoretical decisions, and behaviors. These reports will include: (a) isolation of the causes of the behavior, (b) empirical documentation of the causation of the behavior, (c) an assessment of what causes of behavior can be manipulated by the social worker, (d) an intervention plan, and (e) specification of the evaluation of the intervention plan.

# PART II: MEZZO AND MACRO PERSPECTIVES

## Groups in Human Service Practice

The techniques for the effective use of groups on the social services are reviewed. How groups affect the human service worker and client is explicated. An introduction to the means of altering relevant group process is provided (Yalom, 1985).

## Course Objectives

*Students will:*

1. Develop a conceptual base for dealing with small groups and organizations.
2. Become aware of the issues involved when professional practice occurs in bureaucratic settings.
3. Understand complex organizations and the social worker's position within the organization.
4. Understand the small group experiences that are a part of social work practice.
5. Develop the conceptual tools for identifying various aspects of small group process and the techniques for dealing with the group process.
6. Develop leadership skills in relation to small group processes as these relate to the task of providing social work service to clients.

7. Differentiate between personality, small group, and organizational factors in relation to problem situations.
8. Identify the need for planned change within the group or organization.
9. Develop skills in promoting change:

- use a group as a means of helping clients change their behaviors
- within the constraints of the organization, facilitate more effective utilization of resources
- within the organization, effect changes in the priorities and constraints or facilitate conflict resolution

## Outline of Topics Covered

1. Groups in social services
2. Components of groups
3. Norms and roles
4. Conformity process
5. Power in-groups
6. Leadership
7. Individual and group reward structures
8. Group development and building group cohesion
9. Group problem solving and decision making
10. Group conflict
11. Effective committee groups
12. Planned change in groups and organizations

## Simulation Exercises

*Students may:*

1. Engage in a cooperative task versus a competitive situation (such an exercise will help students see the effects of cooperation on group atmosphere, group problem-solving capabilities, group cohesion, and group productivity).
2. Observe how leaders structure intervention. (The exercise shows how groups need structure to define goals and the subsequent leader facilitation to attain them.)

3. Take a blind walk to build trust. (This exercise helps students observe how dependence on others can facilitate the execution of relevant tasks.)

4. Imagine themselves as astronauts who have crash-landed on the moon and must decide how to reach their mother ship 200 miles away. They only have limited supplies not ruined in the crash. The task of the students is to rank them in order of usefulness in reaching the mother ship. (This exercise, developed specifically for a systematic study of group decision making, helps students assess the merits of using groups to solve problems. A discussion afterward should include the types of problems that are solved more readily by groups as compared with individuals.)

5. Divide into two committees, each dealing with a conflict over an agency's budget; each committee then critiques its behavior in solving the conflict.

## Performance Criteria

Students choose a group process they wish to alter. They assess the variables maintaining the process, base their intervention on a theoretical rationale, and elucidate how they will evaluate whether the intervention was effective. Students present the project to fellow students for feedback and submit a written report.

Deriving a practice principle from a human behavior theory and carrying out the process through logical steps provides students with first-hand experience in the translation of human behavior theory concepts into relevant practice principles. The instructor has a special role in helping the students in the actual translation, choice of practice principles, and evaluation of the transformation. Throughout this process the instructor should provide continuous feedback and offer support and assistance. In a class discussion other students can offer constructive criticism concerning various aspects of the process and point out concepts or transformation linkages that were overlooked.

## SUGGESTED REFERENCES

Bloom, M., & Fischer, J. (1982). *Evaluating practice: Guidelines for the accountable professional.* Englewood, NJ: Prentice-Hall.

Campbell, D. T. (1967). From description to experimentation interpreting trends as quasi-experiments. In C. W. Harris (Ed.), *Problems in measuring change.* Madison: University of Wisconsin Press.

Campbell, D. T., & Stanley, J. C. (1967). *Experimental and quasi-experimental designs for research.* Chicago: Rand-McNally.

Harrison, D. F., Thyer, B. A., & Wodarski, J. S. (1996). *Cultural diversity and social work practice* (2nd ed.). Springfield, IL: Charles C Thomas.

Heffernan, J., Shuttlesworth, G., & Ambrosino, R. (1996). *Social work and social welfare: An introduction* (3rd ed.). St. Paul, MN: West.

Kazdin, A. E. (1975). *Behavior modification in applied settings.* Homewood, IL: Dorsey.

Kazdin, A. E. (1977). *The token economy.* New York: Plenum.

Longres, J. F. (1995). *Human behavior in the social environment* (2nd ed.). Itasca, IL: F. E. Peacock.

Pillari, V. (1998). *Human behavior in the social environment: The developing person in a holistic context* (3rd ed.). Pacific Grove, CA: Brooks/Cole.

Reid, W. J. (1978). The social agency as a research machine. *Journal of Social Service Research, 2* (1), 11–23.

Rosen, A., & Proctor, E. K. (1978). Specifying the treatment process: The basis for effectiveness research. *Journal of Social Service Research, 2* (1), 25–43.

Salkind, N. J. (1985). *Theories of human development.* New York: John Wiley & Sons.

Sigelman, C. K., & Shaffer, D. R. (1991). *Life-span human development.* Pacific Grove, CA: Brooks/Cole.

Thyer, B., & Morris, T. (1997). Is it possible to know when theories are obsolete? In M. Bloom & W. C. Klein (Eds.), *Controversial issues in human behavior in the social environment* (pp. 64–80). Boston: Allyn and Bacon.

Whitaker, J. K., & Tracy, E. M. (1989). *Social treatment: An introduction to interpersonal helping in social work practice.* Hawthorne, NY: Aldine De Gruyther.

Wodarski, J. S. (1975). Use of videotapes in social work. *Clinical Social Work Journal, 3* (2), 120–127.

Wodarski, J. S. (1980). Procedures for the maintenance and generalization of achieved behavioral change. *Journal of Sociology and Social Welfare, 7* (2), 298–311.

Wodarski, J. S. (1981). *Role of research in clinical practice.* Austin, TX: PRO-ED.

Wodarski, J. S. (1997). *Research methods for clinical social workers: Empirical practice.* New York: Springer.

Wodarski, J. S., & Buckholdt, D. (1975). Behavioral instruction in college classrooms: A review of methodological procedures. In J. M. Johnson (Ed.), *Behavior research and technology in higher education.* Springfield, IL: Charles C Thomas.

Wodarski, J. S., & Feldman, R. A. (1973). The research paradigm: A beginning formulation of process and educational objectives. *International Social Work, 16,* 42—48.

Wodarski, J. S., & Feldman, R. A. (1974). Practical aspects of field research. *Clinical Social Work Journal, 2* (3), 182–193.

Wodarski, J. S., & Feldman, R. A., & Pedi, S. J. (1974). Objective measurement of the independent variable: A neglected methodological aspect of community-based behavioral research. *Journal of Abnormal Child Psychology, 2* (3), 239–244.

Wodarski, J. S., Feldman, R. A., & Pedi, S. J. (1976). The comparison of pro-social and anti-social children on multicriterion measures at summer camp: A three-year study. *Social Service Review, 3* (3), 255–273(b).

Wodarski, J. S., & Pedi, S. J. (1977). The comparison of anti-social and pro-social children on multicriterion measures at a community center: A three-year study. *Social Work, 22,* 290–296.

Wodarski, J. S., & Pedi, S. J. (1978). The empirical evaluation of the effects of different group treatment strategies against a controlled treatment strategy on behavior exhibited by anti-social children, behavior of the therapist, and two self-ratings measuring antisocial behavior. *Journal of Clinical Psychology, 34* (2), 471–481.

Yalom, I. D. (1985). *The theory and practice of group psychotherapy* (3rd ed.). New York: Basic Books.

# Index

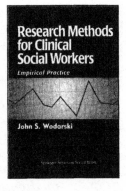

# Social Work Practice and Psychopharmacology

**Sophia F. Dziegielewski,** PhD, LCSW,
and **Ana Leon,** PhD, LCSW

*"Undoubtedly the most comprehensive book currently available to social workers and other human services professionals regarding medications, mental health, and social work practice. It is an invaluable tool for social workers working with clients who are receiving any type of medication. It is well organized and clearly written."*

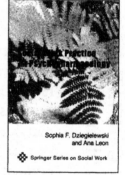

Sophia F. Dziegielewski
and Ana Leon

❖ Springer Series on Social Work

—**C. Aaron McNeece,** PhD
Walter W. Hudson, Professor of Social Work
Director Doctoral Program in Social Work

A working knowledge of psychotropics is a must for all in clinical practice today. This book supplies social workers with a basic understanding of psychotropic drugs, including medication uses and misuses.

### Partial Contents:

2001   352pp   0-8261-1394-X   hard

# Law and Social Work Practice, 2nd Edition

## *A Legal Systems Approach*

### Raymond Albert, MSW, JD

This completely rewritten and updated new edition of a practical text continues to provide a firm introduction to law and legal processes and their relation to social work practice. Using Clinton's welfare reform act of 1996, Albert provides a conceptual framework to illustrate how sociolegal problems emerge in the welfare state, and presents the skills base necessary for effective social work response.

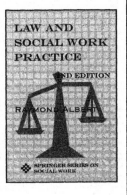

**Partial Contents:**

- An Introduction to Legal Processes
- Law and the Social Environment
- The Judicial Process: The Nature of Case Law
- The Judicial Process: Introduction to Civil Procedure
- The Legislative Process
- The Implementation of Legislation
- The Administrative Process
- The Skills Demension
- Legal Research  Resources and Techniques
- Court Testimony and Evidence
- Socio-Legal Issues in Social Work Practice
- Informed Consent to Medical Treatment
- Imposing the Death Penalty on Juveniles
- Restrictions to Legal Services for the Poor

1999   560pp   0-8261-4891-3   hard

# Multicultural Perspectives in Working with Families

## Elaine P. Congress, DSW, Editor

*"Elaine Congress's new book is an extremely useful text, on the cutting edge of this emerging and critical issue for our field and our world. The book is well-written, thoughtful, and full of practical insights to help therapists develop their work in this area. This book should be read by all students who want to understand the world they will be dealing with as they become professionals for the 21st century."*

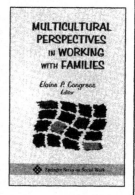

**—Monica McGoldrick,** PhD
Director, Family Institute of New Jersey

### Partial Contents:

* Use of the Culturagram to Assess and Empower Culturally Diverse Families
* Motherless Children: Family Interventions with AIDS Orphans
* Working with Soviet Jewish Immigrants
* Machismo, Manhood and Men in Latino Families
* The Impact of Ethnicity and Race on the Treatment of Mothers in Incest Families
* Multicultural Practice and Domestic Violence
* Working with Culturally Diverse Substance Abusers and Their Families
* Substance Abuse and Homeless Mothers: Multiple Oppression
* Ethical Issues and Future Directions

**Springer Series on Social Work**
1997   376pp   0-8261-9560-1   hard

CPSIA information can be obtained at www.ICGtesting.com
Printed in the USA
BVOW08*0912100516

447378BV00003B/19/P